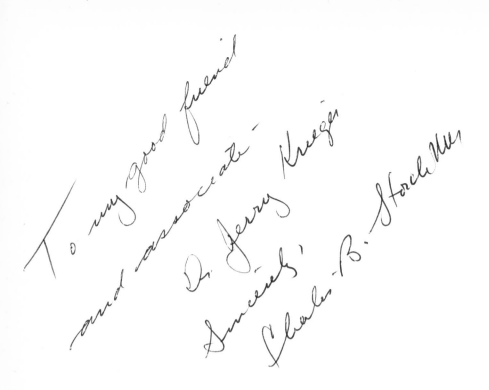

To my good friend
and associate –

Dr. Jerry Krieger

Sincerely,

Charles B. Stockholm

Fundamental Aids in

Roentgen Diagnosis

Emphasizing Spot Filming and Fluoroscopy

By CHARLES B. STORCH, M.D.

Associate Clinical Professor, New York University–
Cineradiology, Radiology, Cleft Palate Research;
Director, Radiology Department, Lefferts General Hospital,
Brooklyn, N. Y.; Associate Attending Radiologist,
Brookdale Medical Center, Brooklyn, N. Y.

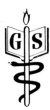 GRUNE & STRATTON · New York · London

Printed in the U.S.A. (W-B)

CONTENTS

Preface

WHENEVER A FILM can give the same information as a fluoroscopic examination, taking the film is preferable. Yet, fluoroscopy with spot filming has particular advantages of its own—direct observation of motion (physiology and pathophysiology) for one, and intelligent planning of positioning for subsequent radiographic filming for another. In these and other ways, the physician called upon to interpret a radiographic film frequently finds his patient can benefit from a fluoroscopic examination. I have discussed the foregoing sentences with a number of radiologists, and there was universal agreement. One of those with whom I conferred put it in apt vernacular: "A radiologist without a fluoroscope can be like a one-armed paperhanger."

With the above qualification and comment, it should be obvious that although not every patient should be fluoroscoped, when a fluoroscopic examination *is* indicated (as frequently it is), that examination should be done correctly. As pointed out in previous editions of the book on which this new volume is based, fluoroscopy must be learned at the side of an experienced examiner. But publishable guides and references can assist and re-enforce that experience, and in this respect I hope that this book will be of aid.

These remarks are obviously addressed to the roentgenologist, particularly the young man in the field, but as much also to interns, residents and students with a special interest in roentgenologic diagnosis, and perhaps even more to the physician nonspecialist in roentgenology—the thoracic surgeon, gastroenterologist, cardiologist, internist and general practitioner—who may want basic background and understanding.

Although an attempt has been made in this present volume as much as possible to bring the diagnostic fluoroscopic and filming material up to date, the main purpose is not to discuss new developments. It is intended,

rather, to give the reader an intelligent, practical and meaningful approach—in logical sequence—to the study and application of roentgenologic diagnosis, with emphasis on fluoroscopy and spot filming. The bulk of the material stems from personal experience. It is the material I have found to be basic and necessary in performing an efficient examination. In addition, occasional reference is made to the literature as it was found applicable to this particular text.

As in my personal teaching methods and previous writings, the Socratic question-and-answer technique has been applied here as far as possible. This is especially evident in the legends to the various figures, and it is hoped that this practice will encourage the reader to picture himself at the examination proper and thereby forced to *work out* both the appropriate form of the diagnostic question and its logical answer.

Thus, in the belief that one picture is worth a thousand words, I have tried wherever possible to tell the whole story with the various illustrations in the book. To me, the picture becomes valuable only insofar as the legend succeeds. I have tried to make the legends succeed. In this respect I wish to thank the numerous interns and residents at the Brookdale Medical Center who were asked to pass on each legend. They, *without my help*, had to evaluate and express to me the *full* meaning of a picture and legend before it could pass—that is, they discussed and criticized until each picture *and* legend told just the *right* story.

It is due to these interns and residents that the name of this book was changed. Although this is actually a revision, updating and enlargement of my earlier FUNDAMENTALS OF CLINICAL FLUOROSCOPY, it was they who informed me that the previous title did not convey the character of the roentgenographic information found in the book. I well remember, for example, a resident enquiring as to why a certain configuration of the stomach appeared on a film. I informed him that it was governed by the position of the patient, and pointed out that this information could be found in my book. He was surprised to find that a book on fluoroscopy could offer information valuable in interpreting a *film*.

It seemed to these interns and residents that a book on fluoroscopy was simply a manual of fluoroscopic technique. They were not aware that—allowing for the usual positive-negative transfer—the picture which appears on the fluoroscopic screen is the *same* picture viewed on the film, and that the understanding of that fluoroscopic image meant understanding the film. Further, that in order to get a good film, i.e., a film properly delineating a lesion, *the examiner must first know what he is looking for and next know how properly to prepare and position the patient to demonstrate that which he is looking for.*

This book attempts to teach all of these, that is, to understand and interpret the fluoroscopic image—and hence the film—, and in this respect why certain positions and techniques are best for demonstrating certain lesions, and how to obtain these positions and use these techniques. It is frequently only through the fluoroscopic examination that the examiner can arrive at the proper position and take the film himself (spot film), or, having performed the fluoroscopic examination, tell the technician how best to take the film. This book is intended to inform the novice or non-roentgenologic specialist on all these matters. Its

former title did not seem to convey this information.

Since fluoroscopy in itself is often not adequate and spot filming of one's findings is *integral* to an efficient fluoroscopic examination, in this book I have tried to describe *how* to examine that spot film—a technique which is applicable also to conventional films. I have pointed out that a film must be examined in its *entirety*. The eye must not be directed *only* to the point or region demonstrated, but the *entire* field covered by that film must be examined. I have tried to demonstrate that which many a seasoned examiner knows well, that often the answer to the patient's problem may be found on the film and yet *not* particularly where it was originally suspected. For example, a study of the colon, in an attempt to discover a hepatic flexure lesion, may instead reveal the patient's symptoms as due to gallstones seen in the upper right quadrant of the abdomen.

In conclusion, although it is not recommended that the fluoroscopic examination be carried out with the formal completeness described in each chapter, yet such descriptions must be included in texts that honestly propose to guide and assist the examiner. The physician who performs a roentgenographic study of a patient, if he is to be efficient, must know how to do a complete examination. It is only through this knowledge of the *complete* examination procedure that he can select *that part* which is suitable for the particular case at hand.

Acknowledgments

As in my previous books, I am grateful to the many who helped in the creation of the present one. First, I wish to thank Dr. William Stambro, Professor of Radiology, George Washington University Medical Center, Washington, D.C., for reviewing much of the new material. Dr. Maxwell H. Poppel, Professor of Radiology, New York University-Bellevue Medical Center, reviewed many of the figures and legends. Dr. Sol M. Unger, Chief of Radiology, Kingsbridge Veterans Hospital, Bronx, New York, made valuable suggestions and reviewed the section on larynx. Dr. Irwin Bluth, Chief Radiologist, Brookdale Medical Center, Brooklyn, New York, reviewed much of the material and made valuable suggestions. Mr. Gerald Shapiro, physicist at the Queens General Hospital and New York University, reviewed the first chapter, mainly on protection. Mr. Stanley Schwartz, the artist, was extremely cooperative and helpful. Mr. Massy Nakamurah did the new photographs and spared no effort to turn out a good job. My publisher and his editor-in-chief, Mr. Duncan Mackintosh, as with my earlier books, offered invaluable assistance.

Finally, I am indebted to my dear wife for her long hours of typing and continued encouragement, and to my children, Carole and Michael, who in their own ways assisted in the creation of this book.

TO MY DEAR WIFE

When a film can offer the same information as a fluoroscopic examination, the film is preferable. Yet, fluoroscopy is still essential in clinical roentgen diagnosis. Together with the "spot film," its value is often decisive. This book attempts both to make the fluoroscopic examination efficient and to help in the interpretation of the film.

CHAPTER I

Basic Concepts: Mechanics, Protection, and Dark-Adaptation

Mechanics

PRODUCTION OF THE FLUORO-SCOPIC IMAGE

FLUOROSCOPY is the direct examination of the patient by means of x-rays bombarding a fluoroscopic screen in a darkened room. Because it permits instantaneous visual observation of the part of the body under examination, fluoroscopy is extremely valuable for diagnostic purposes.[1]

The fluoroscope consists essentially of an x-ray tube properly housed and mounted so that x-rays from it strike a screen. The screen is a cardboard sheet covered with fluorescent material and protected by a pane of lead glass.[2] These fluorescent substances on the screen (e.g., barium plastinocyanide, calcium tungstate, or other crystals) convert x-ray radiation into visible light. The fluoroscopic screens in use today are mainly of the zinc cadmium sulfide variety. These chemicals are subject to discoloration by bright daylight, and for this reason the screens should be shielded.

In the passage of x-rays through matter, the beam is modified, being absorbed and scattered by the material traversed. These processes are dependent upon the energy of the radiation (a function of the applied kilovoltage) and the type of material traversed. In general, different thicknesses of material absorb different amounts of radiation. At the voltage used for diagnosis, tissues containing elements of high atomic numbers (such as calcium) will show a much greater absorption per gram. As a result, when a patient is placed between an x-ray tube and a fluorescent screen, a shadow image of the part of the body under examination will be produced on the screen. The dense parts of the body as well as organs of higher atomic number will absorb more radiation and so produce a darker shadow on the screen. This is because less x-ray will pass through to reach the screen and therefore produce less illumination. The parts which are less dense absorb less x-ray, thus permitting more of the x-rays to pass with resultant increased illumination.

SIGNIFICANCE OF CONTROLS ON THE FLUOROSCOPIC MACHINE

Certain controls on the fluoroscopic machine are essential for achieving the best results with a minimum of hazard to the patient and physician. These include. control of kilovoltage or penetrability; control of milliamperage or illumination; control of fluoroscopic shutter mechanism, and the use of grids.

The kilovoltage controls the penetrability of the x-ray. The higher the voltage applied to the x-ray tube, the smaller is the dose delivered to the patient for the same screen illumination (the absorption of radiation in tissue decreases with increasing kilovoltage). As a result, as the voltage is increased, the current (ma.) can be reduced substantially with no loss of screen illumination and a sizeable reduction in patient dosage. It is important to remember to reduce the current as the voltage is increased, for otherwise there will be a very bright image on the screen, but there will also be a sizeable increase in the radiation delivered. For example, increasing the voltage from 60 kv. to 85 kv. will double the roentgen output at the panel; however, for the same screen illumination, the current would be reduced to about one-third, resulting in a 40 per cent reduction in skin dose.

The milliamperage controls the amount of illumination. It should be as low as possible without sacrificing satisfactory fluoroscopic vision, and should in no case exceed 5 milliamperes (ma.). Beyond 5 ma. is unwise and may not be safe for the tube.

It is common practice to use no more than 3 ma. at 85 kv.p. for abdominal fluoroscopy; 3 ma. at 70 kv.p. for the chest, and 3 ma. at 60 kv.p. for the extremities.

The shutter mechanism enables the operator to limit the size of the field. The field should be as small as possible because radiation received is in proportion to the volume of tissue irradiated.[3] By reducing the field, more protection is given to the examiner as well as to the patient; also, the image becomes more sharply defined.

A grid or arrangement of parallel lead strips around interstices is used to prevent the screen being struck by diffuse secondary radiation from the patient. It is placed between the patient and the screen. It has the advantage of increasing contrast, especially in the examination of heavy parts. The use of such a stationary grid requires an increase of approximately 10 peak kilovoltage over the non-grid examination. Non-focus grids are designed specifically for use in fluoroscopy and have been found useful for examinations where a limited shutter is employed, i.e., use of small field. For the examination of large areas such as chests or intestinal tracts, a focused grid can be used. This is one where the lead strips have been focused for a fixed target-screen distance.

The size of the focal spot used for fluoroscopy should be known. The sharpness of the image on the fluorescent screen is dependent, to a marked degree, upon the size of the focal spot used. A focal spot of 1.5 mm. is recommended; with focal spots larger than 2.5 mm. the fluoroscopic detail is poor.

The Dangers of X-ray and the Need for Protection

THE DANGERS OF X-RAY

The biological effects of x-rays may be manifested by skin changes, by changes in the development of finger or toe nails, by changes in the blood and other deep-seated tissues, and possibly by genetic effects. The x-ray output ("r" or roentgens) at the surface of a fluoroscopic table is often as great as that delivered to the skin by a deep therapy machine in the treatment of cancer. Further, the soft radiation from the fluoro-

us to the
ion of a

changes
re itch-
hening,
eration
Severe
e also
fortu-
with-

in-
may
rtly
ter
rs.
ay
nd
st
d

... be or interest.[4]

... patients, or exactly half of the total, were physicians or other persons professionally engaged in x-ray work. Only 3 of the entire number were radiologists. The small number of radiologists is of particular interest, since these men, working at their specialty, had been exposed to radiation for periods ranging from twenty to forty years—which could easily account for their injuries. These figures are significant and are confirmed by the experience of others.[5, 6]

The following conclusions may be drawn: First, the number of radiologists involved is small. This is as would be expected because of their special training and more thorough knowledge and familiarity with the biological effects of x-rays and the need for taking precautions. Second, the majority of the injured physicians received their injuries following x-ray diagnostic work. Uhlmann[4] further indicates that of the non-

professional group who came to the hospital for treatment, in every instance where injuries occurred during diagnostic procedures, physicians other than radiologists were responsible.

NEED FOR X-RAY PROTECTION

Various standards and terms employed in x-ray work need brief discussion before we proceed further.

Today protection from the hazards of x-rays is regarded in terms of permissible dose in roentgens. A roentgen ("r") is a universally accepted unit of x-ray exposure.[7] The maximum permissible dose (M.P.D.) is the total dose that any part of the body of a person may receive continuously or intermittently in a given period of time. This has been determined as 0.1 r per week for a worker in radiation. It is advised that every individual piece of equipment used for fluoroscopy should be calibrated by a qualified physicist in order that the amount of radiation or r unit output received by both the patient and the physician may be clearly known and taken into consideration. The dosage rate measured at the panel should not exceed 10 roentgens per minute. Braestrup[8] describes one installation he calibrated in which, using the settings at which it was normally operated, the r/min. at the panel was 127; that is, an erythema dose would be reached in about 3 minutes! Such a unit could be classified as a lethal diagnostic weapon, and yet there are some like it still in use.

In a recent study, only two of eighty-one fluoroscopes met all the design and performance recommendations of the National Bureau of Standards Handbook 76.[29] These authors state that over 90 per cent of the fluoroscopes could be made acceptable by simple modifications. These included adding aluminum filtration, decreasing maximum milliamperage settings, decreasing maximum shutter openings, and adding accessory shielding. In a few machines, it may also be necessary to increase the distance between the panel and the x-ray tube. In some machines, new fluorescent screens were necessary.

Using these standards, what do we learn regarding need for x-ray protection?

A comparison of permitted exposure, as measured in roentgens, and the amount of radiation, also measured in roentgens, received by fluoroscopists, patients and other individuals present during fluoroscopic examination has been made by Cowing and Spalding.[9] A review of their findings makes the need of x-ray protection evident. An instance was demonstrated in which a physician performed fluoroscopic examinations without a lead apron. The time required per examination was four minutes. The patients were examined in the horizontal position. The total amount of radiation in roentgens received by this physician per examination was such that if he were to protect himself adequately, he could examine only 7 patients per day before exceeding the permissible dose. When this physician performed the same examinations wearing a lead apron, he was permitted thirty-nine examinations before the maximum permissible dose was reached.

The observers referred to above also demonstrated the importance of protection to the bystander. At one institution the amount of stray radiation per examination received by an intern nearby at fluoroscopic examinations who was not protected by a lead apron was such that it limited the number of patients he was allowed to observe to 6 per day before the permissible dose was reached. Another intern who wore an apron received only a negligible amount of stray radiation, permitting him far more observations. During one survey a student nurse standing beside her patient was permitted to assist with only 5 patients per day before receiving her permissible dose. With the installation of a suitable barrier, in this case a lead rubber apron hung between the nurse and the x-ray tube, she could assist with thirty-three examinations. In a more recent study, it was shown that the stray radiation in the worst installations was in the order of 700 times the stray radiation in the best installations.[29] Thus the need for x-ray protection is evident.

In summary, a survey by Hanson Blatz for the New York Department of Health has shown that of the radiographic equipment in use in New York City in 1962, 85 per cent was improperly used or installed and that of the fluoroscopy being done, less than 15 per cent was in the hands of radiologists.

With the use of a fluoroscope, properly installed and operated, a man can do all the examinations required of a busy hospital practice without needlessly exposing the patient or himself and without exceeding the Radiation Protection Guide Limits as listed (Federal Radiation Council Report #1 September 1961).

X-Ray Protection

METHODS FOR PROTECTING THE FLUOROSCOPIST

(a) Control of shutter opening.

There are various procedures at the disposal of the fluoroscopist to protect him from excessive radiation. The diaphragmatic shutters should never be opened to their limit, since when the distance between the screen and the tube is very great the oblique rays may be projected outside the frame of the fluoroscopic screen, and the fluoroscopist will consequently receive too much exposure. This can be prevented by remembering always to keep the outline of the diaphragmatic shutter edges visible on the screen.[7]*

* Since opening the diaphragmatic shutters to their full limit is a dangerous procedure and is not

The National Bureau of Standards Handbook **76** recommends that diaphragms should be installed to limit the radiation field and should be so constructed that there will be an illuminated margin on the screen regardless of the position of the screen during use. With older equipment one often finds the fluorescent screen sagging, so that the x-ray beam is no longer properly aligned, often resulting in the unattenuated x-ray beam striking the fluoroscopist.

(b) Use of filters.

Cowing and Spalding[9] demonstrated that when a piece of aluminum one mm. thick was placed within the lead cone which was located between the tube and the table-top, the scattered radiation was diminished by 35 per cent. The addition of this aluminum filter did not affect the brilliance of the screen or impair its detail. The filter recommended by the National Bureau of Standards is 2.5 mm. aluminum, i.e., total filtration.

The addition of such a filter is a simple procedure, and every physician should make certain his machine has it.

It should be stressed that added filtration is used to preferentially absorb the low energy radiation which contributes to the over-all patient dose but does not penetrate deeply enough to materially affect the fluoroscopic image. The use of sufficient filtration is one of the most important methods of reducing patient dose without affecting the fluoroscopic image.

(c) Use of hands.

It is emphasized that the examiner should never have his hands in the direct beam between the tube and the patient during fluoroscopy, even though his hands are protected

advocated in this book, the term "large" shutter opening must be taken in a relative sense. It means opening the shutters to the fullest limit which still allows the shadows of the shutter edges to appear as a visible frame on the screen. The physician rapidly scans the image at this "large" opening for diagnostic clues, then narrows the field with a "small" shutter opening for examination of more specific areas.

by lead-rubber gloves.[1] Palpation in direct beam but on the side of the patient opposite the tube is obviously much less dangerous but still to be avoided wherever possible by the use of compression cones, wooden spoons and palpation outside the shutter opening. When manipulation is essential, the beam should be reduced to strike as small an area as is practicable. Care must also be taken that the gloves on which the fluoroscopist relies for protection are discarded before they become old and cracked and no longer serve their purpose.[10]

(d) Time employed for fluoroscopy.

Another serious radiation problem is produced by the long period of fluoroscopy some physicians seem to require for examination of the alimentary tract. Preliminary investigations indicate that almost all of the intelligence recorded on the fluoroscopic screen can be appreciated by the observer within a few seconds after the image has first appeared on the screen. Protracted periods of scrutiny are usually of little value in obtaining additional diagnostic information. While the speed of intelligent appreciation depends to a great extent on the observer's experience, there seems little reason why the majority of gastro-intestinal examinations need be prolonged by the average radiologist beyond a period of five minutes of actual fluoroscopy. As Carman once said: "The longer one looks, the more one is apt to see what does not exist." The examination can be regarded as complete the moment the examiner forms a definite idea as to the significance of the manifestations presented.[11]

A manually reset cumulative timer should be installed to indicate the elapsed time and to turn off the equipment at a predetermined limit. This timer should have a maximum range of five minutes.

(e) Lead protective devices.

Lead rubber aprons, lead rubber gloves and where applicable lead-protected chairs as well as other lead protective devices should be employed. Whenever possible their adequacy should be checked periodically.

Apron: The lead rubber used for the apron should have a lead equivalent of at least 0.4 mm. measured at 80 kilovolts.

Gloves: The gloves should have a lead equivalent of 0.5 mm. and must cover the whole hand, fingers and wrist.

Chairs: A protective chair with a 1.0 mm. lead shield device built into the back and a lead rubber curtain to protect one's legs is a useful device for vertical fluoroscopy.

Protective curtain: Whenever possible the flexible lead-impregnated protective curtain attached to the fluoroscopic screen should be used, since it is effective in reducing scatter arising from the patient.

Where a bucky slot is present, a suitable shielding should be added.

Lead rubber flaps suspended from the screen between the patient and fluoroscopist should also be employed.

(f) Distance between tube and screen.

Added protection can be secured if the distance from the x-ray tube to the screen is increased, since the intensity of the rays varies inversely with the square of the distance. At no time should the table panel be closer than 12 inches to the tube; 18 inches is preferable.

Increasing the distance between target and patient will always result in a reduction in patient dose *for the same screen illumination.* For example, increasing the target panel distance from 8 to 12 inches will result in a 33 per cent reduction in skin dose.

(g) Exposure rate at panel.

The exposure rate at the panel should be as low as possible and should never exceed 10 r per minute.

(h) The fluoroscopic screen.

The fluoroscopic screen should always be kept as close to the patient's body as is practical. In this way, the fluroscopist is protected from exposure to radiation both primary and secondary that might be projected beyond the sides of the screen frame. Furthermore, less distortion occurs at the closer screen-patient distance. The fluoroscopic screen should be covered with a transparent protective window having a lead equivalent of at least 2.0 mm. for 100 peak kilovoltage.

For average settings it would be wise to measure the dose rate above the screen, i.e., radiation transmitted through the screen without a patient in position. With the screen at a distance of 15 cm. from the panel surface, 20 mr or less is acceptable.[29] In a recent study, 17 per cent of machines exceeded this dosage.

The National Bureau of Standards Handbook recommends that the tube and screen should be so linked that under normal use the screen always intercepts the radiation emitted through the aperture of the x-ray tube.

(i) Dark adaptation.

It cannot be too strongly emphasized that the fluoroscopist should allow his eyes to become fully adapted to the darkness before beginning his fluoroscopic examination. Otherwise, there may be unsatisfactory fluoroscopic vision which may tempt the operator to increase milliamperage, kilovoltage or the time beyond the maximum recommended value. In this way he may expose the patient, and under certain conditions himself and his assistant as well, to amounts of radiation which may be dangerous.

(j) Intermittent exposure.

The make and break or the intermittent type of exposure, as made possible by the foot switch, is also advantageous. The intermittency of the exposures helps to protect the skin of the patient. It also reduces the amount of heat generated in the target of the x-ray tube.

(k) Bucky slot.

Whenever possible a shield of 0.25 mm. lead equivalent should be placed between patient and fluoroscopist and over the bucky slot. These shields should not substitute for the wearing of a protective apron.

(1) Periodic checkups.

It is advisable that the examining physician and those working with radiation should be checked on the radiation they have received. This is done by using a small ionization chamber capable of totaling up the radiation received over a period of time. Such an instrument, which looks like a fountain pen, is carried during the time spent in the locality of the fluoroscope. At the end of any convenient period, the instrument is checked to see how much radiation it registers. There are also ionization instruments which give a quick indication of the stray radiation at any given point. In the absence of such instruments, rough checks may be made with x-ray film of the type generally used for dental radiography. Such dental film, employing a filter to indicate the penetrability of the ray, is carried on the person for a specified period and then developed. This is the basis of the film badges which are used as a type of dosimeter in appraising the amount of radiation received by the wearer. It is efficient and recommended. Tests such as these serve two purposes: they check on the adequacy of protective measures, and they check also on the safety habits of the individual involved. Any indication of excessive exposure should lead immediately to an investigation of the protective measures used in the particular office or laboratory, as well as of the conduct of the particular individual.

Blood counts are also used for checking on excessive radiation. Changes in the blood count are usually the first conveniently obtainable biological indication of extensive overexposure to radiation.[12] However, there are no blood changes which dependably indicate incipient damage to personnel from radiation exposure, i.e., before real damage has occurred. Blood counts should be repeated periodically. Emphasis should be placed upon trends in serial blood counts rather than on one blood examination. A reduction of the white cell count by 2,000 may indicate radiation injury and should be investigated.

Summary.

Again and again it has been emphasized that experience and training of fluoroscopists are as important as mechanical protection with regard to safety during fluoroscopy. Experienced examiners adapt their eyes fully to darkness, work rapidly, use a small beam and keep the examining hand out of the field of illumination on the screen.[13] In other words, training, common sense and experience are probably the three most important protective devices with which the operator can fortify himself.[14] *It should be remembered that while lead aprons and gloves are cheap and time for accommodation is cheap, the hands and health of the physician are without price.*[10]

METHODS FOR PROTECTING THE PATIENT

A few words should be added in describing protection to the patient. Of the various diagnostic x-ray applications, fluoroscopy probably presents the greatest radiation hazard, not only to the examiner but also the patient.[8] The dose or number of r received by the patient for a given illumination depends upon a number of conditions: (a) The target panel distance; (b) the extent of filtration; (c) the size of the field; (d) the voltage of the tube; (e) the sensitivity of the screen. In large part, these points have already been discussed under "Methods for Protecting the Fluoroscopist." Here the discussion will concern itself specifically with the patient.

(a) The target panel distance: The distance between the target of the x-ray tube and the patient's skin must be *at least 12 inches.*[8] Greater distances are preferable since they reduce the likelihood of overexposure and also improve the fluoroscopic image.[15] The intensity of the x-ray radiation reaching the patient's skin varies inversely with the square of the distance from the target of the x-ray tube. For example, the intensity of the x-ray radiation at ten inches distance is four times that at twenty inches distance, all other factors remaining the same.

(b) The extent of filtration: The best practice is to use a minimum of 2.5 mm. aluminum filter or its equivalent between the x-ray tube and the patient. This filter equivalent should be determined at the maximum kilovoltage of the x-ray machine.

(c) The size of the field: To prevent needless exposure of other parts of the patient's body and to improve the sharpness of the fluoroscopic image, the shutter mechanism should be adjusted to the *smallest size field* necessary to cover the part being examined.[8] The small field sizes imposed by screens of thirty to fifty square inches have done much to reduce the radiation exposure of patients under examination.[16]

If a "high-low switch" is available on the fluoroscopic machine used, then the low intensity should be used to locate the area of interest and the high intensity only momentarily to explore that area.

(d) The voltage of the tube: The milliamperage should be as low as possible without sacrificing satisfactory fluoroscopic vision. The milliamperage should in no case exceed 5 ma. The kilovoltage should be set in accordance with the thickness and density of the part being examined. Though the rating of the machine may be 100 peak kilovoltage or more, as already noted, no more than 85 kv.p. for abdominal fluoroscopy, 3 ma. at 70 kv.p. for the chest, and 3 ma. at 60 kv.p. for the extremities should be used.[8, 16]

(e) Sensitivity of screen: The more sensitive the screen, the less radiation need be used, thus aiding in the patient's protection. The type of screen in common use is the Patterson B2 screen.

Further Precautions for the Patient's Protection

After outlining the various factors involved in the dose of radiation received by the patient, further precautions for the patient's protection can be suggested.

The exposure in roentgens should be measured at the table-top for the maximum voltage and minimum filter used in both fluoroscopy as well as radiography. The product of roentgens per minute and the number of minutes consumed for an examination is the number of roentgens received by the patient during examination. A synchronous clock in series with the foot switch will enable the fluoroscopist to keep an exact record of the amount of time x-rays are being generated. This information will also be valuable in calculating the dose he himself has received.

CORRECT INSTALLATION AS AN AID TO PROTECTION

Safety against the harmful effects of x-ray implies a safe installation. For practical purposes, the average fluoroscopic installation today needs no further check beyond making sure that the equipment is shock-proof and that there is no radiation to any unwanted point, as for example, to adjoining rooms, or rooms above or below the installation. This can be tested by exposure of film left in these places and periodically checked for control. The original installation and the periodic check-up should be done by a trained physicist.

Clear and specific information about safety requirements is available in such publications as the National Bureau of Standards Handbook 76[12] and should be consulted without fail.

A Safe Fluoroscopic Room

A stationary *upright* unit located in the corner of the room presents no hazardous condition for the roentgenologist, but when the technician is present and standing at the side next to the wall, he receives a large amount of radiation scattered back from the wall.

Assuming that both the roentgenologist and the assisting technician are fully protected by lead aprons and gloves and that a *horizontal* fluoroscope is used, drawing on the data gathered by Cowing and Spalding[9] we can conclude that the minimum room dimensions should be twelve by fourteen feet. At least six feet of clear space should exist between the roentgenologist and the closest wall regardless of the type of examination carried out.

SUMMARY: RULES FOR PROTECTION

The actual rules for the protection of patient and physician during fluoroscopy and radiography are not complicated. Strict obedience to these rules will obviate most of the hazards to which writers have called attention for over two decades. They are especially important to keep in mind for physicians *who do not* specialize in radiology and whose main interest is in the diagnostic result. Such physicians are traditionally apt to give too little consideration to the need for protection.

The fluoroscope should be operated only by those physicians who have had special training in its use and who have proved to the satisfaction of a qualified roentgenologist that they have sufficient knowledge of the physics, uses, and—in particular—the dangers involved in the use of this apparatus.

Here are the simple rules for the use of the fluoroscope:

Don't start to fluoroscope until your eyes are dark-adapted. (See next section, on "Dark Adaptation.")

Don't fluoroscope while other patients are free to move about the room.

Don't use more than 5 milliamperes of current and 85 peak kilovoltage.

Don't use any but a red electric bulb of small wattage for illumination during the time necessary for change of patients; thus adequate dark adaptation is carried over from one patient to another.

Don't use any but the smallest possible shutter opening at any time.

Don't fluoroscope without wearing proper protective gloves and apron.

Don't permit any attendant to remain during fluoroscopy unless he has proper protective materials.

Don't keep the current on for a fraction of a second more than necessary; learn to interrupt the current while moving the tube about, turning the patient, and other maneuvers.

Don't fluoroscope any patient for more than four to five minutes during any one week.

Don't repeat within two weeks any fluoroscopic or permit any radiographic examination of a patient who has received a tolerance dose.

Don't energize the tube for more than 20 seconds continuously. Frequent make and breaks should be routine.

Don't leave the fluoroscopic room without turning off the main switch.

Don't abuse the apparatus.

The tragedies wrought by x-rays in the past were caused by ignorance; today the injuries are caused by folly. Radiation injuries have been greatly reduced because operators know today with what they are dealing, and what precautions must be taken. Under excessive exposure, the rays themselves are just as deadly as they ever were.[17] But now there is practically no excuse for anyone ever being injured by x-rays or radium. The great majority of x-ray installations are as safe as designing can make them. What injuries occur arise from ignorance, carelessness or haste.

It has been urged that the recommendations of the Safety Committee should be published once a year, and should be more widely circulated in the non-roentgenologic medical literature, which is read by those who "do a little x-ray work." One must distinguish clearly and emphatically the fact that the physician who occasionally does some x-ray work has an entirely different risk outlook from that of the expert roentgenologist. It is the physicians in the first group who *need* protection.[18]

Dark Adaptation

Since fluoroscopy takes place in a dark room, the subject of dark adaptation is of great importance. It is incumbent upon the fluoroscopist to understand the basic retinal physiology, for with a knowledge of the limitations of his own visual apparatus the examiner will not attempt to fluoroscope a patient without full dark adaptation.

BASIC PHYSIOLOGY

Dark adaptation can be defined as increased retinal irritability. The increase in retinal irritability after dark adaptation is truly amazing. It has been calculated by various investigators to be as much as 50,000 to 100,000 times as great as the irritability existing in the eye which is not dark-adapted.[19] Chamberlain quotes authorities who demonstrated an increased irritability up to 40,000 times as great in the dark-adapted eye as compared with the eye which is not dark-adapted.[14]

Dark adaptation is a function of the rods, and the basic physiology can be stated thus:

Retinene + Vitamin A + Colloid (Protein)
darkness Rhodopsin (Visual purple).

It is the presence of *rhodopsin* (visual purple) within the rods[19] which in the main is responsible for vision in the dark, and without it a state of night blindness exists— i.e., inability to see in a dark room which makes fluoroscopic vision impossible. The examiner who proceeds with his fluoroscopic examination immediately after turning off the light should at least be acquainted with this basic physiological fact.

In the light the disintegration of rhodopsin takes place in this manner:

Rhodopsin (Visual purple) + Light → Retinene
$$\downarrow$$
Vitamin A

The disintegration of *rhodopsin* in the presence of light takes place far more rapidly than its formation in the dark. The retina after exposure to bright light for three minutes loses its sensitivity 40,000 fold,[14] and it bears repetition that it is this sensitivity that is so necessary for adequate vision on the fluoroscopic screen.

Normally, in bright light a perception of different degrees of brightness as well as visual acuity is a function of the cones rather than the rods.[20] When the eye is dark-adapted and the rods are functioning at peak efficiency, perception of these qualities is markedly diminished. The light-adapted human eye is able to distinguish differences in brightness when these differences are of the order of 1 to 2 per cent. The same eye, in the dark, even though completely dark-adapted, requires a 20 to 40 per cent difference of brightness for discrimination.[14] Upon a moment's reflection, the fluoroscopist will realize that since such a diminution in visual acuity occurs in a dark room, *even when his eyes are completely dark-adapted*, certainly *when he is not dark-adapted his vision must be tantamount to blindness*. This is best illustrated by the familiar experience of walking into a dimly lit room from the bright sun.

METHODS OF INDUCING DARK ADAPTATION

Dark adaptation is brought about by the formation of rhodopsin (visual purple). This is synthesized in the dark, i.e., the absence of light stimulation. Dark adaptation is more precipitate *after* the use of red goggles.[30] On the average, the examiner should remain in complete darkness for four minutes after red goggles have been worn for twenty minutes. This is especially important when thick parts are to be viewed. After the first patient has been fluoroscoped and red goggles are again put on, succeeding patients can be examined after one minute of darkness, providing strong light sources are avoided.[30] The achievement of efficient dark adaptation will vary in time in different individuals up to a half hour.

TESTING DARK ADAPTATION

A means of testing dark adaptation is desirable, if not indispensible. A wristwatch with its luminous hour marks has been found by one observer to be a reliable test object.[11] When the numerals become more clearly visible in the dark, one can consider himself well adapted. Other, more detailed, means of testing dark adaptation have been described at length by Chamberlain[14] and Harvey.[21] The latter suggests arranging a series of film strips in steps (in a darkened room), corresponding to a progressive increase in density. The observer who is properly dark-adapted will be able to see a greater number of these strips than when not dark-adapted.

FLUOROSCOPIC VISION

If, when one has been outdoors for some minutes on a dark night, a feeble star is seen, and the gaze is then turned slightly to one side, it will be noticed that the brightness of the star appears perceptibly greater. This can also be demonstrated with an ordinary luminous watch. When the face of the luminous clock is looked at directly in a darkened room, the figures are blurred and less noticeable. Directing the gaze a trifle to the side will make the watch dial appear more luminous and the numbers sharper. This is because in a dark-adapted eye perception is shifted from the central fovea to the more peripheral area of the retina where the rods are located. It is thus evident that if the fluoroscopist can train himself to look with a scanning type of vision, his perception will be greater than by observing with a direct gaze.

To observe rapidly moving objects, peripheral vision is abandoned.[32, 33] This is because the perception of motion in these cases rests partly on the kinesthetic impulses from the extraocular muscles. Pe-

ripheral vision is not useful in following this type of motion. In the study of such motion, i.e., movements of the diaphragm or of the heart, it is valuable to use certain landmarks to gauge the movements. The use of shutters and/or other devices (fig. 73) as reference points (figs. 28, 29, 30) to gauge this motion is valuable.

It is recommended that during fluoroscopic examination, short intermittent exposures be made rather than long-continued ones. Since at low brightness levels vision is cumulative[31] and since the full stimulus is not perceived by the eye for about one-fifth of a second, the intermitence of the exposures is not confined to one- or two-second bursts of fluoroscopy. Instead, the examiner should rapidly view the field and get as much information as the image on the screen can offer and then take his foot off the switch. The examiner should train himself to gain the information in as short a time as possible, averaging between five and ten seconds per exposure. This will reduce the amount of radiation the patient receives and prolong the life of the x-ray tube.

The rate of replenishment of visual purples depends upon age, physical fitness, vitamin sufficiency and other factors. For normal eyes, the time required for complete replenishment, or dark adaptation, ranges from twenty to thirty minutes.

Persons who normally wear glasses should not remove them when doing fluoroscopy.[17]

SUMMARY OF DARK ADAPTATION

It cannot be too strongly emphasized that the fluoroscopist must allow his eyes to become fully adapted to the darkness before beginning his fluoroscopic examination.

If this rule is not observed the following dangers may result:

There may be *unsatisfactory fluoroscopic vision*, which may tempt the operator to increase the milliamperage, the kilovoltage, or the time, beyond the maximum recommended value. In this way, he may expose the patient and under certain conditions himself and his assistant as well to an amount of radiation that may be dangerous.

Wrong interpretation may be put on the fact that things are *not* seen on the screen. A fluoroscopist who begins an examination before an appropriate degree of dark adaptation has been achieved owes it to himself and to his patient to know precisely what is involved when he makes this misinterpretation: unless he has an understanding of his own visual apparatus and the way it works,

he is apt to be deceived into believing that what he does *not* see has great significance. Great care must be taken in every case to avoid the danger that *absence of fluoroscopic evidence* may be given too much weight. Even when the fluoroscopist is completely dark-adapted, there are inherent limitations in fluoroscopy. If to these is added the further limitations growing out of inadequate dark adaptation, the deficiency may be considerable.

Vitamin A has been observed to help in dark adaptation. This is especially true with advancing years.[39]

New Developments in Image Intensification

Recently, electronic aids have been devised to intensify the brightness of the fluoroscopic image.[22-25] During conventional fluoroscopy, the human eye utilizes about 1 to 5 per cent of the diagnostic information produced by the *roentgen ray photons* at the fluoroscopic screen.[26] The purpose of intensifying the brightness of the fluoroscopic screen is to improve the efficient utilization of these roentgen ray photons, thereby considerably improving the diagnostic clarity of the fluoroscopic image. With *conventional fluoroscopy*, the eye depends upon rod vision, which is capable of *gross* detail discrimination. The image produced by these newer methods of intensifying the brightness of the image (*image intensification*) is suitable for cone vision and reveals much more *detail*. Prolonged dark adaptation is not necessary. More rapid examinations made possible by a brighter image reduce the amount of radiation rereived by both patient and physician. The obvious advantages of this new type of equipment will undoubtedly result in increased use as it becomes more generally available, and thus it warrants some discussion here.

HOW IS BRIGHTNESS INTENSIFICATION OBTAINED?

The basic factors responsible for the intensification of image brightness are:

1. X-rays, after passing through the patient, impinge upon a fluorescent screen similar to the conventional fluoroscopic screen. The x-rays, acting on the fluoroscopic screen, release *photo-electrons* from a photo surface deposited on the back of the screen. Thus, the fluoroscopic image is transformed into an *electronic* image. This electronic image is intensified by accelerating the photo-electrons through a 25 to 30 kilovolt potential difference. The *accelerated electrons* then strike an output fluorescent screen, releasing *more light* than from the original fluorescent screen. The more energy an electron possesses on its arrival at the screen, the more fluorescent light will it produce. By this method the energy is increased.

2. Another important factor is the gain in brightness produced by *reduction of the size* of the image. Since *all* the electrons contribute toward the final image, an increase in brightness is obtained by *all of the*

electrons being *concentrated* in a smaller area. By employing a reduction factor of 5 to 9 times, the electrons are concentrated in a much smaller area.[27] The reduced image, when viewed through an optical system, is again magnified without loss of any of the brightness gained.

3. Special type television intensifiers are also employed. Here a photosensitive tube, an image orthicon, is used. The light from the conventional fluoroscopic screen is focused on this photosensitive tube, which in turn produces an electrical signal. This signal is amplified and is impressed on the control grit of the cathode ray tube. Eventually there appears on the surface of the cathode ray tube a fluoroscopic image of the patient.[28]

VALUE OF IMAGE INTENSIFICATION

By means of the intensification of the fluoroscopic image, fluoroscopy will become altogether a more valuable and more widely used diagnostic weapon than ever before. Improvement in the actual visualization of the image on the screen can open new fields in diagnostic fluoroscopy and radiography. Examination of the heart, for example, can reveal calcification of valves and even coronary arteries, previously seen with difficulty. The ease with which the pathologic or normal physiology of the gastrointestinal tract can be observed will result in more exact and gainful diagnosis. The small bowel will undergo increased study.

The radiation necessary to produce a diagnostic image with an image intensifier, e.g., for chest fluoroscopy, involves .05 r for 15 seconds. With conventional fluoroscopy, the same image would use .75 r.[35]

Further, the image from the screen can be photographed. The resulting cineradiography appears to be the future of diagnostic radiology. Televising the image from the screen is also already a fact, and useful at this time especially in teaching. Televised images recorded on tape are among the new technics being developed.

CHAPTER II

Examination of the Chest

General Fundamentals

THERE IS A growing tendency to avoid use of the fluoroscope wherever possible. If a film can give as much information as a fluoroscope screen, the film study is preferable. Yet, the physician who depends on the roentgenographic film for his diagnosis *must* often resort to fluoroscopy. A radiologist without a fluoroscope can be likened to the proverbial one-armed paper hanger. It is with this realization in mind that this chapter is approached. A description of a complete examination of a chest by fluoroscopic means will be given. This is rarely indicated and ordinarily is not recommended. Yet, such a description has a two-fold purpose. First, the physician who undertakes to do a good and efficient radiographic examination should understand the basic essentials involved in the full fluoroscopic examination of the chest. Secondly, with such a knowledge of the *whole* examination, he can readily select any applicable portion and use it as needed in meaningful and productive fashion.

No diagnosis should ever be arrived at from fluoroscopic examination alone. Information derived from the fluoroscopic procedure constitutes but a single link in the chain leading to final diagnosis. Where necessary and in the interests of efficiency and completeness a routine for fluoroscopic examination should be adopted and adhered to. The procedure recommended here, when done completely, is: (1) General survey of the chest; (2) positioning; (3) localization; (4) detailed examination, and (5) diaphragmatic and mediastinal movements.

PREPARATION

The examination is valueless unless the physician's eyes are properly accommodated. This has been considered in greater detail in Chapter I. For chest fluoroscopy, accommodation can be considered adequate when the middle-sized pulmonary vessels can be seen. As shown in figure 1, these vessels are adjacent to the hilar shadow, approximately in the middle lung field. On the fluoroscopic screen these vessels appear as a fine, reticulated pattern.

The patient should be asked to strip down to the waist. It is permissible for him to wear an ordinary light-weight gown. He is made to stand (or sit, if very weak) behind the fluoroscopic screen, facing the examiner.* The anterior chest wall should touch the screen.

A glassful of barium mixture, two heaping tablespoonfuls of barium to eight ounces of water, should be at hand.

---

* This is the "frontal" position, a term used frequently in this book. It should be taken to mean the postero-anterior position, i.e., the pa-

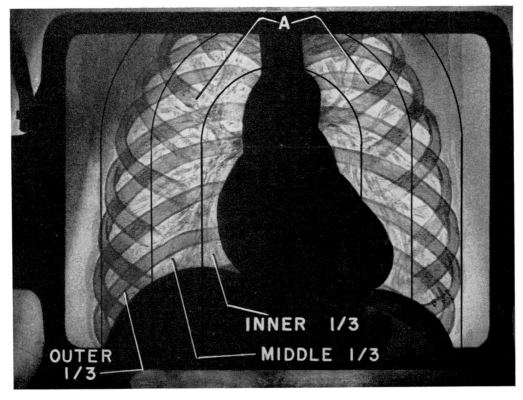

1

Structures making up and radiating from the hilum consist in the main of the various divisions of the pulmonary artery. The prominence of these vessels is greatest in the inner third and diminished in the middle third and finally disappear in the outer third. If markings are evident in the outer third, they must be considered as increased.

EXAMINATION

GENERAL SURVEY

The fluoroscopic shutters are opened wide,* and the entire chest and mediastinum are examined. Both lung fields normally should be equally illuminated (fig. 2). On

tient facing the examiner or screen, with the x-ray tube behind the patient. (See also note, page 42.)

Regarding positioning, it is important to remember that—unless otherwise specified—in every position, whether back or front, the chest or abdomen (depending on the part being examined) should be touching the screen or should be as close to it as possible; this is to avoid undue magnification, which causes distortion.

* Throughout this book, reference to wide opened shutters always implies use of a lead frame as described in Chapter I.

either side of the mediastinum the butterfly-like hila are seen, the right being slightly lower than the left (fig. 3). The various vascular markings radiating from them should be noted. It should be understood that the pattern in the lung fields making up the hila and the reticulated lung parenchyma consists, in the main, of the various divisions of the pulmonary artery. The caliber and prominence of the pulmonary vessels are greatest in the inner third of each lung field, and become less prominent in the middle third of the lung fields. The peripheral third has a paucity of markings and is relatively clear (fig. 1).

Next, a search is made for any abnormal opacities within either lung field. A lesion usually cannot be seen on the fluoroscopic

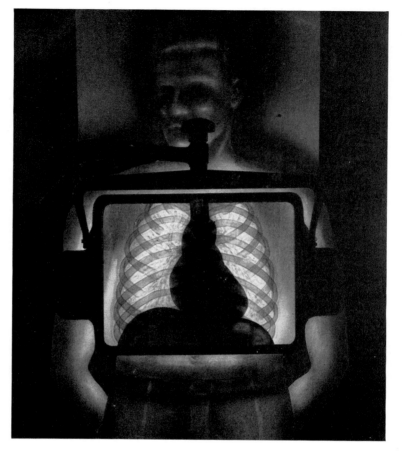

2

The first step of the general survey should reveal both lung fields equally illuminated.

screen unless it has grown to about one-half inch at its greater diameter. It should be noted in this connection that it is entirely possible for a lesion to have become far larger than one-half inch and still not be visible on the fluoroscopic screen because the very structure of the abnormality is not sufficiently dense. This may occur in the presence of either pneumonia, tuberculosis, or metastatic neoplasms. However, the disease process will be demonstrated on the radiographic film.[1]

As part of this gross survey, the mediastinum is observed. In order to distinguish an abnormal shadow in this region, it is important to know and understand the normal structures comprising the mediastinal shadow. Figure 4 illustrates this.

Normal Shadows Which May Cause Confusion

During this *general survey* the fluoroscopist may be confronted by certain possibly confusing, normal shadows. These will now be described.

In women the position of the nipples and breasts must be defined to prevent the misinterpretation of their shadows as changes in the lung. The breasts are seen usually as hazes at both bases. The nipple may be seen as a nodular shadow within the lung field closely simulating a true pathological lesion (fig. 5). If such an abnormality is suspected in these regions, moving of the breasts will help determine it—the nipple will move when the breast is moved, while an abnor-

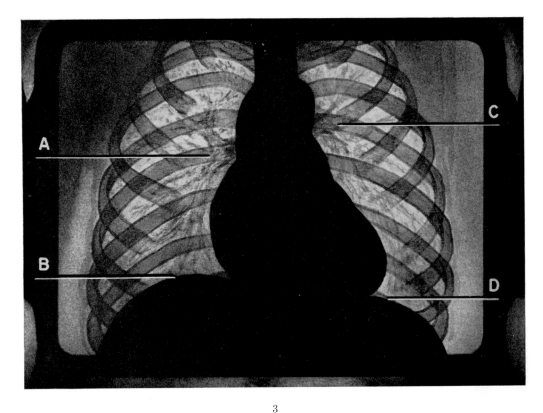

3

A. Right hilus lower   C. Left hilus higher
B. Right diaphragm higher   D. Left diaphragm lower

mal shadow within the lungs will remain stationary.

The nipple in men may also cause a similar difficulty. The same maneuver is applicable as in the female.

The vertebral borders of the scapulae are seen in the upper lung fields, and their outline must be defined to prevent errors in diagnosis. The inexperienced observer may occasionally mistake them for lobar consolidations (fig. 5).

The apices of both lungs may occasionally be clouded because of the overlying neck muscles (fig. 6). An attempt should be made to move these muscles with the hand, in order to clear these shadows. If the examiner finds this impossible, special apical roentgenographic procedures should be carried out.

On occasion, when a calcification is noted in the lung apex, the observer should try to displace it with his finger. A lesion present in the neck may be projected into the lung apex by the obliquity of the x-rays.[1] By palpating in the neck the examiner may find this opaque shadow and move it about.

Calcifications in the chondral cartilages joining the ribs to the sternum are occasionally seen (fig. 7). They are usually multiple, in line with the ribs, and situated in the inner third of each lung field. They follow the ribs, and move with respiration.

The mediastinum may appear to be widened by scoliosis of the dorsal spine. When such is the case, a bulge is usually seen on the convex side of the curve (fig. 8). Fluoroscopically, scoliosis is often detected from the abnormal widening of the intercostal spaces on one side, and narrowing on the other. Confirmation, if necessary, should be secured either by raising the kilovoltage

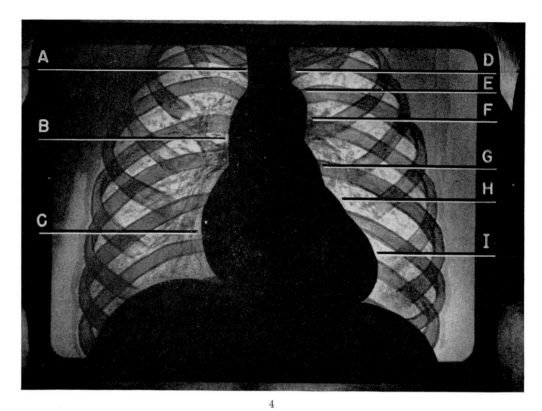

4

A. Inominate artery
B. Ascending aorta
C. Right auricle

D. Subclavian vessels
E. Aortic knob
F. Descending aorta
G. Pulmonary artery
H. Left auricular app.
I. Left ventricle

during fluoroscopic visualization or by securing an overpenetrated film of the chest.

Abnormal Shadows

In the majority of examinations, since no abnormality is discovered, the examiner can proceed, as recommended, to the *detailed examination*. However, in those instances when an abnormality is discovered, the next procedures to be followed are *positioning* and *localization*.

Positioning. When an abnormal shadow is found during fluoroscopy, a roentgenogram is the next essential procedure. The radiographic film is superior to the fluoroscopic examination in that it allows more time for study, and gives sharper delineation of the image. The x-ray provides the examiner with a clearer, more permanent record of the lesion.

A radiographic film taken without previous fluoroscopy may not show the abnormality to its greatest advantage. During the fluoroscopic examination the patient can be rotated until the apparent lesion is cleared of overlapping shadows. Subsequently, when taking the roentgenogram the patient should be placed in the same position in reference to the radiographic film as he previously occupied in relationship to the fluoroscopic screen.

Localization. When an abnormality has been discovered, its localization is important. This can be accomplished with either

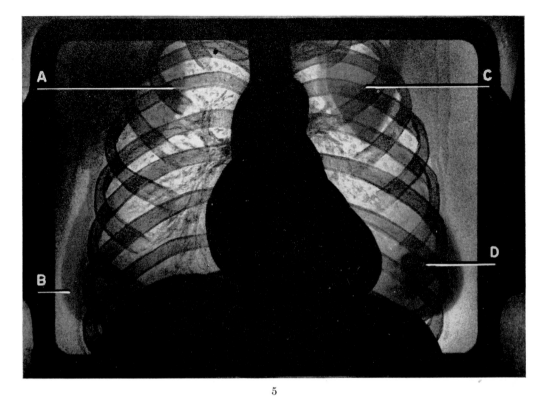

5

A. Scapula
B. Haze at base may be due to breast

C. Scapula shadows (not to be confused with a lobal consolidation)
D. Nipple may be seen on one or both sides. Hazes at base due to breast.

Note: If doubt exists as to the origin of the nodular shadows, moving the breast will clear the dilemma. The breast and nipple will move. A true pathological entity will remain stationary.

multiple radiographic films or fluoroscopically. Two procedures useful for fluoroscopic localization will be described.

As in figures 9 and 10, it is seen that the farther away an object is from the surface upon which its shadow is projected, the larger and more indistinct the shadow becomes. The converse of this naturally follows. The closer the object is to the surface on which its shadow is projected, the smaller and more sharply delineated it becomes.

During fluoroscopy this principle may be applied to the localization of a pathologic lesion. The pathological process is studied first with the patient facing the fluoroscopic screen; next, the patient is turned so that his back is towards the fluoroscopic screen. The size and sharpness of the shadow is observed. The position in which it is smaller and more clearly demarcated will be the cue to the examiner as to whether the lesion is in the anterior or posterior lung field. (See figure 11 and compare with figure 12.)

The second method of localization is based on the "law of the circle." When the circle is rotated in a clockwise direction, objects posteriorly located (i.e., 12 o'clock position) will rotate from left to right. An object anteriorly located (i.e., 6 o'clock position), on the other hand, will travel from right to left. This is an important concept. It, too, can be applied to the fluoroscopic localization. If, when rotating the

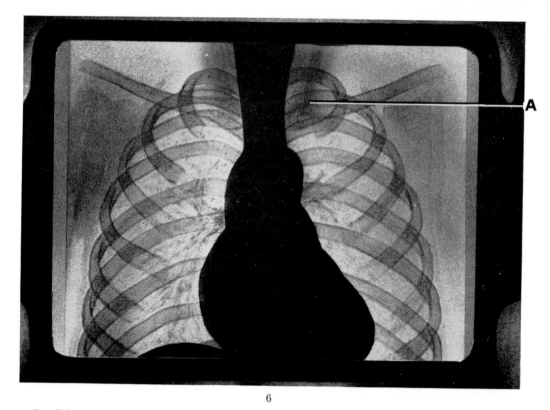

6

Overlying neck muscles (A) may simulate infiltration in both apices. Hooking the fingers into the lateral margin of the sterno-mastoid muscle and moving them about will solve the dilemma.

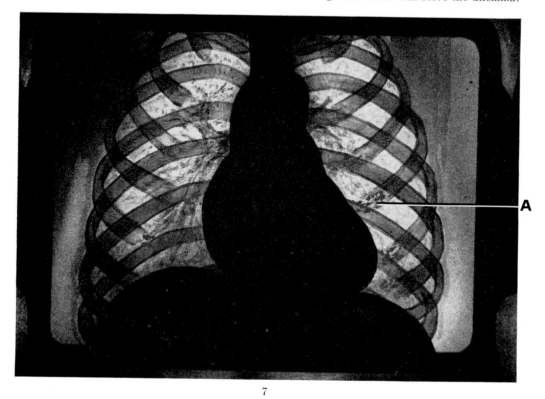

7

Calcification in chondral cartilage (A) may cause confusion. These usually are in line with ribs and move with respiration.

chest, the abnormal shadow rotates in the same direction as the spine (or the patient's back), the lesion is situated posteriorly. If the abnormality rotates in the same direction as the sternum, it must be located anteriorly (figs. 13 and 14).

In practice, the "law of the circle" as described here is simple. Yet, it does happen occasionally that as the patient is being ro-

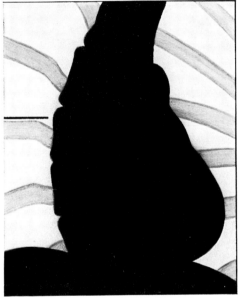

8

An apparent widening of the mediastinum may be produced by a scoliotic spine. The abnormal widening of the intercostal spaces on one side and closer approximation on the other side should be a clue to proper diagnosis. Confirmation can be secured by raising the kilovoltage or securing an overpenetrated film and thus visualizing the spine.

tated towards one side or the other, it is difficult to determine in which direction the abnormal shadow travels. As in figures 15–19, an opaque marker can be used as a reference point. One margin of the abnormal shadow is placed in a direct line with a marker fixed to the anterior chest wall. When the patient is rotated, the movements of the margin of the shadow in question can easily be determined by its changing relationship to the marker.

Approximately how far anterior or posterior the lesion is situated can often be gaged by observing the rate of speed at which the lesion travels. We are all familiar with the fact that a spoke of a rotating wheel will travel more rapidly at the periphery than at the center. This can be applied directly to observing the speed at which the abnormal shadow rotates in reference to a coin pasted on the posterior or anterior chest wall, depending upon which of the two is closer to the lesion. If, in rotating the chest, the lesion and coin travel at the same rate of speed, we may assume that they are close together. Should the coin travel much more rapidly than the lesion, we can assume more separation. With a little experience the approximate depth of the lesion can be determined.

Because of overlapping shadows, lateral fluoroscopy of the chest is not as useful as the equivalent roentgenogram of the chest in the lateral position.

Having established a lesion within the lung to be adjacent to a rib, it becomes im-

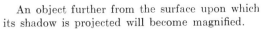

Source of Light   Object

Shadow large and hazy

9

An object further from the surface upon which its shadow is projected will become magnified.

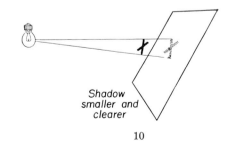

Shadow smaller and clearer

10

An object closer to the surface upon which its shadow is projected will become smaller and more clearly delineated.

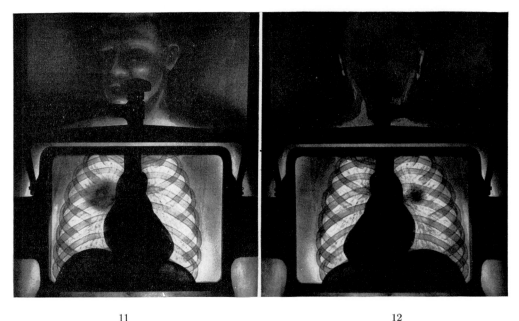

11

12

Patient facing examiner. Shadow large and hazy.

Patient with back to examiner. *Same* shadow as figure 11 now appears smaller and sharper. Shadow thus located in posterior chest.

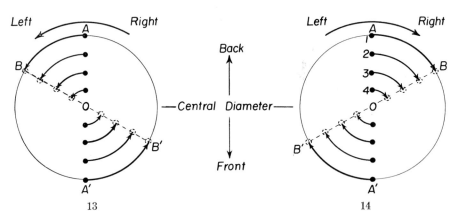

13

14

Circle (or patient) rotated from right to left (counterclockwise). All structures in back will move from right to left (A to B). All structures anteriorly move from left to right (A' to B').

Circle or patient rotated clockwise. All structures posteriorly travel from left to right (A to B). All structures anteriorly travel from right to left (A' to B').

portant to determine whether or not the lesion is free, or adherent to this bony structure. A simple principle which will prove of great aid in making this determination is as follows: During respiration, air entry into the lung is accomplished by the barrel-like action of the ribs moving upward, causing the lungs to *expand*. The diaphragm, traveling downwards, causes the lung to *descend*. When a lesion is present and free from the rib, it will manifest itself as a descending shadow following the diaphragm downward with inspiration, while simultaneously the ribs are traveling upwards. When, on the

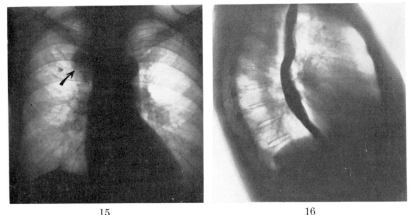

15
A mass is seen (arrow).

16
The lateral study does not
help to place the lesion.

The law of the circle is employed to place the lesion.

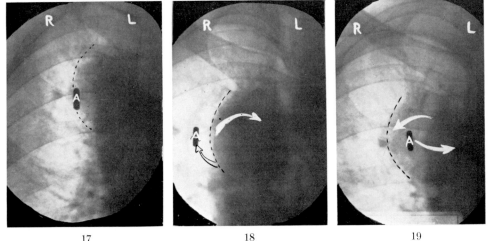

17

The patient is placed be-
hind the fluoroscopic screen in
the frontal position. The lesion
is found (dotted line) and
opaque marker A, fixed to the
anterior chest of the patient,
is placed at the periphery of
the shadow.

18

Opaque marker A is used as
a reference point. The patient
is turned so that the anterior
chest is directed toward the
patient's right (lower arrow).
The margin of the lesion travels
towards the left (upper arrow).

19

The patient is turned so that
the anterior chest is directed
towards the patient's left
(lower arrow). The margin of
the lesion travels towards the
patient's right (upper arrow).

Comment: The opposite movements of the marker, fixed to the anterior chest wall, and the
lesion indicates the position of the lesion as being posterior.

other hand, the abnormal shadow is due to
a lesion adherent to a rib, it will follow the
movements of this latter structure. These
opposite movements of the ribs and lesion
are easy to perceive and valuable for the information they yield.

DETAILED EXAMINATION

Following the general survey, the chest
is now gone over in fine detail. The tube
diaphragm is closed down to a suitable size
in order to gain contrast. A transverse slit
is often useful. The screen is carried up to

the lung apices, and the chest is studied from above downwards, section by section, one side being compared with the other (figs. 20–23). Starting high up in the apical portions of the lung, air entry with result-ant increased illumination of the lung fields is observed when the patient is asked to breathe in deeply. Occasionally, air entry is more clearly discernible when the patient is asked to cough. After proper observation

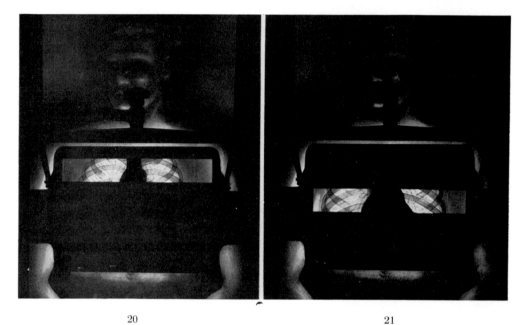

20   21

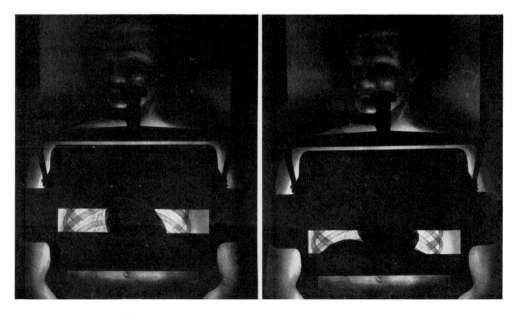

22   23

Chest examined section by section from above downward.

of the supraclavicular regions, the fluoroscopic screen, with the slit still the same size, is moved down and the subclavicular areas studied with the same degree of care as the lung portions above. The same procedure is carried out for the mid-lung fields, and, lastly, for the bases of both lungs.

In observing the lung bases the diaphragms are brought into view. The right, being pushed up by the liver, is normally slightly higher than the left. Elevation of the right diaphragm up to 2.5 cm. above the left diaphragm may often be regarded as within normal limits. It normally lies at a height equivalent to the sixth rib anteriorly. Certain divergent configurations of the diaphragm are entirely within normal limits, and should be understood as such. A band may occasionally divide the right cusp into an inner and outer half (fig. 24). The inexperienced observer may sometimes consider this pathologic. The left diaphragmatic cusp may at times be pushed up by the splenic flexure of the colon or the magenblase of the stomach (fig. 25). This must be distinguished from eventration of the diaphragm or diaphragmatic paralysis. As will be shown presently, the observation of the respiratory excursions may aid in arriving at a proper diagnosis.

It would be wise to gain the habit of always looking just below the diaphragm. The stomach air bubble on the left should be studied. The true magenblase, when distended with air, is thin-walled and situated immediately beneath the diaphragmatic cusp. If any considerable space exists between the top of the stomach and the left leaf of the diaphragm (in the upright position), an explanation on a pathologic basis must be considered (fig. 26 and figs. 227–230). In studying the stomach air bubble,

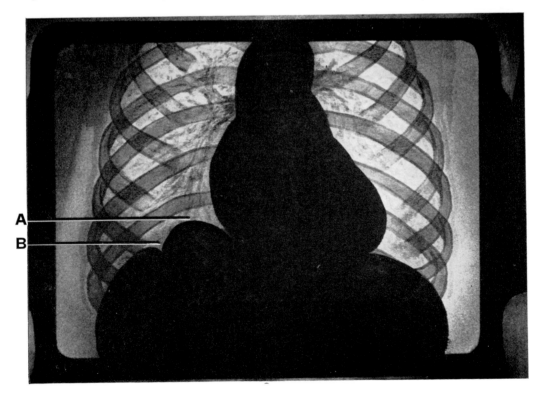

24

(A) is a normal cusp, caused by a fibrotic band (B) dividing the right hemi-diaphragm.

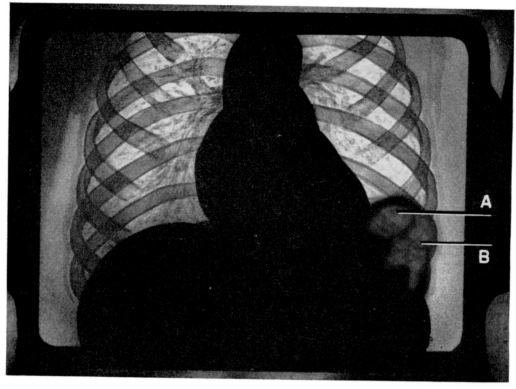

25

The diaphragm may be raised by gas distention below it.

A. Stomach air bubble, recognized by its round contour and absence of haustral markings within.

B. Splenic flexure distention is recognized by presence of haustral markings within air-distended loops.

any encroachment on the round "distended" lumen should be especially noted. Such an invasion often is due to a carcinoma of the cardia of the stomach. Before a diagnosis of an abnormal encroachment into the stomach air bubble can be made, the normal structures that may impinge and deform it should be known and understood (fig. 27). These include: the thickened mucous membrane of the stomach; the liver; the heart; the splenic flexure, and occasionally the spleen.

Other characteristics of the magenblase should be observed:

Is it pear-shaped and free of fluid level?

Is a fluid level present?

These characteristics are important, especially if the patient presents himself with

a fasting stomach. A fluid level in such a case is significant of hypersecretion. The pear-shaped fundus is usually consistent with a lack of hypersecretion (fig. 27).

Movements of the Diaphragm and Mediastinum

The one contribution that fluoroscopic examination can offer, which can be duplicated in no other type of examination, is observation of the actual movements of the diaphragm and mediastinum. One of the most valuable aspects of chest fluoroscopy is the observation of the movements of these structures. Once seen and properly evaluated, a diagnosis may often be made which would be impossible with any other type of examination. By what better method can

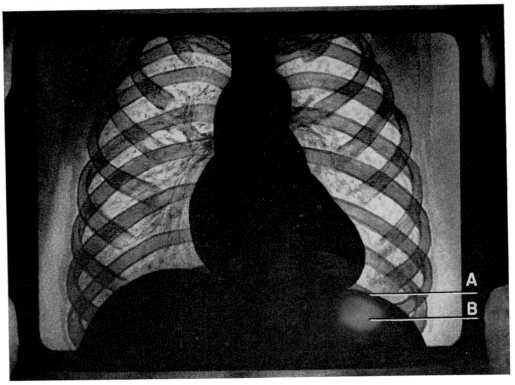

26

The examiner must observe the stomach air bubble (B) and determine it as round. In the erect position, the space (A) between the diaphragm above and the roof of the stomach air bubble must be a thin line.

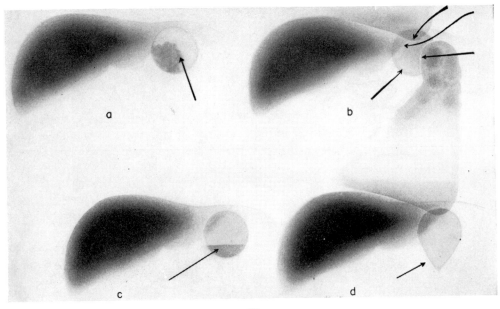

27

(a) Carcinoma (arrow) seen projecting into stomach air bubble.

(b) In order that a projection into the stomach air bubble (b) be labeled as abnormal, the normal impressions must first be known. These latter consist of left lobe of liver, cardiac apex, and splenic flexure of colon. The spleen may also produce a deformity here.

(c) A fluid level (arrow) when found in the fasting stomach can be taken as evidence of hypersecretion.

(d) The stomach air bubble can normally be expected to be "pear shaped" (arrow).

we observe diaphragmatic paralysis or paradoxical movements?

Diaphragmatic Movements. Usually, the
diaphragmatic excursions, i.e., the dome-
shaped structures on either side of the chest,

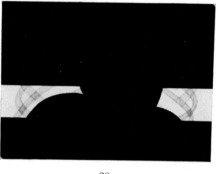

28

Normal amount of air above each diaphragm.

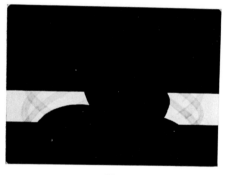

29

With inspiration the diaphragms travel down
and the amount of air above each cusp is greater.

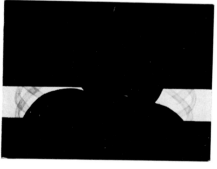

30

With expiration the diaphragms travel up and
the amount of air above the cusps is diminished.

moving up and down with respiration, are
easily observable. Yet at times great difficulty may be encountered. Let us postulate
that one of the diaphragmatic cusps was
paralyzed: It may often prove quite difficult
to discern its lack of up-and-down motion.
For example, we are all familiar with the
motion-picture device of placing a stationary object, such as an automobile, in front
of a moving background. Although the object is stationary, the moving background
makes it appear to be in motion. In the
same way, the ribs moving up and down
with respiration would make it appear that
a stationary or paralyzed diaphragm was in
motion. How, then, can we determine true
diaphragmatic excursions?

To facilitate observation the diaphragmatic shutters are narrowed down to include both diaphragmatic cusps as well as a
small segment of aerated lung above each
cusp. The amount of air in this space is
gaged and observed, and as the patient is
asked to inhale, the examiner's eyes should
be fixed, not on the downward excursion of
the diaphragm, but instead on the air-containing space above. This space should become larger and more air-filled as the diaphragm goes down. On expiration, as the
diaphragm goes up, the air space above becomes smaller (see figures 28, 29, 30).
Should a lack of diaphragmatic movement
exist, no change of size would take place in
this space, bounded by the shutter of the
diaphragm above and the diaphragmatic
cusps below.

Another method of discerning diaphragmatic movements on the fluoroscopic screen
has been referred to as the "peeling off"
phenomenon. The costo-phrenic angle on
either side of the chest is observed, and the
patient is asked to inhale. The diaphragm
can easily be imagined to act as if it were
peeled off the lateral chest wall as it makes
its decent (fig. 32). On expiration, as the
diaphragm ascends, one can imagine the
diaphragm being pasted back to the lateral
chest wall (fig. 33).

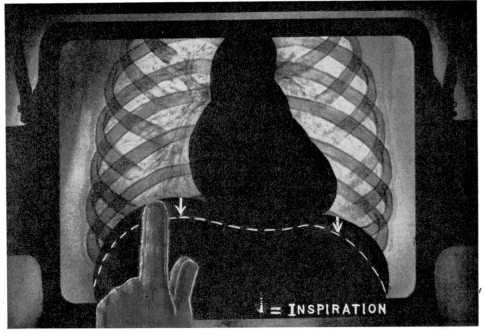

31

Alternate method to figures 28–30 for discerning diaphragmatic movement. Use of the protected finger in this manner may also be used as an alternative to figure 37 for observing mediastinal shift.

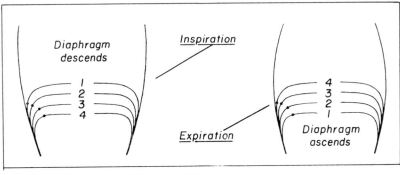

"Peeling Off" phenomenon.

32	33
Inspiration. Diaphragm peeled off lateral chest walls.	Expiration. Diaphragm pasted back onto lateral chest walls.

Perhaps the most efficient and ready method of determining diaphragmatic movements is to place the protected finger at the margin of the cusp to be examined and ask the patient to breathe in and out. With inspiration, the movement of the dia-phragm away from and beneath the fixed position of the finger, and with expiration, the movement of the diaphragm above the fixed position of the finger, are readily discernible (fig. 31).

There are some individuals who breathe

without true diaphragmatic excursions. To demonstrate diaphragmatic movements in such people the patient is asked to "sniff" or cough. The diaphragm will be jerked in a corresponding manner, and diaphragmatic movements are thus easily observed. This has been called the "sniff" sign.

It is often simpler to discern diaphragmatic movements in horizontal, than in erect fluoroscopy. This is due partly to the immobilization of the ribs by the weight of the patient while lying down (in effect, his lying on his ribs inhibits their movement). Since respiration depends upon both diaphragmatic and costal movements, inhibition of the latter is compensated by increased excursion of the diaphragm. This increased upward excursion of the diaphragm is also aided by the fact that in the horizontal position the abdominal viscera push upward.

Normally the right diaphragm is slightly higher than the left. Right diaphragmatic movements are somewhat limited by the liver below, and its normal excursion is approximately 25 per cent less than the left diaphragm.[6]

Diminution in mobility of the diaphragm may be limited to its anterior portion. In order to best visualize this limited mobility the patient may, on occasion, be examined obliquely so that the diaphragm may be seen in its entirety from before backwards.

Increased Movements of the Diaphragm: A hiccough or a spasm is an involuntary, sudden movement of the diaphragm. It is observed on the fluoroscopic screen as a

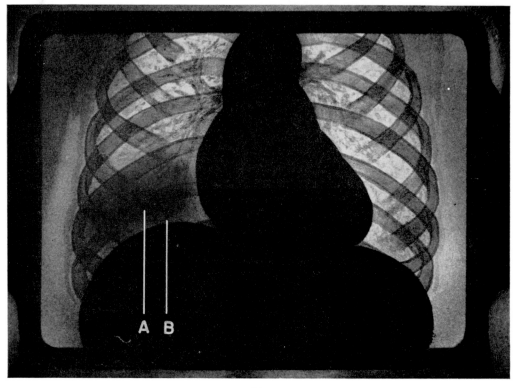

34

A pneumonitis in the lower lung of primary intrathoracic etiology would not be so closely adjacent to the diaphragm (A, haze; B, space separating haze from diaphragm).

The diaphragm here would have more mobility than in the presence of a subphrenic abscess.

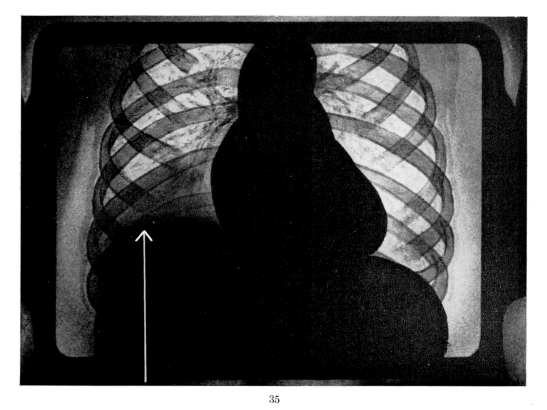

35

Pneumonitis in lung caused by subphrenic pathology (abscess, arrow) is located directly adjacent to the diaphragm. This diaphragm would be immobile.

quick, jerky, spasmodic descent of this structure.

Increased movements of the diaphragm appearing as a persistent flutter[1] have been described as a complication of epidemic encephalitis, influenza, and cardiospasm associated with hypocalcemia.

Diminished Diaphragmatic Movements: Diaphragmatic movements may be diminished on one or both sides in the presence of an adjacent inflammatory process. A radiographic picture often confronting the clinician is the finding of a pneumonic process in the lower lung fields of a postoperative patient. The problem here is etiologic: Is the lower lung field involved as a result of lymphatic extension from a subdiaphragmatic abscess (often abscesses beneath the diaphragm reveal themselves *only* by changes

in the adjacent lung); or is the process as seen a pneumonia of intrathoracic origin?

In such circumstances, the roentgenographic and roentgenoscopic findings can be of real diagnostic value:

1. In a pneumonia of subdiaphragmatic origin, the entire process appears to follow closely the diaphragmatic contours* and tends to remain adjacent to the diaphragm. A primary pneumonia does not generally show such close approximation to the diaphragm (cf. figs. 34 and 35). Also, with a primary pneumonia, the hilar region on the same side will display more involvement.

2. Since the pneumonia with a subdiaphragmatic etiology invades the lung by

* The word "contour" as used throughout this book is to be taken to mean not just the shape of the organ under study, but specifically the profile image.

first passing through the diaphragm and "pleural" lymphatics, a pleural effusion with obliteration of the costophrenic sinus on the same side will be a more common finding than when the pneumonia has a primary intrathoracic origin.

3. Restricted diaphragmatic motility is an early sign of subdiaphragmatic abscess; at a later stage, the diagphragm becomes raised and fixed. It is well to note that although some restriction of diaphragmatic movement can occur in a primary intrathoracic pneumonia, it is not common for the diaphragm to become fixed.

4. An important sign—roentgenographic as well as fluoroscopic—for diagnosis of subdiaphragmatic abscess is the presence of air and a fluid level below the diaphragm.* Fluoroscopic examination in prone, lateral and erect positions (if the patient's condition permits) can determine the exact position in which such a fluid level is best seen. The air beneath the diaphragm associated with a subdiaphragmatic abscess must be distinguished from the air under the diaphragm (with *no* fluid level) following laparotomy, which latter normally disappears in about two weeks.

5. Since most subdiaphragmatic abscesses occur on the right side, an increase in the size of the shadow, due to the liver being displaced downward by the abscess above, is another helpful sign. Normally, the distance from the superior margin of the cusp to the inferior liver margin is 20–22 cm.; when this distance increases, either the liver is enlarged or something else (subdiaphragmatic abscess) must be present. Neoplasm, when it invades the liver, especially the region of the dome, causes an increased elevation of the right diaphragm and also restricts its movement.[6] The distance from the superior margin of the cusp to the inferior liver margin may be greater than 22 cm. If the clinical history cannot clearly distinquish between liver neoplasm and

* Twenty-five per cent of such cases present fluid levels surmounted by air.

subphrenic abscess, it should be borne in mind that, with neoplasm of the liver, there is usually no concurrent overlying parenchymal or pleural involvement.

6. With the patient in the lateral position, if the abscess is under the right diaphragm the normal downward slope of the diaphragm (fig. 49) is reduced, its posterior leaf tending to become horizontal.

Diaphragmatic Paralysis: Paralysis of the diaphragm presents an interesting phenomenon known as Kienbock's sign or paradoxical movements of the diaphragm. Paradoxical movement (fig. 36) is explained as follows: The normal diaphragm will descend with inhalation, and this will increase the intra-abdominal pressure. This increase within the abdomen is distributed with equal force in all directions. However, the

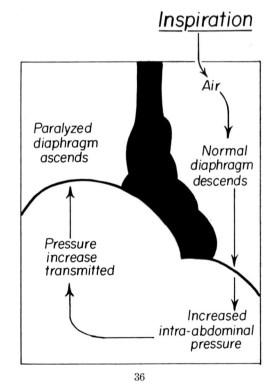

Inspiration

Air

Paralyzed diaphragm ascends

Normal diaphragm descends

Pressure increase transmitted

Increased intra-abdominal pressure

36

Note: With *expiration*, the reverse occurs, i.e., the left diaphragm ascends, intra-abdominal pressure decreases, and right diaphragm falls.

The alternate falling and rising of the opposite sides of the diaphragm is called "see-saw" action.

abnormal diaphragm will be pushed *up* by the transmitted upward pressure. The descent of the normal diaphragm with inhalation and the synchronous rising of the paralyzed diaphragm due to the increased intra-abdominal pressure is known as a paradoxical diaphragmatic movement. On expiration, the reverse of this movement occurs. This condition has also been referred to as "seesaw movement" of the diaphragm.

Paradoxic movement may occur in conditions other than paralysis, i.e., in any case where downward descent of the diaphragm is limited, such as pleuritis or increased negative pressure in the pleural cavity resulting from atelectasis. These paradoxic movements may show mainly with a sniff test (described below). In these cases, movement of the diaphragm in the normal direction may be brought about by forceful inspiration. When the disease no longer exists, the diaphragmatic excursions become normal.[1]

Another maneuver to determine these abnormal diaphragmatic movements is the "sniff" test, referred to earlier. When difficulty is encountered in arriving at a conclusion as to the excursions of the diaphragm, it is advised that the patient be asked to "sniff" instead of performing deep inspiration and expiration. The short jerky movement thus transmitted to the diaphragm allows for better visualization of the movements of this structure. As the patient "sniffs" in, the response of the cusps normally should be the same as with inspiration, but the descent is quick and short.

Eventration of the diaphragm: Eventration of the diaphragm is usually caused by a phrenic nerve paralysis which may on occasion be incomplete. The involved diaphragmatic cusp is thin and atrophic. It is raised high, and diaphragmatic movements may or may not be present (fig. 37). This may often simulate a normal diaphragm pushed up by distention of either the stomach air bubble or other loops of bowel, such as splenic flexure (fig. 25). The close resemblance between diaphragmatic elevation due to air in the stomach or gastro-intestinal tract and diaphragmatic eventration exists particularly since eventration is more common on the left side than on the right. This is so because the intestines, distended with air, cannot push up the right diaphragm—since the liver intervenes. The left diaphragm is in direct contact with the intestines. One of the ways of distinguishing true eventration is to watch for diaphragmatic movements. If present, and normal, they speak for a normal diaphragm; if paradoxical, they suggest eventration.

Mediastinal Movements. A separate chapter (Chapter III) is devoted to cardiac fluoroscopy. For the present, only the shifting mediastinal movements associated with pulmonary disease are considered.

Discerning a mediastinal shift is important in diagnosing a unilateral increased or decreased intrathoracic pressure. Bronchostenosis on one side will not allow as great an air entry there as on the opposite normal side. The lung with normal air content will have a higher pressure than the one with a lesser air content, particularly during inspiration. The shift on inspiration in this instance will be towards the lung with lesser pressure. An emphysematous lung, which does not permit proper exit of air because of some ball-valve obstruction, will contain more air on expiration than the opposite normal lung. In this event, the mediastinal shift with expiration will be again towards the lung with less air pressure, or away from the emphysematous lung.

The mediastinum will shift to the affected side on inspiration when acute marked bullous emphysema exists. The reason is that in the presence of this disease many of the smaller bronchi are obstructed —at least in part—and so do not permit free entry of air with inspiration. The opposite normal lung, properly aerated with inspiration, will push the mediastinum towards the abnormal side.

A shifting mediastinum can be as uncom-

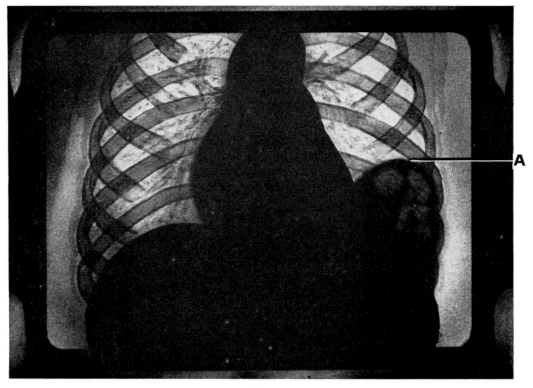

37

The raised diaphragm, as illustrated here (A), can be either eventration or a normal diaphragm elevated by air below it. The difference is distinguished by observing the diaphragmatic movements.

plicated or as difficult to observe as diaphragmatic movements, and for this, too, special technics are helpful. The following technic is especially useful when the shift is to a minor degree only. As in figure 38, the diaphragmatic shutters of the fluoroscopic machine are narrowed, so that the mediastinum, together with a narrow, long segment of lung, is seen on either side. As the patient inhales, the chest elongates from above downwards, and the mediastinal shadow becomes narrower. *But the normal mediastinum will not be displaced to either side.*

Mediastinal shift is discerned by observing the amount of lung on each side. When the mediastinum shifts to the right, the amount of lung tissue on the right side becomes proportionately smaller, and on the left proportionately larger. The reverse of this is true when the mediastinum shifts to the opposite side. The mediastinum shifting back and forth has been compared to a pendulum (figs. 39, 40, 41). The pendular movement of the mediastinum toward the side of the lesion in complete or partial bronchial stenosis is accentuated by the patient's taking short, deep breaths.[2]

In studying the mediastinal shadow, it is often valuable to distinguish whether or not a mediastinal mass pulsates. When an abnormal mediastinal shadow is noted, the shutters should be narrowed to avoid secondary radiation, and the pathological lesion be closely observed. Careful observation should be made for pulsation of this structure. The difference between expansile and transmitted pulsation, although described, has rarely been seen with certainty.

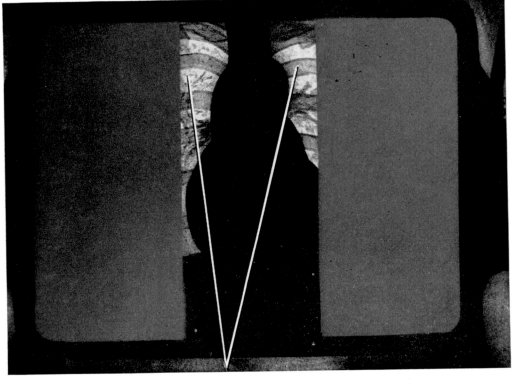

38

Shutters narrowed down to show only a narrow section of lung on either side of the mediastinum.

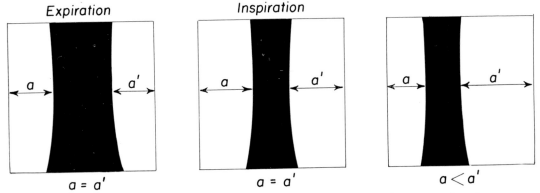

Normal relationship of mediastinum (central black shadow) and lungs at either side.

39

With *expiration*, mediastinum broadens symmetrically from side to side so that air space on either side is equal; i.e., a = a′.

40

With *inspiration*, the mediastinum narrows symmetrically so that the air space on either side increases equally in size; i.e., a = a′.

41

Shifting mediastinum. With inspiration and expiration the changes in the lung field on either side are not equal; i.e., a < a′.

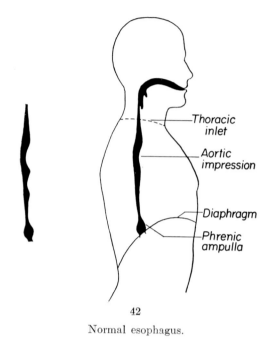

42

Normal esophagus.

No examination of the mediastinum can be considered complete without an esophagogram, which is simply an x-ray examination of the esophagus. Fuller details of such a study will be discussed under gastro-intestinal fluoroscopy (see Chapter IV), but a few words will be included here, sufficient for chest fluoroscopy.

The normal esophagus (fig. 42) is somewhat narrowed as it passes through the thoracic inlet. The first, most common, and often the only indenture seen will be observed at the level of the arch of the aorta. The esophagus then courses down, directly behind the left pulmonary bronchus and, beneath this, the left auricle. The left auricle causes a slight smooth, curved indenture in its anterior aspect. The descending thoracic aorta often causes a transmitted pulsation to the esophageal column. The pulsations of the esophagus will receive more attention presently.

At the lower end of the esophagus where it passes through the diaphragm a dilatation is frequently seen. This dilatation is normal, and is referred to as the phrenic ampulla.

Fluoroscopy of the Pathological Chest

Very often shadows seen on the roentgenogram require the aid of a fluoroscopic examination for complete interpretation. In addition, the fluoroscopic procedure can save the examiner a great amount of time and effort. Various diagnostic procedures, as will be shown, can be performed instantaneously on the fluoroscopic screen, whereas when radiographic film examination is used alone it is often necessary to recall the patient and to take many repeat films.

Pulmonary infarct is a case in point. A conventional film may not reveal any abnormality when the latter is hidden behind the cardiac silhouette. If possible, the patient should first be fluoroscoped, and by rotating him, hidden shadows may reveal themselves. To make a roentgen diagnosis of infarct, the examiner will look for the shadow to be peripheral; behind the fluoro-

scopic screen, obvious shadows as well as those not readily apparent can be tested by rotating the patient, and thus it can be determined whether or not the shadow is peripherally located. Other signs of infarction, such as wedge-shaped areas of density and a small amount of fluid within the pleural cavity, can also be more easily discovered and positioned to best advantage through this fluoroscopic procedure.

It would be wise to precede our discussion with a note of warning as well as of encouragement. After one of his lectures, the author was once approached by a physician who asserted that only a man with special training was able to observe the various findings as described. Indeed, that is true. But the training period can be markedly shortened if this single rule is adhered to: One examination with the observer's eyes propery accommodated is worth innumerable examinations when the eyes are not properly prepared. One other bit of advice: Take advantage of every examination performed, and carry it out properly. Experience and acquaintance with the normal will prove invaluable in recognizing the abnormal.

TRACHEAL DEVIATIONS

A deviation of the trachea from its normal position is significant. During the course of any examination the trachea should be carefully sought for and determined as being in the midline, remembering the normal slight deviation to the right as it passes behind and to the right of the aortic arch. Occasionally, an abnormal position or angulation of this air column may be seen more readily on the fluoroscopic screen than on the roentgenogram. A substernal thyroid is a potent cause for such an abnormal configuration.

Softening of the Trachea.[5] Ascertaining any displacement and change in shape of the trachea is only part of the information roentgen examination can give regarding this structure. In addition, it offers further knowledge as to the condition of the tracheal walls, i.e., their powers of resistance and firmness. Softening of the tracheal rings is caused by pressure from a long-existing goiter or mediastinal tumor. In some cases the cartilage may disappear, causing sudden death due to tracheal collapse. Therefore, softness of the trachea is an absolute indication for operation.

Thus, having diagnosed a deviated or stenosed trachea, the next step would be to test for tracheal cartilage softness. This can be accomplished (1) by *increasing* intratracheal pressure, i.e., making use of the Valsalva experiment (deep inspiration, closure of nose and mouth, and attempt to exhale), with malacia demonstrated if the narrowed region dilates widely; (2) by markedly *decreasing* intratracheal pressure, i.e., use of the Müller experiment (complete exhalation, closure of nose and mouth, and attempt to inhale), with "soft trachea" demonstrated if the involved area becomes markedly narrowed.

This dilatation with increased intratracheal pressure, and collapse with decrease in intratracheal pressure, is usually not only marked but often eccentric; i.e., one wall, being weaker and more softened than the other, will respond more vigorously than its less involved mate on the opposite side.

A simple method of increasing intratracheal pressure is to have the patient cough (instead of the Valsalva maneuver); to decrease intratracheal air the patient might "sniffle" (instead of the Müller experiment).

SUBSTERNAL THYROID

A superior mediastinal mass may confront the examiner as a diagnostic problem (fig. 43). Since a variety of pathological processes can produce such a configuration, any aids that can be secured from the fluoroscope are of value. Deviation as well as softening of the trachea, as discussed above, can be produced by substernal thyroid. The patient is placed behind the fluoroscopic screen and asked to swallow. The superior mediastinal mass is carefully observed.

If during the act of deglutition the mass is seen to rise, the examiner can assume that the abnormal shadow is both adjacent and adherent to the trachea. The most common disease process which fills these requirements is a substernal thyroid.

ATELECTASIS

Various observations can be made by the examiner during fluoroscopy which will be of great assistance in arriving at a diagnosis of atelectasis.

Normally with inspiration, as air enters into the lung alveoli, the various pulmonary arteries which in the main make up the radiating shadows emerging from the hila fan out and become greatly separated.

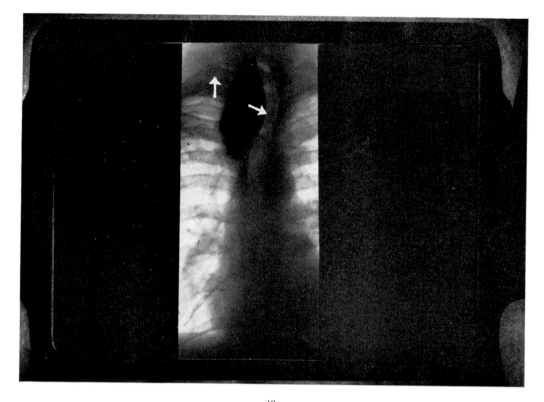

43

Question:
   What is the density in the superior mediastinum?
Fluoroscopic Examination:
   1. The trachea, being deformed (lower arrow) indicates proximity of mass to the trachea.
   2. When the patient was asked to swallow, the dense shadow was noted to rise (upper arrow).
Answer:
   A density in the superior mediastinum fulfilling these requirements is most likely due to a thyroid tumefaction.

When a lobe or any portion of a lung is atelectatic, this fan-like separation will fail to take place with inspiration. If doubt exists as to the interpretation of this observation a comparison of the abnormal side with the normal should be made. With expiration, the vessels on the normal side should come together like a closing fan. With atelectasis this approximation will not occur.

Various disease processes, such as bronchial tumor, which may cause obstructive emphysema, will produce the same phenomena as described above for atelectasis. (It should be noted that the portion of the lung involved with emphysema, because it is distended with air, is radioluscent, whereas the paucity of air in that portion of lung which is atelectatic renders its shadow more opaque.)

Atelectasis of the right middle lobe is frequently not easily visible in the frontal projection. Anteriorly it is overlapped and hidden by the upper lobe (figs. 44, 45), posteriorly it is covered and hidden by the lower lobe. In addition, these lobes above and below, because of compensatory emphysema, are hyperilluminated. As a net effect, instead of the increased density that is expected to be produced by the atelectatic

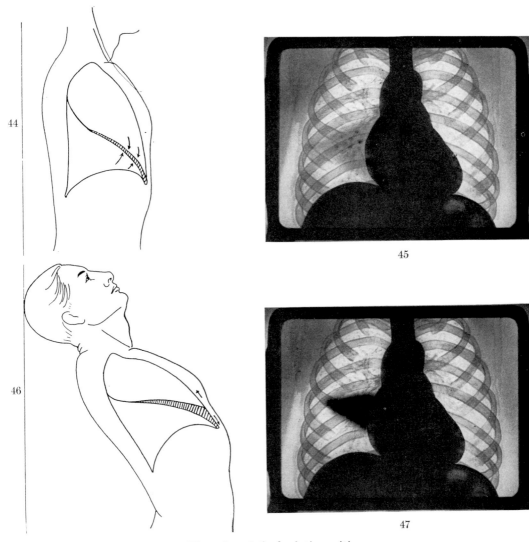

The value of the lordotic position.

44

The patient is erect and facing the examiner. The upper and lower lobes overlap (arrows) the atelectatic lobe. The middle lobe itself is disposed in a more or less vertical fashion.

45

A slight haze is noted in the right middle lobe region. The density of the haze is not sufficient to make *any* diagnosis.

46

The same patient now steps forward six inches and leans back so that the back of his head touches the back panel. (Lordotic position.) Upper and lower lobes tend to separate (arrows) and allow middle lobe to appear. The atelectatic middle lobe also becomes disposed in a more horizontal fashion, thus presenting more atelectatic lung tissue in the path of the x-rays.

47

In this position (lordotic) a dense middle-lobe atelectatic shadow is seen.

middle lobe, the examiner may find what appears to be a normal lung field. To demonstrate this middle lobe atelectasis, the lordotic view, as in figures 46 & 47, is useful because it separates the lung above from the lung below and allows the middle lobe to creep out from between its covers, and so renders the shadow more evident.

Another important reason for the value of the *lordotic view* is that with the patient in this position the atelectatic middle lobe is thrust out in such a fashion that the x-rays pass through more thicknesses of atelectatic tissues, and so register the atelectatic shadow more definite on the screen. The rationale of this statement can be illustrated by a simple hypothesis. If the reader, for example, were to place his hand in front of him in vertical position and visualize it pierced with a sharp instrument, the blade would, at most, pass through about one inch of tissue. If instead the fingers and palm were thrust out horizontally, the blade, entering in the *same* plane as formerly, would pass through many inches of tissue, starting with the fingers and ending behind the eminences of the palm.

In summary, the atelectatic middle lobe can be demonstrated on the roentgenogram only by the use of multiple views but is an instantaneous maneuver during fluoroscopy.

The lordotic position is also useful in demonstrating an interlobar effusion.

The lordotic position can easily be attained during a fluoroscopic procedure by asking the patient to step forward six inches and then lean backwards, so that his shoulders come to rest on the back wall of the fluoroscope.

An additional sign of bronchial obstruction is reported by Golden.[2] To recapitulate, the pulmonary markings fan out and separate with inspiration; during expiration they come closer together. When air cannot escape from a portion of a lung, this closer approximation of the lung markings is not permitted. Instead, the upward movement of the diaphragm in expiration will push these markings up. This upward movement, together with the loss of closer approximation of these lung markings, is stressed when the lung cannot expel its air. Following the same reasoning a rule can be stated: *Whenever the middle lobe is obstructed and the short fissure is visible on the fluoroscopic screen, this short fissure will move up and down with the diaphragm.*

Further fluoroscopic findings which would enable an examiner to reach a diagnosis of atelectasis—such as shadows with concave margins usually being atelectatic, as opposed to bulging margins indicating fluid—can more properly await film examination.

Differentiating infiltrations or lymph nodes from blood vessels: The radiating structures from the hilum are caused in the main by the pulmonary vessels. The influence of the intra-alveolar pressure on the filling up of these vessels is indeed interesting. In Valsalva's maneuver, when intra-alveolar pressure increases, a considerably decreased vascular pattern can be seen in the hilum and the lungs. These changes are due in great part to the increased intra-alveolar pressure, compressing the blood vessels and causing the degree of filling of the vessels to decrease.[3]

By employing this Valsalva maneuver and so compressing the central branches of the pulmonary artery we are enabled not only to make small lymph nodes in the hilum stand out more clearly, but also to confirm the presence of a blood vessel by the very fact that its shadow narrows and tends to disappear. When the intra-alveolar pressure is raised and the hila blood vessels tend to disappear or thin out, large glands formerly covered over and hidden may emerge more distinctly and become easier to define. On the other hand, many a time it may be difficult to decide whether a particular shadow is caused by a hilum gland or whether it is a dilated vessel which is present and probably seen on end. In these cases, the diagnosis may also be facilitated if high pressure studies are made; the gland is not affected and maintains its size, whereas the vessel becomes compressed (fig. 48).

Another method is useful in determining whether an abnormal shadow is a blood vessel or not: First having located the shadow on the fluoroscopic screen, rotate the patient slightly. When the shadow is due to a lymph node or similar structure, it will maintain itself. A shadow due to a blood vessel may, with rotation, either disappear or elongate, and so demonstrate its true nature.

PSEUDO-CAVITY

All persons who have examined roentgenograms of the chest are familiar with those occasional fortuitous combinations of blood vessel shadows that produce by their accidental overlap what appears as a "true" cavity. To solve this problem the examiner may employ the following simple procedure. After visualizing what appears to be a cavity on the fluoroscopic screen, he then rotates the patient. The fortuitous *overlap* of shadows when due to normal blood vessels is soon separated and a false cavity will no longer be seen.

PNEUMOTHORAX

Different types of pneumothorax cause various respiratory movements of the mediastinum. It should be constantly borne in mind that the mediastinum will shift with inspiration to the side of the chest where the pressure is lower. With the usual closed type of pneumothorax, the mediastinal shadow moves with inspiration towards the side of the pneumothorax and with expiration to the opposite side.

The mediastinum may not only shift with inspiration or expiration, but may also be noted as being displaced. Again, the displacement is towards the side with less pressure on inspiration.

When a patient is being examined for radiographic or fluoroscopic evidence of a

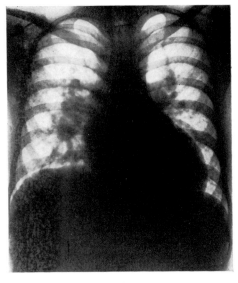

48

Question:

Are the increased shadows adjacent to the heart (hilar densities) lymph glands or dilated hilar vessels?

Fluoroscopic Examination:

1. They were observed to pulsate.

2. With increased intrathoracic pressure (Valsalva) the shadows markedly decreased in size.

Answer:

The increased hilar densities are not lymph glands, but are vascular in nature.

pneumothorax, various phenomena may exist with which the examiner should be familiar. For example, it is entirely possible for an incomplete pneumothorax to be present and yet to be seen only when the patient is placed in a certain specific angle in relationship to the fluoroscopic screen or x-ray film. The conventional postero-anterior film or fluoroscopic examination of the patient in the frontal position alone may not disclose any abnormal shadows suggestive of pneumothorax. A clear space between lung and ribs will establish a diagnosis of pneumothorax, and this finding will often be obtained only through trial and error. For adequate study by film examination alone, the patient may need to be rotated several times. On the fluoroscopic screen the ex-

amination and proper positioning are instantaneous.

In addition, through utilization of the
principle of illumination with inspiration
and dimness with expiration, the examiner
will suspect pneumothorax when on *full expiration* a segment of lung remains hyperilluminated. During inspiration, when air
enters into the alveoli the lung fields become more illuminated. On expiration, as
the air content diminishes, the brightness
will dim. If one lung field remains illuminated on expiration, a pneumothorax (or an
emphysema with a valvular bronchial obstruction) may be present.

Finally, every physician who is familiar
with this disease is acquainted with the peculiar heart flutter observed during a pneumothorax. The explanation for this has to
do with air reaching the mediastinal surface. Once observed it will not be forgotten.

PLEURAL EFFUSION

It should be remembered that there are
posterior and anterior costophrenic sinuses

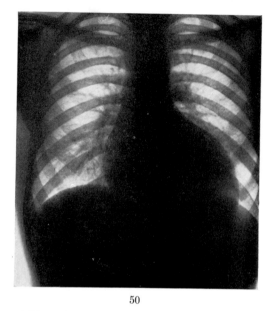

50

This patient was examined for pleural effusion
and none was found in the routine film. (See fig.
51.)

as well as the lateral costophrenic sinuses.
The posterior costophrenic sinus, it should
be noted, is the lowest portion of the thoracic cage and can be considered as the
trough of the chest (fig. 49). When a pleural
effusion is formed, it is in this posterior
trough that it first collects. It should be
carefully noted that it is entirely possible
to overlook an early stage of pleural effusion if frontal examination alone is done.
The importance of lateral and oblique examinations of the patient thus becomes immediately evident (figs. 50 and 51).

Another method of observing the posterior costophrenic sinus which is deep and
obscured by the dome of the diaphragm, or
for that matter, a method of visualizing
lung parenchyma deep down behind the
diaphragmatic dome and not usually seen in
frontal examination, is to place the patient
with his back to the screen and to elevate
the tube. The x-rays radiating out from the
tube in all directions will pass over the
dome and project a lesion downward on the
screen (figs. 52, 53). Subsequent roentgenograms may be made with the patient in a

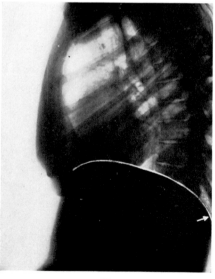

49

The posterior costo-phrenic sinus (arrow) is
the lowest point in the chest. This is important,
since fluid collects here first. Thus, in searching
for small amounts of fluid the examiner must not
neglect to look at this region.

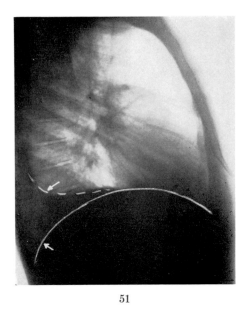

51

Same patient as figure 49, when examined in the lateral position, reveals a filling in the posterior costo-phrenic sinus (between arrows above and below), thus revealing *first evidence of fluid in the chest.*

similar relationship. This same principle can be used in demonstrating lesions at the apex; i.e., with the patient facing the screen, the tube is lowered, projecting apical lesions above the clavicle. Once the examiner understands these principles he may make modifications to suit his needs.

FLUID LEVELS

Occasionally, during the fluoroscopic examination of the patient, a shadow simulating a fluid level may be seen (fig. 54). This can readily be determined as fluid (figs. 55 and 56) by having the patient alternately shift his position by leaning to the right side and then to the left. If indeed a fluid level exists, the horizontal line during these maneuvers will remain horizontal or maintain its parallelism to the floor (figs. 55, 56). On the other hand, if the line bends, leans over, or in any way loses its parallelism to the floor, it is probably not fluid. The best example of this principle can be obtained by performing a simple experiment: If the reader should half-fill a glass with water and then tip this glass at various an-

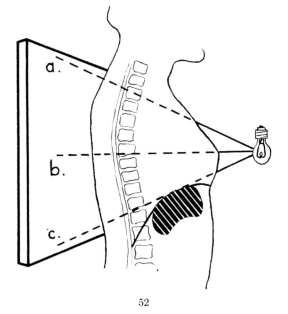

52

With the tube low, "ray c" cannot project the posterior costo-phrenic sinus on the fluoroscopic screen (liver projected).

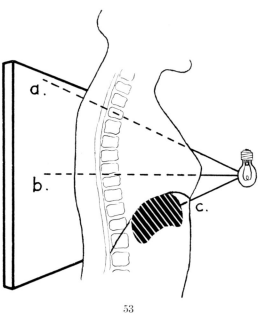

53

By raising the tube the posterior costo-phrenic sinus is projected.

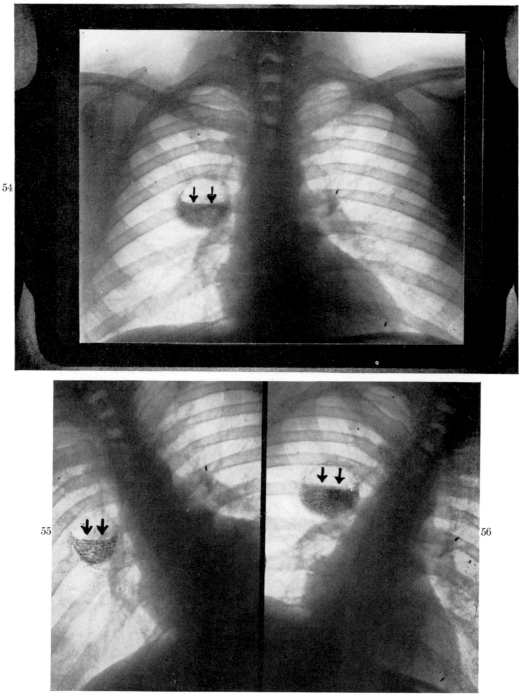

Proof of existence of fluid level in abscess cavity.

54

Does abscess cavity contain fluid?

55   56

Patient tilted to right; fluid level remains   Patient tilted to left; fluid level maintained
parallel to floor.   parallel to floor.

Note: If the density within the cavity were not fluid, when patient was tilted to the right or left,
the *level* would tilt to the side the patient was bent.

gles to the horizontal, it will be observed that no matter the angle of the vessel, the level of the fluid contained in it is always parallel to the floor; on the contrary, a ring in an empty glass, caused, say, by a crack in the surface, will tilt at the same angle as the glass is tilted. *The same principle applies to the behavior of fluids inside the body.* If the surface of the shadow remains consistently parallel to the floor, this is justifiable evidence that the shadow is being cast by fluid; if the shadow tilts as the patient changes his angle from the vertical, it is not fluid.

PULMONARY FIBROSIS[4]

Those fibrous reactions occurring within the lungs which are multifocal and general in character are termed here "pulmonary fibrosis." Tuberculosis, bronchiectasis or syphilis have been described as etiological factors in some such cases. Radiation therapy, asthma, pneumoconiosis and scleroderma are also causes.

Fluoroscopic examination is of considerable help in reaching the diagnosis when this condition exists. During normal respiration, the ascent of the diaphragm with expiration is slower than descent is with inspiration. This slowing has been described as a lag. In the presence of pulmonary fibrosis the lag is accentuated. Indeed, when the lung involvement is of sufficient severity, the diaphragm may become absolutely immobile. It is likely that the associated emphysema is largely responsible for the diaphragmatic immobility.

Other fluoroscopic findings in this condition are paradoxical movements of the mediastinum. It appears wider with inspiration and narrower with expiration. (Cf. figs. **68** and **69**.) Widening of the tracheal air space, when found, is an important factor in arriving at an accurate diagnosis.

PROCEDURES REQUIRING FLUOROSCOPY[4]

Fluoroscopic visualization has been helpful not only in passing a tracheal catheter between the vocal cords so that opaque material can then be injected during bronchography, but, more recently, under direct fluoroscopic observation the various bronchi within the lung have been entered into and medicated. Similarly, the location of a lesion with reference to a bronchoscope which has been passed into one of the main bronchi may be observed when bronchoscopy is performed with fluoroscopic control. In difficult cases it may be necessary to make use of fluoroscopy in two planes, which is done by use of the biplane fluoroscope. Finally, the fluoroscope has been found useful in the aspiration of small loculated empyemas and tumors. It should be remembered that when this is done a horizontal fluoroscope should be used in order to obviate danger of air embolus to the brain.

CHAPTER III

Examination of the Heart

Fundamentals

Fluoroscopy of the heart supplements other clinical information and can thus be considered a useful weapon in the armamentarium of the physician. It has been found useful not only in determining various chamber enlargements but, as detailed below, it has proved an extremely important link in the chain of information leading to an exact diagnosis.

Before passing on to actual fluoroscopic examination it would be wise to review various fundamentals.

ANATOMY

Frontal Projection (patient facing the screen)

In the frontal projection the anatomic structures which make up the mediastinal and cardiac contours are detailed in figures 57 and 58. The right side consists, from below upwards, of the right auricle, the ascending aorta and the innominate vein.

In young subjects the superior vena cava often forms part of the right mediastinal contour instead of the aorta.

The left heart side from below upwards consists of the left ventricle, left auricular appendage,[1-2] pulmonary artery and aorta. Higher up in the mediastinum the subclavian vessels are found.

Oblique Projection*

The fluoroscopic observation of the heart in its oblique projection seems a difficult

---

* The *frontal* position has already been defined. (page 14n). When we speak of the right (or left) anterior (or posterior) *oblique* position, the first word refers to the side of the patient brought forward (i.e., right or left); the second word indicates whether the involved plane of the patient faces the screen or film (anterior) or is directed away from the screen or film (posterior); the third word gives the angle (i.e., oblique, rather than frontal or lateral). In the oblique and lateral positions, the hands should be over the head (out of the field).

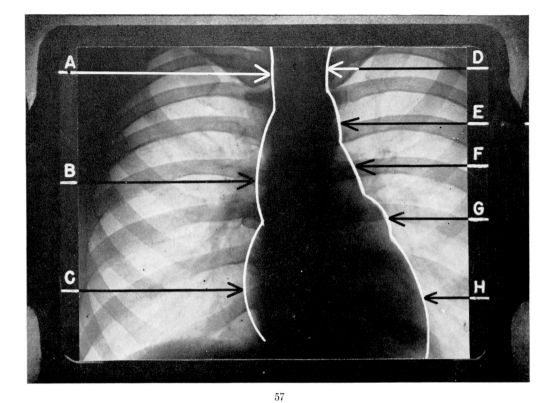

57

A. Inominate vein
B. Ascending aorta
C. Right auricle

D. Subclav. vessels
E. Aortic knob
F. Pulmonary artery
G. Left auricular appendix
H. Left ventricle

task for the novice, in contradistinction to the relatively easy understanding of the frontal contours.

When observing either diagram or film or an image on a fluoroscopic screen the observer must train himself to think in terms of depth, i.e., third dimension. If the diagram as illustrated (fig. 59) is constantly kept in mind, visualization of the heart in any projection will easily be understood.

(1). *Right Anterior Oblique (Right shoulder close to screen, with patient facing the screen)*. The right anterior oblique projection is the rotation of surface B (fig. 60) toward the examiner.

The standard amount of rotation to the right is about 45 degrees but this may be varied according to the need. The required degree of rotation depends to a great extent upon the patient's habitus, i.e., sthenic, hypersthenic, or asthenic. It also depends on the degree of cardiac chamber enlargement.

(2). *Left Anterior Oblique (Left shoulder closer to the screen with patient facing the screen)*. The left anterior oblique is the rotation of surface A toward the examiner (fig. 61). The two ventricles are seen with the interventricular groove separating them. This latter groove is usually best visualized with the patient taking a deep breath and the heart in systole.

TYPES OF HEART

The habitus of an individual will, as with other organs, determine the heart shape.

The Vertical Heart. This heart is usually

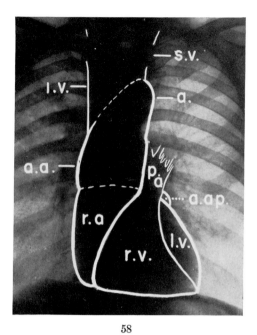

58

r.a.—right auricle   l.v.—left ventricle
i.v.—inominate vein   a.a.—ascending aorta
a.—aorta   s.v.—subclavian vessels
a.ap.—auricular app.   p.a.—pulmonary artery
                      r.v.—right ventricle

associated with asthenic individuals. It is long and narrow. The pulmonary artery and conus segment are prominent and form the greatest portion of the left border below the aortic knob. The left ventricular segment forms less than one-half of the cardiac contour below the aortic knob, sometimes even less than one-third of this distance.

In the right anterior oblique position the pulmonary artery conus segment is prominent. This information is important and should be noted since, if it is not appraised properly, it may cause difficulty, as will be demonstrated.

During the phase of expiration, or in recumbency when the diaphragm is higher, a vertical heart may resemble the oblique or even transverse type heart.

The Horizontal Heart. The horizontal heart is usually found in hypersthenic individuals with broad, short chests. In these people the diaphragmatic leaves are usually elevated and the heart is transverse in position. The left ventricular contour forms more than one-half of the left cardiac border below the aortic knob.

In the right anterior oblique position the pulmonary artery conus segment is not prominent.

The Oblique Heart. The oblique heart is usually found in sthenic individuals and is intermediate between the vertical and the horizontal. The length of the pulmonary artery conus and of the left ventricular segments are approximately equal.

FRONTAL

Surface "B"

Surface "A"

59

Frontal diagram of the heart.

The heart, for diagnostic purposes, may be considered as two ice cream cones lying adjacent to each other in a box. Each ball of ice cream represents an auricle. Each cone represents a ventricle. (Cf. fig. 58.)

R.A.—right auricle   R.V.—right ventricle
L.A.—left auricle   L.V.—left ventricle

RIGHT ANTERIOR OBLIQUE

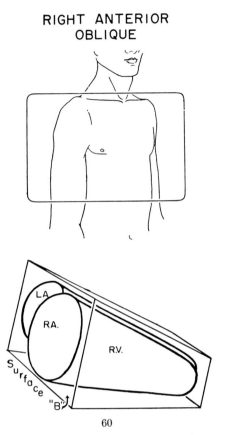

60

Right anterior oblique diagram of the heart.

The right anterior oblique position turns the box so that the two balls of ice cream are turned toward the examiner.

R.A.—right auricle   R.V.—right ventricle
L.A.—left auricle

Infant Heart.[20] The main difference between adult and infant pictures is that in the infant the chest is rounder, the diaphragm higher, and the vertical axis of the heart more nearly horizontal than in the adult. Consequently, in the infant the chest is wider than it is long, in the child approximately as long as it is wide, and in the adult longer than it is wide.

MISCELLANEOUS CONSIDERATIONS

Extrapericardial Fat Pad. The examiner, in observing the cardiac contours in the frontal projection, may on occasion see an *area near the apex of the heart wherein pulsation is diminished or absent.* At other times this same area may cause confusion and lead him to suspect he is dealing with an enlarged cardiac shadow. It is therefore important to become acquainted with this extrapericardial fat pad (fig. 65) situated at the apex of the heart just above the left diaphragmatic leaf. With careful observation the true apex may be discerned as a separate shadow within this fat pad. In order to demonstrate the true apex on the fluoroscopic screen it may be necessary to reduce the size of the fluoroscopic field with the shutters and increase the penetrability of the ray by raising the kilovoltage.

LEFT ANTERIOR OBLIQUE

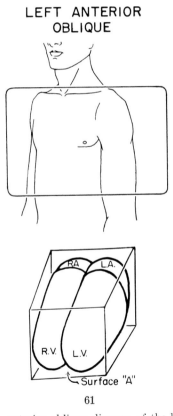

61

Left anterior oblique diagram of the heart.

The left anterior oblique position turns the box so that the two cones are turned toward the examiner.

R.A.—right auricle   R.V.—right ventricle
L.A.—left auricle   L.V.—left ventricle

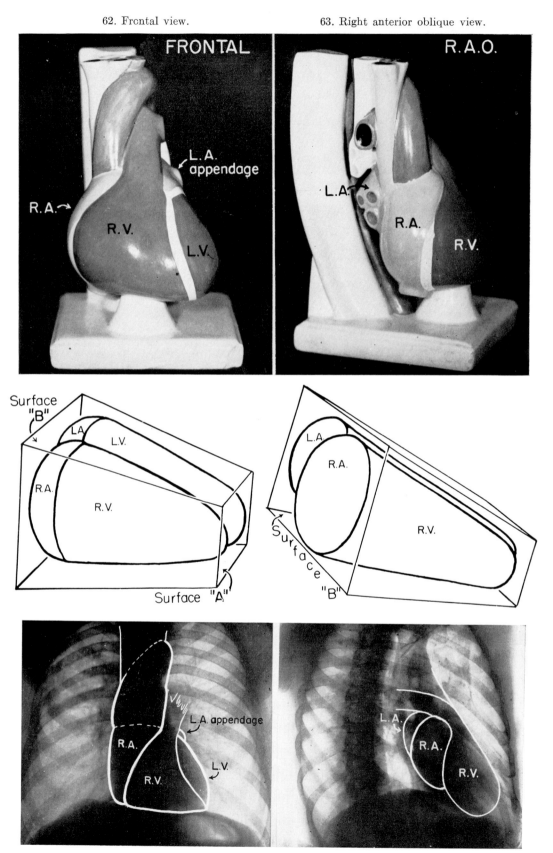

64. Left anterior oblique view.

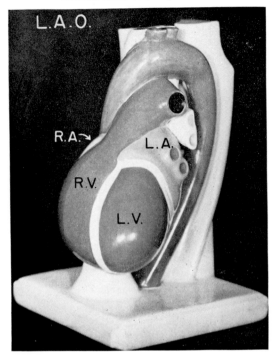

The reader would be wise to understand figures 62, 63, and 64 before proceeding further.

R.A.—right auricle
L.A.—left auricle
R.V.—right ventricle
L.V.—left ventricle
I.V.—interventricular (groove)

Top row: Models of heart in three views.

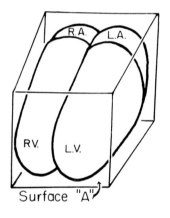

Middle row: Corresponding diagrammatic explanations of same three views.

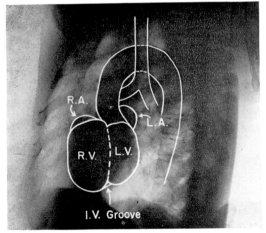

Bottom row: Fluoroscopic projections of same three views.

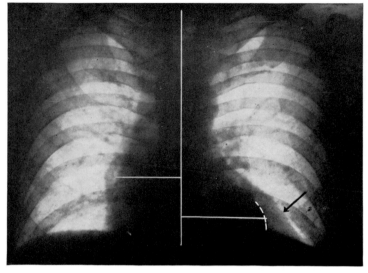

65

The apical pericardial fat pad (arrow) may cause the examiner to suspect cardiac enlargement when none exists.

Question:

How may this difficulty be overcome?

Answer:

Raise the kilovoltage (penetrability of the ray) and look into the shadow for the true apex.

Spinal Deformities. A spinal deformity, such as scoliosis, may so distort the heart and mediastinal shadows that neoplastic disease, aneurysm, or other conditions are closely simulated. To determine the true state of affairs, the examiner should rotate the patient and examine the spine. Often, proof that the enlarged shadow on the right or left side of the mediastinum is caused by the spine can be secured only by over-penetrated films (figs. 8 and 66).

Having determined the apparent deformity produced by the spine, the next problem is how to examine the heart.

Scoliosis with a convexity to the right will rotate the heart so that in the frontal projection of the patient, the heart itself is viewed in the right anterior oblique. Conversely a scoliosis with a convexity to the left will rotate the heart so that it is apparently viewed in the left anterior oblique.[3] To overcome these difficulties the heart should be positioned behind the fluoroscopic screen in a true frontal plane—with no re-gard to the actual position of the patient. Once the heart is seen in its true antero-posterior contours, the examination can then proceed as detailed below. All further necessary rotations (keeping figures 62–64 in mind) should be performed with respect to the heart only and no attention paid to the actual position of the patient.

Size of Heart and Body Position. The heart size increases when the patient changes from the erect to the horizontal position.[2a] An actual volumetric change occurs especially if there is a slowing of heart rate.[2] However, the change as visualized is to a greater extent caused by the elevation of the diaphragm. In the recumbent position the diaphragm is elevated, carrying the heart with it. The heart therefore assumes a more transverse position and its transverse diameter appears to increase. The mediastinal shadow, compressed from below upwards, bulges to either side and appears widened.

Effect of Respiration on the Heart and

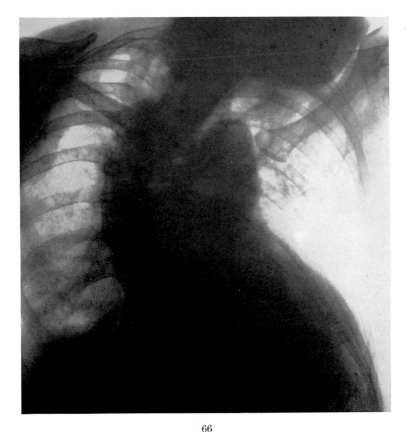

66

Question:

How would the examiner decide whether the bulging shadow on the right side of the mediastinum is due to the spine?

Answer:

1. Raise the kilovoltage, thus increasing the penetrability of the ray, enabling one actually to see the vertebrae.

2. Rotate the patient and bring the spinal column clear of the heart.

3. A valuable clue can be secured by seeing the wider separation of the ribs on the right side and closer approximation of the ribs on the left side.

Mediastinal Shadows. With deep inspiration the heart descends with the diaphragmatic leaves, causing an elongation of the great vessels within the mediastinum. The result is that the entire mediastinal shadow tends to become narrower (fig. **68**). With deep expiration the diaphragmatic leaves ascend, carrying the heart upwards. The mediastinum, apparently compressed in a smaller space from below upwards, bulges widely (fig. **69**). With normal respiratory movements the changes as detailed are not as marked.

This knowledge has proved especially useful in examining infants. Often a routine chest film of an infant taken in the usual supine position may present a perplexing problem. The mediastinal shadow may appear to be unduly widened because of two factors. First, since one cannot control the phase of respiration in the infant it is likely that the film may be exposed during the wrong phase of respiration, i.e., expiration with the ascent of the diaphragm. The heart may therefore be pushed upwards and the mediastinum may bulge widely. The

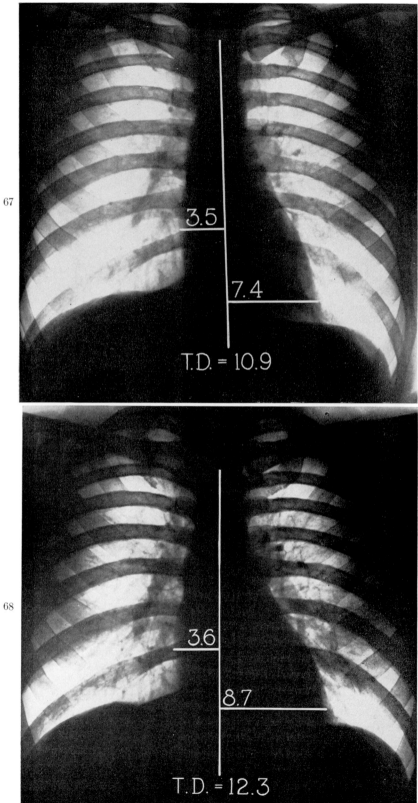

67

3.5

7.4

T.D. = 10.9

68

3.6

8.7

T.D. = 12.3

See legends, facing page.

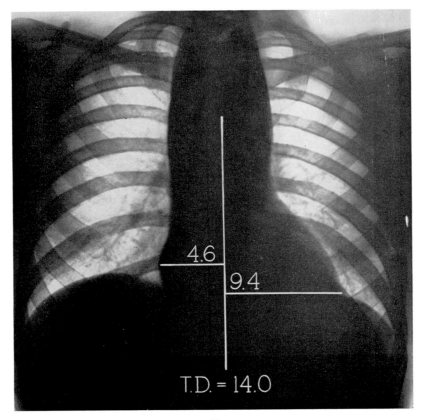

69

Effects of respiration on the heart and mediastinal width.

67	69
(Top, p. 54)	*(Above)*

With the Valsalva maneuver the heart and mediastinal shadow are *smallest*.

With expiration the diaphragm ascends. The heart becomes transverse in type and is broadened. The mediastinal shadow also becomes wider.

68

(Bottom, p. 54)

With deep inspiration the heart and mediastinal shadow are small as *compared with their size during expiration.*

second factor is the expected elevation of the heart in the infant's supine state, which again causes a widening of the mediastinal shadow. A differentiation must therefore be made between the normally widened mediastinum and the pathologically widened mediastinum, the most important cause of which in the infant is an enlarged thymus gland. By observing the crying infant be-

hind the fluoroscopic screen and paying close attention to the change in mediastinal width, a diagnosis may be made. With each sigh (deep inspiration) the diaphragm descends, pulling the heart with it and, if the mediastinum is indeed normal, it will become narrower. When, with each sigh and subsequent descent of the heart the widened mediastinal shadow maintains its

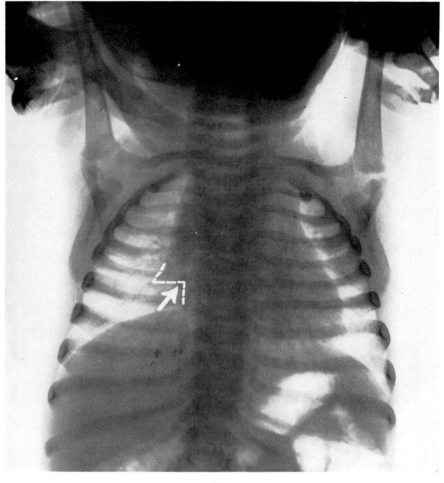

70

Question:
    What are some important fluoroscopic signs in diagnosing an enlarged thymus gland?
    Answer:
    1. A widened superior mediastinum which maintains its same width with deep inspiration.
    2. The characteristic thymic angle found on the right border of the mediastinum (arrow).

width and does not become narrower—some underlying pathological process must be suspected by the examiner.

Another useful method of differentiating an enlarged thymus gland is to place the infant in the left anterior oblique position. If the shadow is caused by the thymus an indenture will almost always be seen above the heart shadow (fig. 70). Such a configuration is never produced by a vascular abnormality.[20]

(Other marked changes in the heart shadow produced by certain respiratory efforts are demonstrated by the Valsalva and Müller experiments and are described later.)

CARDIAC PULSATIONS

Viewed on the fluoroscopic screen, the left border of the heart will be seen to have a "see-saw" action. The fulcrum of this "see-saw" is called the "point of opposite pulsations." The "see-saw" movement for practical considerations may be considered caused by the contraction of the ventricles, chiefly the left, and the almost simultaneous expansion of the aorta and pulmonary artery. The alternate contraction of one as blood is being emitted and the expansion of the other in which the blood is being received, and the reversal of this during diastole is the explanation for this "see-saw" action (fig. 71).[1] In cases where the point of opposite pulsations may be difficult to find, it is recommended that the examiner alternately look for aortic pulsations and then ventricular pulsations. Each of these should then be followed towards each other; the fulcrum will be found at the point where they meet.

The point of opposite pulsations, as described above, is a useful tool in helping to determine right and left ventricular enlargement. With hypertrophy and dilation of the right ventricle the fulcrum descends towards the apex, because of enlargement of the shadow produced by the pulmonary artery segment. With dilatation and hypertrophy of the left ventricle and resultant elongation of the left ventricular segment on the left heart border, the point of opposite pulsations moves upwards.

It should be noted that in the frontal view the inthrust of the apex lags slightly behind the upper left ventricular wall, as in figure 72,[5] and also that, as seen in the left anterior oblique projection, the pulsations of the left ventricle are generally greater than those seen in the frontal view. In the later study of disease processes this information becomes important. Thus, in reaching a diagnosis of a pericardial effusion, the absence or existence of pulsation is important, and should be looked for. In the presence of an effusion the pulsation movements of the heart are tamponaded

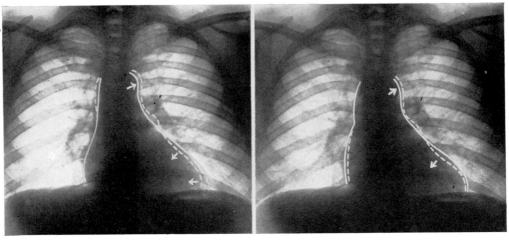

| 71 | 72 |

Normal "see-saw" pulsation with no apical lag.   "Normal see-saw" pulsation with apical lag.
Intersection in both figures between dotted and solid lines is the fulcrum of the "see-saw."
Question:
With right ventricular hypertrophy and dilatation, in which direction does the fulcrum move?
Answer:
Down.
Question:
With left ventricular hypertrophy and dilatation, in which direction does the fulcrum move?
Answer:
Up.

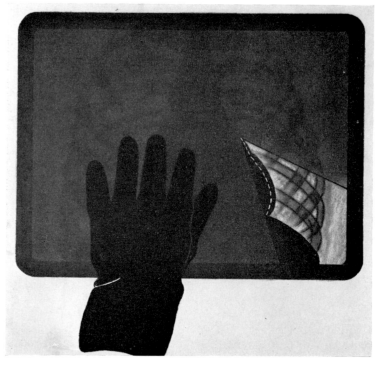

73

"V"-shaped cutout placed on fluoroscopic screen. Each side wall of the "V" is used as an indicator to note the approach or departure of the cardiac contour during the pulsation of the heart.

and tend to disappear. But since pulsations are normally more obvious in the left anterior oblique position, it would be wise, when in doubt as to the existence of pulsations, to examine the patient in this latter position.

The pulsation of the right cardiac contour is neither as easy to see nor as important as the left. Two types of movement are seen here. The more vigorous is transmitted from the right ventricle. The other, a fine ripple, is purely auricular.[4]

A word regarding auricular pulsations: Although theoretically, sufficient time (about 0.15 sec.) elapses between auricular and ventricular contraction to allow separate study of these chambers, yet in actual practice this is not generally possible. When the auricle is enlarged, however, and its pulsations vigorous, if the examiner observes carefully in the frontal or preferably the

left anterior oblique position it is possible to see a contraction (auricular systole) of the left auricular border ahead of the left ventricle. This becomes more and more marked with increased delay in auriculoventricular conduction time.

For better observation of cardiac pulsation, the following suggestions should be kept in mind:

(1). Full adaptation of the eyes is of utmost importance—a rule clinicians commonly do not live up to.

(2). On occasion when it is difficult to visualize these pulsatory movements on the fluoroscopic screen, a magnification can be secured by moving the screen a greater distance away from the chest wall of the patient.

(3). An important factor in securing improved observation of cardiac pulsation is the controlled respiration of the patient. He should be instructed to take only a moderately deep inspiration and then voluntarily stop breathing. The examiner thus benefits by a slowing of the heart rate since it is easier to observe these pulsations in a heart that is not beating rapidly and filling more adequately. Further, the patient should be instructed not to strain, since by increasing intrathoracic pressure—the venous return to the heart is reduced with resultant diminished amplitude of pulsation.

(4). The apical pericardial fat may simulate noncontraction of the apex. The examiner must increase the kilovoltage and look into this shadow to find the true cardiac apex.

(5). When the heart rate is rapid, pressure on the carotid sinus not only slows the rate, but also increases the magnitude of pulsation. (This should not be used with old people since it interferes with cerebral flow.)

(6). A sheet of steel, from which a "V" has been cut can be used as a special shutter (fig. 73). Watching the heart pulsate, the changing shape of the lung space and the arms of the "V" used as reference points, the examiner may more readily observe cardiac pulsation. This has proved especially valuable in arriving at a conclusion of contrapulsile or other abnormal pulsations.[26]

(7). The "see-saw" action of the heart can be exaggerated by increasing the fullness of contraction by having the patient exercise.

Fundamentals of Specific Chamber Enlargement

Before starting this section, the reader should thoroughly understand figures 62–64.

RIGHT VENTRICLE ENLARGEMENT

Outflow Tract. In order to understand how the heart shadow is distorted by right ventricular enlargement, it is necessary to know the directional flow in this chamber.[6] Figure 74 illustrates the inflow and outflow tracts of the right ventricle. The inflow tract extends from the auriculo-ventricular valve to the apex; the outflow tract, from the apex up to the pulmonary artery. The latter is the more important of these two tracts. It is the enlargement of the outflow tract which one observes first in right ventricle enlargement.

The enlargement of the right ventricle, following the direction as indicated by the arrow in figure 74 is upwards into the conus and pulmonary artery segments. It is the enlargement and dilatation of this latter structure which is responsible for the filling in of the normal left-sided concavity of the heart in various types of heart disease with right ventricular involvement; cor pulmonale, etc. This filling in of the left cardiac border may be simulated by the asthenic or long heart. Left auricular enlargement also produces a straightening or filling in of this left-sided cardiac concavity (fig. 81).[19]

With enlargement of the right ventricle the heart rotates so that more of the conus and pulmonary artery segment comes to occupy the left heart border. This causes a displacement of the "point of opposite pulsations" downwards (figs. 71, 72).

The right ventricle, being a three-dimensional organ, enlarges in height, width and depth. The depth enlargement is in a plane toward the observer, and when viewed with the patient in the frontal position this dimension cannot be determined. How to determine this third dimensional anterior enlargement may be answered upon a moment's reflection. To ascertain the length of a man's nose one would look at him from the side. To observe anterior enlargement of the right ventricle, the lateral or oblique

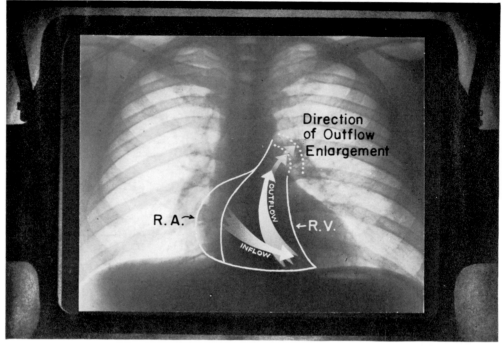

74

Inflow and outflow tract of the right ventricle. Note the direction of outflow tract enlargement.
Because of this enlargement, a filling in of the left-sided cardiac concavity takes place.

projections of the heart are used. From the normal anatomy (fig. 63) the profile of the anterior margin of the right ventricle is seen in the right anterior oblique position and it is usually straight (except in the asthenic heart). With anterior right ventricular enlargement this straight line will be changed to a convex bulge (fig. 82).

For practical purposes, outflow tract enlargement is all one need know in regard to right ventricular enlargement.

Inflow Tract. The inflow tract of the right ventricle, situated on a line extending from the A-V valve to the apex, when enlarged, will also bulge forward. This too requires the lateral or oblique projections for adequate visualization. For this purpose the left anterior oblique position is used and is demonstrated in figure 64. The anterior bulge of the right ventricle in this view (fig. 83) when due to inflow tract enlargement will not become straight upon deep inspiration.[1]

LEFT VENTRICLE ENLARGEMENT

Again we encounter inflow and outflow tracts, the former stretching from the mitral valve to the apex, the latter from the apex to the aorta (fig. 75). Again, for practical purposes all we need know is outflow tract enlargement.

Enlargement of the left ventricle is demonstrated by increased length of the left ventricular segment (fig. 84). This lengthening is manifested either by the apex of the heart extending beyond the mid-clavicular line or downward into the air bubble of the stomach. This chamber also enlarges in a third dimension, i.e., backwards. It would be wise to look in behind the left ventricle and to search for an index that would be useful to gage backward enlargement. To do this the patient is turned to the left anterior oblique position. The spine in this view is situated behind the heart and normally is separated from the left ventricle by a clear

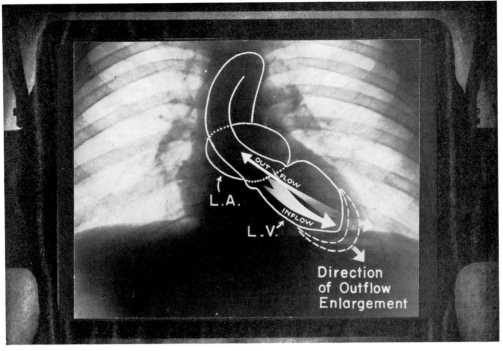

75

Inflow and outflow tract of the left ventricle. Note the direction of outflow tract enlargement, thus producing enlargement of the left ventricle in this direction.

space (see fig. 64). When the left ventricle enlarges backwards, it soon bulges into this clear space, obliterates it and overlaps the spine (fig. 86). Thus, the posterior component of left ventricular enlargement may be visualized by turning the patient into the left anterior oblique position and searching for this clear space, separating the heart shadow from the spine. Normally, this space appears with about 60 degrees of rotation but with considerable posterior left ventricular enlargement, the patient may have to be rotated to a greater degree of obliquity before the clear space between the heart and the spine is visualized. In the normal child, according to Wilson,[8, 9] the angle of clearance is 50 degrees plus; an angle of 55 degrees or more is considered abnormal.

The following are objections to this method of gaging posterior enlargement:

(a) It is cumbersome, and involves special apparatus for measuring degree of obliquity.

(b) Normal variations for the type of heart and chest have not been determined.

With left ventricular enlargement the heart is so rotated that not only is the segment of the left ventricle elongated, but the conus and pulmonary artery occupy less space on the left cardiac profile. The net result of both is an upward displacement of the point of opposite pulsations (figs. 71, 72).

LEFT AURICULAR ENLARGEMENT

Frontal Position. Three possible manifestations of left auricular enlargement can be seen on the fluoroscopic screen when the patient is in the frontal position.

1. As the left auricle becomes enlarged the normal concavity on the left side of the heart becomes filled in (fig. 81). This filling in is caused by the left auricular appendage. It is thus evident that two different chambers of the heart may be responsible for a

filling in of the normal concavity on the left
heart border, i.e., left auricular (appendage), and the pulmonary artery secondary
to right ventricular hypertrophy and dilatation. Distinguishing one from another is
usually quite simple and will be described
presently.

2. The left auricle when it is enlarged
contains more blood and is thus seen as a
ball-like area of increased density situated
within the heart shadow (fig. 76). This increased density is better demonstrated on
the radiographic film but may, on occasion,
be demonstrated on the fluoroscopic screen
by increasing the penetrability of the ray,
or raising the kilovoltage.

3. With considerable enlargement of the
left auricle, the right border of this chamber
creeps out from behind the heart and is
visible to the right of the right auricle (fig.
87). This is, in the main, a late sign.

Left Anterior Oblique Position. The left
anterior oblique position also presents evidence of left auricular enlargement.

A manifestation of upward enlargement
of this chamber is an obliteration of the
infra-bronchial space with elevation of the
left main bronchus (fig. 89).[10, 11] The observation of this elevation is not useful for

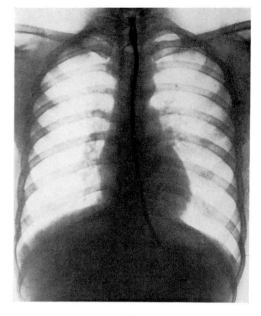

77

The esophagus passes down in a more or less
straight line behind the heart. Left auricular enlargement may deviate it to the right.

early diagnosis, since it is late in its appearance. The closure of the infra-bronchial
space is relatively early in appearance.[26]
This earlier sign can often be best demonstrated on the roentgenogram.

Right Anterior Oblique Position. The
backward enlargement of this chamber is
most important, and is best demonstrated
in the right anterior oblique position. This
is so since the esophagus lies directly behind
the left auricle and it is this structure which
acts as the principal index of left auricle enlargement. Such enlargement will compress
and distort the normal contour of the esophagus (fig. 82) and may go on to close in the
retrocardiac space.

Esophagogram: Normally in the right
anterior oblique view, when the esophagus
is made visible by a swallow of barium
(fig. 117), it presents a shallow curve be-

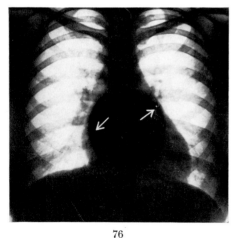

76

Frontal projection. Left auricle when enlarged
may be seen as a ball-like density behind the
heart.

hind the heart. It is especially evident if
the patient has not taken a deep enough
breath. Occasionally, this shallow curve

may be present even at the height of inspiration.

When the left auricle enlarges backwards (fig. 82) it will bulge into the esophagus, deform and compress it. These changes in the esophagus can be considered diagnostic of left auricular enlargement.

In attempting to diagnose early posterior left auricular enlargement a few words of warning about the type of mixture used and exactly when to make observation are important. Minimal left atrial enlargement is best detected by administering a thick barium paste which adheres to the esophageal mucosa, outlining it for some length of time after swallowing. It is inadvisable to make observation during swallowing of a thin barium mixture such as is used in gastro-intestinal study, for the thin barium bolus may not be indented by the left atrium during deglutition, and lesser degrees of retro-displacement of the esophagus will therefore escape observation.[14] Another maneuver, which may help in discovery of early enlargement of this chamber, is observation of the esophagus in the posteroanterior view. In this view (fig. 77) the esophagus courses downward in a more or less straight line behind the heart. A short distance above the diaphragm it deviates to the left in order to pass through this latter structure and enter the stomach. The normal left auricle not infrequently causes a shallow impression on the frontal contours of the esophagus, deviating it only slightly to the right. When the left auricle is enlarged this deviation to the right becomes much more marked and can be useful as a confirmatory sign.

On occasion the barium-filled esophagus in frontal view may be deviated to the left. This may occur especially when adhesions exist between an elongated aortic arch and the esophagus; or it may occur in an eccentric position of the esophagus (fig. 96).

It is noteworthy that scoliosis seldom causes a displacement of the esophagus. Therefore, if posterior displacement of the esophagus is found in a patient with scoliosis, the probability is that the deviation of the esophagus is not due to scoliosis, but is caused by enlargement of the left auricle.

RIGHT AURICULAR ENLARGEMENT

When the right auricle enlarges it increases the frontal diameter of the heart to the right (fig. 90). In the left anterior oblique position, a bulge will be seen as indicated in figure 91. With the patient in the right anterior oblique position the space behind the heart is encroached upon—but since the esophagus is not related to the posterior wall of the right auricle, the esophagus will neither be deviated nor compressed.

Procedure for Cardiac Fluoroscopy

The fluoroscopic rule regarding the handling of the diaphragmatic shutter is applied here, in the study of the heart, as elsewhere. The entire field is first viewed through as large an aperture as the screen permits, remembering, as described in an earlier chapter, that for adequate protection a thin border formed by the shutters should be kept framing the screen. Subsequently, when only certain portions of the cardiac silhouette are under study, the aperture should be reduced to such a size so that only the particular part being viewed is exposed. By thus reducing the field the examiner not only secures finer detail on the fluoroscopic screen, but also helps protect both the patient and himself.

For practical purposes, *every heart should be examined in at least three positions*. The *purpose* for each position is all important here: through a logical sequence of examination to hunt for clues in the first position, then to follow up these leads, cross-checking the examiner's suspicions and confirming or disproving the tentative diagnosis by examination in the subsequent positions. Such a sequence means thorough examination through depth studies, the gaining of the complete picture through true three-dimensionality. If the examiner can train himself in such a pattern of examination he will find that he must rely less and less on rote memory and that the sequential development of information will become more meaningful; the examination, incidentally, becomes a more interesting procedure for the examiner with this method.

Should the reader be confronted in the descriptions directly following with terms or procedures with which he is not completely familiar, he need not be alarmed, since many of these details will be discussed more extensively in a following section. The immediate purpose here is to detail a method of examination

As discussed above, a *complete* fluoroscopic cardiac examination is described. The physician who resorts to the roentgen film as his aid in cardiac diagnosis should know and understand this complete procedure. In actual practice, certain problems may require no part of the fluoroscopic procedure outlined. However, to really understand a part of the over-all roentgen examination, the whole must be known.

FIRST POSITION

Position. Standing or sitting frontal view, patient facing the screen (see also figure 59).

Purpose. The examiner not only desires to make a general fluoroscopic survey of the chest and abdomen, but seeks to answer certain specific questions regarding the heart and mediastinal shadows.

With the patient in this position, then, what information does the examiner seek, and what information can the picture give him?

A. General Cardiac Enlargement. For this, the principles of orthodioscopy and magnification are useful, and will be described presently.

B. Specific Chamber Enlargement.

1. Left ventricular enlargement: (a) Is the apex of the heart beyond the midclavicular line (fig. 84), or does it extend into the stomach air bubble? (b) Is the point of opposite pulsations (the fulcrum) displaced upwards (figs. 71, 72)?

2. Right ventricular enlargement: (a) Is the concavity of the left border of the heart filled in (fig. 81)? (b) Is the point of opposite pulsations displaced downwards (figs. 71, 72)?

3. Left auricular enlargement: (a) Is there filling in of the left heart border? (b) Is a soft bulge noted on the right side of the heart just above the right auricle (fig. 87)?

4. Right auricular enlargement: Is the heart enlarged to the right side in the region of the right auricle (fig. 90)?

5. Finally, are the vascular contours normal (figs. 57, 58)?

Procedure. A suggested routine for cardiac fluoroscopy is to examine the patient first in the postero-anterior position. After a brief preliminary inspection of the lung parenchyma, movements of the diaphragmatic cusps and abdomen, the heart and mediastinal shadows are studied.

The various cardiac and mediastinal contours are studied in their frontal projections. If the examiner wishes, he may now determine heart size (detailed below). Any abnormal configurations are noted. The normal cardiac pulsations are studied. Carefully observing the left border of the heart, the "see-saw" action of this margin is determined. It will usually be found at a point midway between the apex of the heart and the aortic knob. In the transverse type heart the "fulcrum" will be a little closer to the aortic knob, whereas in the tear-drop type or asthenic heart, the "fulcrum" will normally be located a little closer to the apex.

A swallow of barium may be given and its vertical course behind the heart noted. Any deviations should not go unexplained.

SECOND POSITION

If any abnormalities are found, the examiner will seek further aid in establishing an exact diagnosis by making use of "depth studies" of the right and left anterior oblique positions of the heart.

It might be well to re-emphasize here the sequential nature of the examination. The structures being examined are physical objects and cannot be thoroughly understood if viewed from one angle only. They are three-dimensional and must be examined three dimensionally; hence, the second position is assumed to follow up the clues developed in the first position.

Position. Right anterior oblique position (see also figure 60), patient standing or sitting facing screen and so "obliqued" that his right shoulder is closer to the screen.

Purpose. In this view the examiner can gauge depth. If in the first position, then, the examiner received some hint of right ventricular or left auricular enlargement (filling in of the concavity of the left side of the heart, etc.), he now seeks to confirm or disprove his suspicions by using the second position for further examination:

1. Right ventricular enlargement. Does the anterior, or retrosternal, contour become convex and tend to bulge (fig. 82, in contrast to the normal, approximately straight line, fig. 63)?

2. Left auricular enlargement: Is there a tendency toward filling in of the space between heart and spine (fig. 82)? Together with posterior deviation and compression of the barium-filled esophagus, this would confirm left auricular enlargement.

Procedure. The patient is next rotated into the right anterior oblique position, that is, with the patient facing the screen and his right shoulder towards the screen. In the right anterior oblique the appearance

of the pulmonary conus and the anterior wall of the right ventricle is observed. The normally straight segment of this ventricular wall (fig. 63) is to be ascertained. Unfortunately, in hyposthenic individuals this may bulge forward normally and thus in these cases not be as useful a sign in diagnosing right ventricular enlargement. The posterior auricular cardiac contour is next examined and a swallow of barium paste given. The normal esophagus as already described must be seen (fig. 117).

THIRD POSITION

Position. Left anterior oblique (see also figure 61), patient standing or sitting facing screen, and so "obliqued" that his left shoulder is closer to the screen.

Purpose. The purpose of the third position is chiefly confirmatory; the examiner looks for corroborative evidence. He searches the critical outlines, constantly keeping in mind the information already obtained, referring back as necessary and, in a logical synthesis, consolidating the new data with that yielded by the previous positions. Specifically, if the first two positions have indicated any chamber enlargement, depth studies of the left anterior oblique position will yield additional clues to an accurate diagnosis.

1. Left ventricular enlargement: Is the retrocardiac clear space evident with the patient rotated 60 degrees or less? Is the intraventricular groove dislocated toward the right side (fig. 86)?

2. Right ventricular enlargement: Is there an undue bulge in the anterior cardiac contour (fig. 83)?

3. Left auricular enlargement: Is the infra-bronchial space obliterated, or is the left main bronchus elevated and compressed (fig. 89)?

4. Right auricular enlargement: Is the typical contour depicting right auricular enlargement seen (as in fig. 91)?

Procedure. In the left anterior oblique

position one notes anteriorly the contours of the right ventricle and the ascending aorta; posteriorly, the left ventricle and the descending aorta. In this view the "clearing of the spine" is noted, and an approximation made of the degree of rotation—bearing in mind that up to 60 degrees is considered normal. (Acquaintance with the normal pulsations of the left ventricle in this view will indeed prove valuable when trying to diagnose the abnormal, as in pericardial effusion.) The patient in this view should be asked to take a deep breath and the straightening of the anterior right ventricular wall should be noted. Familiarity with the normal here again will be valuable in diagnosing an abnormal bulge signifying enlargement in this region. Finally, the normal position of the interventricular groove should be studied in the left anterior oblique. It is best seen on deep inspiration with the ventricles in systole (fig. 64).

Fluoroscopy of the Pathological Heart

As a preface to this section it is not unwise to repeat that no diagnosis can be arrived at on the fluoroscopic screen alone. The full clinical acumen of the clinician is needed. In addition, many if not all of the findings made in fluoroscopy must be proved and checked by subsequent radiographic films. With this in mind the following pathological processes will be discussed.

DETERMINING HEART ENLARGEMENT

Principles of Orthodioscopy and Magnification. Orthodioscopy is a procedure rarely if ever used today. Yet, its principles should be understood. This would not only serve as a useful exercise in the understanding of the x-ray beam, but it also has historic significance.

Because of the *obliquity* of the rays emitted from the tube, the image on the fluoroscopic screen becomes magnified (fig. 78). It will be noted, however, that only the central ray *travels a straight line* parallel to the floor, has *no obliquity* and thus no resultant distortion. To capture this central beam and trace the outline of any structure with it gives the true size of an object. Such is the principle of orthodioscopy.

This is accomplished by screening off with the diaphragmatic shutters all the rays emitted from the x-ray tube except the central beam. A small lead marker is next fixed on the tube so that it is exactly in the center of this central beam. On the fluoroscopic screen this "central ray" is now seen as a small illuminated field with a black central dot. The shadow of an object in its path will not be distorted since the ray is traveling with no obliquity.

The patient is next placed behind a stationary fluoroscopic screen and one border of the heart found with this central beam. The entire cardiac contour is next traced directly on the screen by moving the tube and following the heart margins. It should be noted that the greatest dimension, i.e., the diastole, is measured.

When the magnification of the cardiac contour is understood, another method useful in measuring heart size would be to magnify a lead-marked measuring stick in exactly the same proportions as the heart shadow itself. This is accomplished by pasting with adhesive tape a lead scale vertically on the anterior axillary line of the patient. On the fluoroscopic screen the lead marker will be magnified and distorted in exact proportion to the heart and the size of this organ may be thus determined (fig. 79).

Measuring Heart Size. For this, a radiographic film taken with a tube-(target)-film distance of 6 feet is preferable to the fluoroscopic examination. Of the many measurements that have been advocated, it

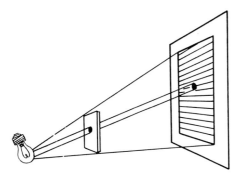

78

(Left)

Principle of orthodioscopy. Oblique rays cause magnification. Central ray causes no magnification.

79

(Below)

The ruler and chest are proportionately magnified. Thus divisions of the ruler can measure structures in the chest.

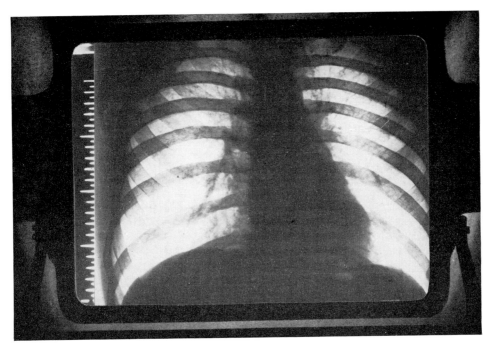

is advisable to make use of the transverse, longitudinal and broad diameters. These suffice to determine whether the heart is enlarged. The transverse diameter which is the sum of the greatest extension of the right border to the right and of the left border to the left of the midline is most widely employed (fig. 80). The cardiothoracic ratio, which is the ratio of the transverse diameter as indicated, to the diameter of the chest taken at the level of the right diaphragmatic cusp, has been widely popularized as being within normal limits if it is less than 50 per cent, but this is crude and inexact. Body build has a most important determining influence on the size of the heart and the correlation of heart size with various factors such as weight and height has been proved important.

Accurate standards based on weight and height have been established by Hodges and Eyster[15] as well as by Ungerleider and Clark.[16]* These latter have had their work confirmed both by Comeau and White,[17]

* "Heart Size Measurements by the Nomogram Method" has been prepared by the Medical Department of the Equitable Life Assurance Society of the United States, and published by Picker X-Ray Corporation.

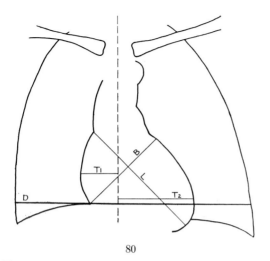

80

Transverse cardiac diameter T1 + T2
Long diameter, L
Broad diameter, B
Transverse thoracic, D

Cardio-thoracic ratio, $\dfrac{\text{T1} + \text{T2}}{\text{D}}$ (normal < 50%)

as well as by Sherman and Ducey.[18] As noted, the predicted transverse diameter for any body build (weight and height) can be compared with the actual. Any deviations greater than 10 per cent may be considered abnormal. Deviations in excess of 15 per cent are definitely considered abnormal.[14]

The long and broad diameters of the heart are important not so much by themselves but for their product—determining the frontal area of the heart. As in figure 80, the long diameter extends from the junction of the cardiac and vascular silhouette on the upper part of the right heart border to the apex of the left ventricle. The broad diameter is the greatest diameter perpendicular to the long diameter. If the heart is placed transversely, it may be necessary to extend the lower part of the right border slightly below the diaphragm in its natural curve in order to delineate the limit of the broad diameter.

Tables predicting the surface area for any given broad and long diameters have been

worked out.[*] Here again, the predicted values can be compared with the actual and a deviation in surface area greater than 10 per cent may be considered abnormal.[14]

Measuring Heart Enlargement: Summary: To recapitulate, it is evident that by the use of either the transverse diameter or the nomographic determination of frontal area, there are two simple and accurate methods which suffice to determine whether cardiac enlargement is present.

DETERMINING CHAMBER ENLARGEMENT

Enlargement of the Right Ventricle. In the postero-anterior view, enlargement of the right ventricle is manifested on the fluoroscopic screen first by a filling in of the normal concavity on the left border of the heart (fig. 81). Secondly, because of the rotation of the heart, causing the pulmonary artery and conus to occupy more of the heart border, the point of opposite pulsations is apparently pushed downwards.

Enlargement of the right ventricular outflow tract is in an *upward* direction (see fig. 74). Also, when one considers the direction of cardiac rotation during right ventricular predominance (i.e., its thrust being towards the interventricular septum and *upwards*), it can be seen that the apex of the heart travels upward.

The examiner, being alerted by these signs, seeks for further proof of right ventricular enlargement. He now wishes to make evident anterior enlargement of this chamber. To determine this he turns the patient to the right anterior oblique position and in this projection the anterior border, which normally should be straight, is instead found rounded and bulging into the retrosternal clear space (fig. 82).

In the left anterior oblique position the intraventricular groove is noted as being displaced towards the left.[1] Also, if the inflow tract of the right ventricle is involved,

Ibid.; see footnote, page 67.

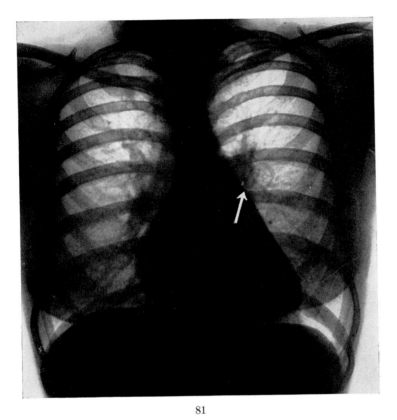

81

Question:

What are the important pathological causes for a straightening (arrow) or filling in of the left side of the cardiac silhouette?

Answer:

1. Enlarged left auricle (auricular appendix presents itself).
2. Enlarged right ventricle (pulmonary artery conus segment presents itself).
3. Dilated pulmonary artery.

the anterior contour of the heart in this projection will bulge beyond the normal (fig. 83).

In summary, the following signs are observed in right ventricular enlargement:

1. The point of opposite pulsations is moved down.

2. The concavity of the left border of the heart is filled in.

3. The retrosternal clear space in the right anterior oblique is filled in by the bulging anterior wall of right ventricle.

4. There is deviation of the interventricular groove towards the left in the left anterior oblique.

Enlargement of the Left Ventricle. On the fluoroscopic screen, enlargement of the outflow tract of the left ventricle is observed by noting in the frontal projection of the heart an increase in the length of the left ventricular segment from the point of opposite pulsations down to the apex. Normally the apex of the heart is situated above the level of the dome of the diaphragm and within the nipple line. With elongation of this segment the apex may extend down beneath the diaphragm and into the air bubble of the stomach. It usually is also displaced beyond the nipple line (figs. 84, 85). (Note: occasionally the normal heart may extend below an elevated diaphragm and this may simulate elonga-

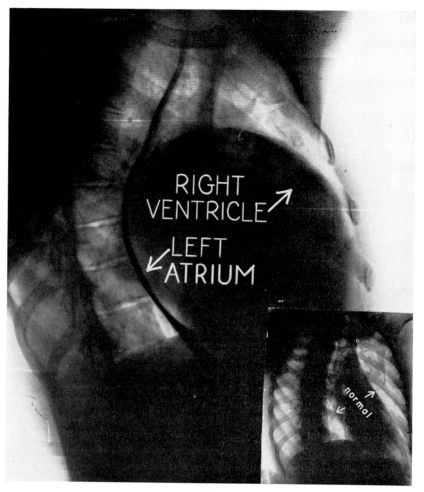

82

In the right anterior oblique position, right ventricle enlargement is indicated by a bulge of the anterior contour. Inset demonstrates anterior contour in normal individual as straight.

The same position is valuable in diagnosing left auricular enlargement, since the left auricle progressively closes in the retro-cardiac space and pushes the esophagus backwards. Inset demonstrates posterior cardiac contour as straight with retro-cardiac space clear and open.

tion of the outflow tract, but in true elongation there is an increase beyond the normal limit of variation of the absolute distance between the point of opposite pulsations and the radiologic apex.) Another feature of left ventricular enlargement to be sought for is the upward displacement of the point of opposite pulsations.

Further proof of left ventricular enlargement is next sought and secured by placing the patient in the left anterior oblique position. In this view the spine should clear the apical shadow of the normal left ventricle in approximately 60 degree rotation. If this is not attained the examiner can assume that there is posterior enlargement of this chamber (fig. 86). Also, in this position, visualizing the intraventricular groove as being pushed away from the left ventricle towards the right and anteriorly is still another sign of left ventricular enlargement.

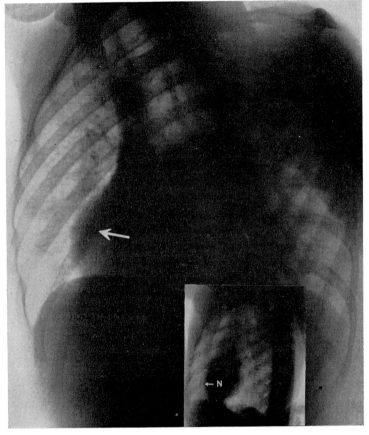

83

A maneuver useful to confirm right ventricular enlargement.

The left anterior oblique position reveals the anterior wall of the right ventricle in profile. In the normal individual (inset-N) this wall is straight. With right ventricular enlargement, the anterior wall bulges (arrow).

The following is a summary of the signs of left ventricular enlargement:

1. The point of opposite pulsations is moved up.

2. The apex of the heart is displaced downwards and outwards beyond the midclavicular line.

3. In order to clear the spine in the left anterior oblique view, the rotation is usually greater than 60 degrees.

4. The intraventricular groove is dislocated towards the right ventricle.

Enlargement of the Left Auricle. On the fluoroscopic screen with the patient in frontal position, the enlarged left auricle is oc-

casionally seen as a separate bulge on the right cardiac contour situated between the normal convexities of the right auricle and ascending aorta (fig. 87). However, since this is a late manifestation, unless the dilatation of this chamber is considerable, it is not evident.

Left auricular enlargement should also be suspected in the frontal view when the normal concavity on the left side of the heart becomes filled in and straightened (fig. 81). This can be caused by enlarged left auricular appendix.[19] When in the postero-anterior view the examiner sees a straightened left cardiac contour, it will be evident from the

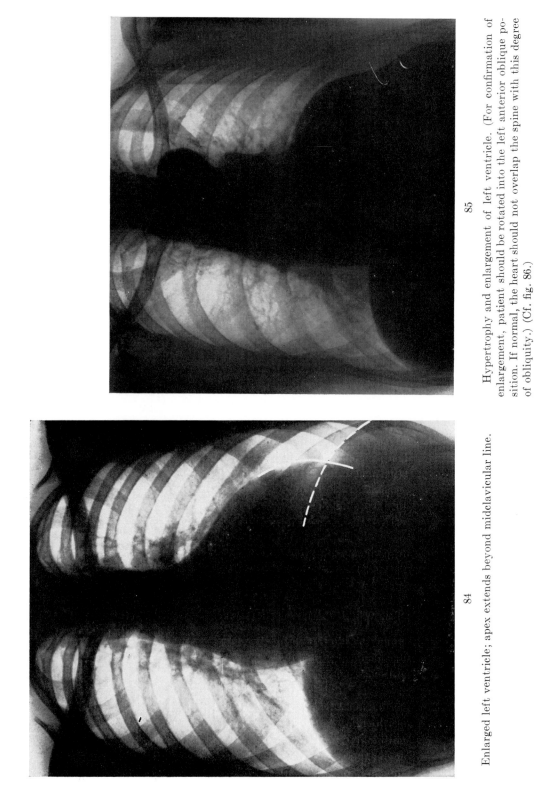

85

Hypertrophy and enlargement of left ventricle. (For confirmation of enlargement, patient should be rotated into the left anterior oblique position. If normal, the heart should not overlap the spine with this degree of obliquity.) (Cf. fig. 86.)

84

Enlarged left ventricle; apex extends beyond midclavicular line.

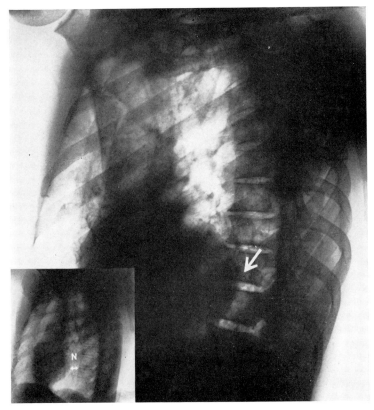

86

The left anterior oblique position can be used to confirm left ventricular enlargement. The patient should be rotated 60 degrees. The enlarged left ventricle (arrow) will overlap the spine. The normal left ventricle (inset) will clear the spine, as indicated by the clear space (N) between the heart and the spine.

evidence presented that he need determine whether this is due to an enlarged left auricle or to a dilated pulmonary artery with possible enlargement of the right ventricle. The latter may be diagnosed, as already described, by placing the patient in the right anterior oblique and looking for the straight line of the anterior surface of the right ventricle being replaced by a round bulge (fig. 82).

The best gage by which to appraise left auricular enlargement is secured by placing the patient in the right anterior oblique position and giving the patient a swallow of barium paste. In this position a posterior deviation as well as compression of the esophagus in the region of the left auricle is pathognomonic of enlargement of this chamber (fig. 88). If the patient now is turned to face the examiner and the opacified esophagus seen during full inspiration, it will also be deviated to one side, usually to the right (fig. 77). This latter deviation, although helpful in arriving at a diagnosis, can sometimes occur with other conditions such as adhesions between the esophagus and aorta, with resultant displacement of the esophagus. An abnormally mobile esophagus may also be seen deviated to the right in the frontal examination of the patient. For this reason a few words of explanation should be given.

Thus it should be emphasized that on *deep inspiration* in the frontal projection,

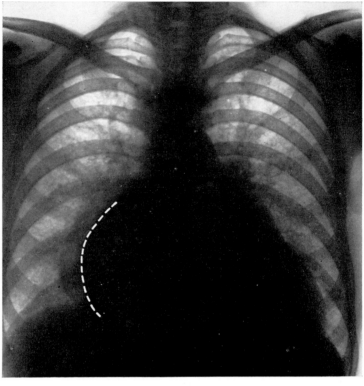

87

"Double Festoon" as produced by left auricular enlargement (frontal view).

Question:

Is this an early or late sign of left auricular enlargement?

Answer:

A left auricle large enough to bulge beyond the right cardiac contour (dotted line) is sufficiently large for this to be a late sign.

the esophagus descends in a more or less straight line behind the heart. On *expiration*, the normal esophagus may be displaced to the right by a *normal* left auricle. This latter is more marked in a stocky individual. As described above, a deviation of the lower esophagus to the right with the patient in *full inspiration* and in the frontal projection should suggest left auricular enlargement. In certain cases, however, the lower esophagus may become sufficiently *mobile* to be displaced to the right when no left auricular enlargement is present. This is especially true when such a patient is in a supine position.[35] The examiner should be aware of this unusual mobility of the lower esophagus and exclude it when using esophageal displacement to diagnose left auricular enlargement. With the patient in the supine position he may be able to test for such esophageal mobility by rotating the *esophagus* from the right side to the left side by rotating the patient, i.e., bringing his right side up, thus throwing the esophagus downwards towards the left. If during this maneuver the esophagus does not shift from right to left, mobility of the esophagus may be excluded.[35]

A comparatively early sign of left auricular enlargement is an obliteration of the infrabronchial space (fig. 89). This is best observed by placing the patient in the left

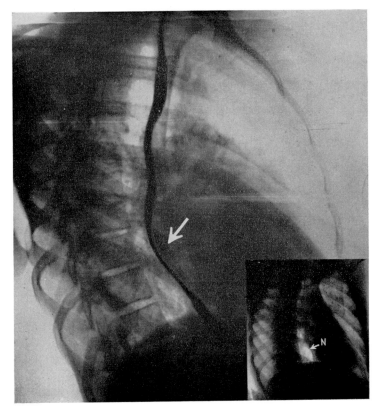

88

The right anterior oblique position can be used to confirm left auricular enlargement.

Enlarged left auricle (arrow) bulges posteriorly and produces narrowing and posterior deviation of the esophagus. With further enlargement the retro-cardiac space becomes closed.

Inset: Normal left auricle (N) does not bulge posteriorly.

anterior oblique position. In a later stage, the pulmonic window may become closed and the bronchus becomes elevated and compressed.

In summary, these are the signs of left auricular enlargement:

1. Posterior deviation and compression of the esophagus occurs.

2. There is a filling in of the concavity in the left heart border.

3. A soft bulge may be noted on the right side of heart, above shadow of right auricle.

4. The infra-bronchial space in the left anterior oblique position is obliterated with occasional elevation and compression of the bronchus.[14]

Enlargement of the Right Auricle. En-largement of the right atrium is conspicuous in tricuspid valvular disease. Enlargement of this chamber occurs usually as part of a generalized cardiac enlargement, almost never as an isolated clinical entity.

For practical purposes a few words only need be mentioned concerning dilatation of this chamber. On the fluoroscopic screen, a bulging or sagging of the right cardiac contour as demonstrated in figure 90 is highly suggestive. Prominence of this contour, however, is not specific, since a prominent right heart border may result from enlargement of any of the cardiac chambers, particularly the right ventricle, displacing the right atrium to the right. It may be simulated by an aneurysm of the ascending

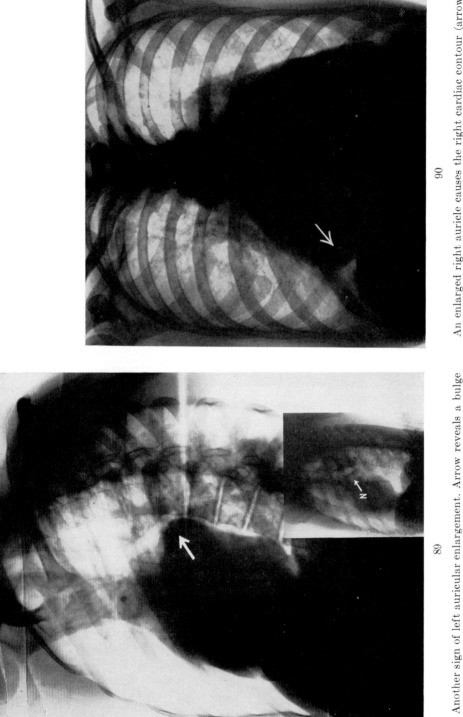

90

An enlarged right auricle causes the right cardiac contour (arrow) to bulge and sag.

89

Another sign of left auricular enlargement. Arrow reveals a bulge due to the left auricle filling in the infra-bronchial space. Inset for normal individual (N) reveals clear space between left auricle and bronchus.

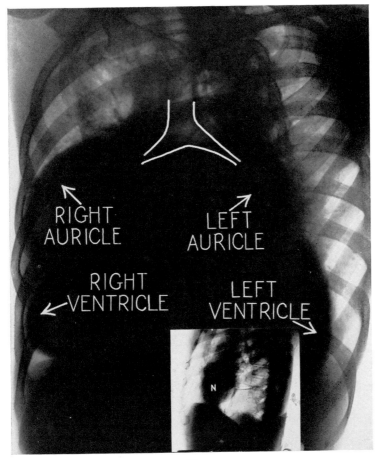

RIGHT
AURICLE

LEFT
AURICLE

RIGHT
VENTRICLE

LEFT
VENTRICLE

91

The left anterior oblique position can be used to confirm *any* chamber enlargement. Note the characteristic bulge of the right auricle. (This picture demonstrates all chamber enlargement. Compare with normal inset.)

aorta reaching down towards the diaphragm, by an arteriosclerotic dilated descending aorta, and by paraesophageal hernia. In the left anterior oblique view the enlarged segment as demonstrated in figure 91 will help prove such an enlargement. In the right anterior oblique position the enlarged right atrium encroaches on or obliterates the lowermost portion of the retrocardiac space, but it does not displace the esophagus.

In summary, the following occurs in right atrial enlargement:

1. Enlargement of the heart takes place to the right. (Fig. 90)

2. Enlargement of the right atrial segment is seen in the left anterior oblique position. (Fig. 91)

3. The retrocardiac clear space is encroached upon, but the esophagus is neither compressed nor indented.

ENLARGEMENT AND DILATATION OF THE AORTA AND PULMONARY ARTERIES

An enlargement of the ascending aorta is evidenced in the frontal view by a prominence of the *right border* of the vascular pedicle and by a forward bulge of the an-

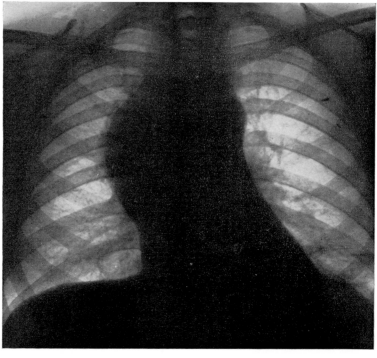

92

Question:

A bulge is seen on the right mediastinal contour. What can produce such a configuration?

Answer:

Abnormalities of any of the anatomical structures in this region (spine, esophagus, ascending aorta, etc.) may cause this.

Question:

How could this bulge be proved to be caused by an ascending aortic aneurysm?

Answer:

The patient should be rotated into various positions. Any shadow blending with the aorta and which rotates with the aorta in all its positions may be assured to be part of the aorta (see fig. 93).

terior border of the aorta as observed in the left anterior oblique view (figs. 92, 93). An arteriosclerotic aorta (fig. 94) is seen in the frontal projection as a characteristic pulsating *bilateral* widening of the vascular pedicle. In the left anterior oblique projection, the aortic shadow is prominent. When aortic regurgitation is present, the observer will see a marked systolic expansion and diastolic collapse. When viewed together with the pulsation of the left ventricle, the "see-saw" action becomes prominent. Other abnormalities of the aorta will be discussed in relationship to the esophagus.

Dilatation of the pulmonary artery is also of great significance. It usually indicates increased blood flow to the lungs. The dilatation of the pulmonary artery causes a pronounced pulmonary artery segment (fig. 95) with resultant straightening or filling in of the concavity on the left side of the heart. Usually the main branches of the pulmonary artery are also distended, and cause conspicuous widening and prominence of both hilar shadows. The fluoroscopist, when his eyes are well accommodated, should seek active pulsations of the hila. This when evident appears as a "hila dance" and is characteristic of pulmonary vessel dilatation (fig. 95).

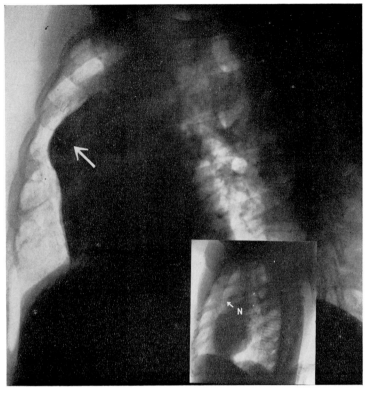

93

In the left anterior oblique position, the bulge (cf. fig. 92) rotates with the ascending aorta (arrow). Inset demonstrating ascending aorta of the normal heart in the left anterior oblique position (N) presents no bulge.

Comment: Any shadow which follows the aorta in all its positions presents evidence of being part of the aorta.

2. To distinguish with certainty whether the bulge is due to aorta, angiocardiography must be performed.

3. The presence or absence of expansile pulsation, practically, is of no importance.

Other causes of increased hila pulsation are: (1) dilated pulmonary artery, (2) pulmonary regurgitation, (3) thyrotoxicosis. A slight to moderate increase in pulmonary artery and hila pulsations are seen with increased exercise.

The shadow of the pulmonary artery can be studied in left anterior oblique as it crosses the "aortic window." In pulmonary atresia this space is abnormally clear.[21]

Normally, pulsation of the great veins (superior vena cava) is not seen, except occasionally in the recumbent position. Vigorous systolic pulsation and diastolic collapse may be seen with a dilated superior vena cava in tricuspid regurgitation, or even often with congestive failure.

Esophageal Distortion Caused by the Aorta. In truth, it would be wise to consider the relationship of the esophagus to any pathological mediastinal involvement. *When an abnormal shadow produces a widening of the mediastinal shadow, it is important to establish its relationship to the esophagus.* For this purpose the patient is placed in the right anterior oblique position and a barium swallow is given. The various normal indentations into the opacified col-

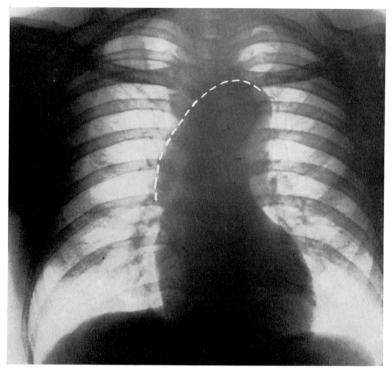

94

Bilateral bulge of the aorta usually indicates an unfolded aorta. Unilateral bulge would make the examiner suspect an aneurysm. Compare with figure 92.

umn are first searched for. These are described elsewhere. Any abnormal impressions, indentures or displacements are noted. The patient should then be examined similarly in the other positions.

It is a fact that abnormalities of the transverse and descending portions of the aorta may cause abnormal impressions on the esophagus, but such impressions are not pathognomonic of a specific lesion within the vessel. Other mediastinal involvements by either tumefaction, lymphoblastoma, etc., may produce the *same* distortions and impressions. The examiner, having found an abnormal mediastinal shadow, and wondering whether this may or may not be an aneurysm, should observe the abnormal shadow for pulsations; determining whether or not it is expansile is an important observation and clue in diagnosing whether this shadow is vascular in nature. To distinguish expansile from transmitted pulsation is indeed difficult. In order to diagnose an aneurysmal bulge with accuracy, angiocardiographic procedures must often be adopted.

When the aorta becomes arteriosclerotic, unfolded and tortuous, and adhesions come to exist between this structure and the esophagus, the latter may follow a devious path through the chest (fig. 96). This, once recognized and evaluated, will cause no difficulty.

Congenital abnormalities of the aortic arch and its branches have been described and classified.[21a] In the vast majority of cases, these abnormalities produce no recognizable effects, but when they do, such effects are produced mainly through distortion and compression of the esophagus and trachea. When a congenital anomaly of the aorta or its branches is suspected, the pa-

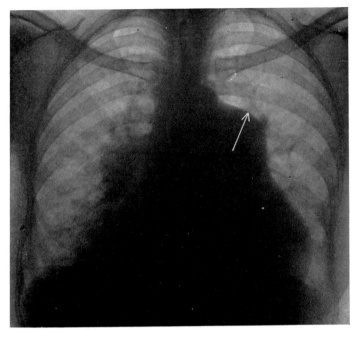

95

Question:
What are some of the important causes for a filling in or *bulging* of the left cardiac concavity?
Answer:
Such a configuration may be produced by
   1. Pulmonary artery dilatation.
   2. Right ventricular enlargement with conus of pulmonary artery enlargement.
   3. Enlarged left auricle.
This case is due to pulmonary artery dilatation.

tient should be given a swallow of barium mixture. *Abnormal* indentures into the esophagus (fig. 117) are important clues to a diagnosis of the condition. Deviations in the trachea also should be sought, and when found are important diagnostic evidence. Angiocardiography is a valuable adjunct in discerning the abnormal course of the various vessels when such conditions exist.

Relationship between trachea, bronchus and aorta. The left bronchus passes *under* the aortic arch and thus the trachea and bronchus may act as a hook-like mechanism capable of pulling the aorta upwards. During ordinary swallowing, the trachea rises and the left bronchus (i.e., the hook) travels up with it. The attachment of the left bronchus to the aorta is wide and *loose* so that ordinarily the aorta remains stationary.

If, for any reason, the fibrous attachment between the trachea, bronchus and aorta is made *taut*, the rising movement of the trachea and bronchus, during swallowing, is transferred to an upward pulling movement of the aortic arch and the aorta will be seen to rise. This may occur in arteriosclerosis or other inflammatory process in the mediastinum which will transform the loose areolar tissue to a firmer fibrous tissue with resulting adhesions between the aortic arch, trachea, and the left main bronchus. These adhesive processes may also be caused by an invasive neoplasm. This sign is also of value in con-

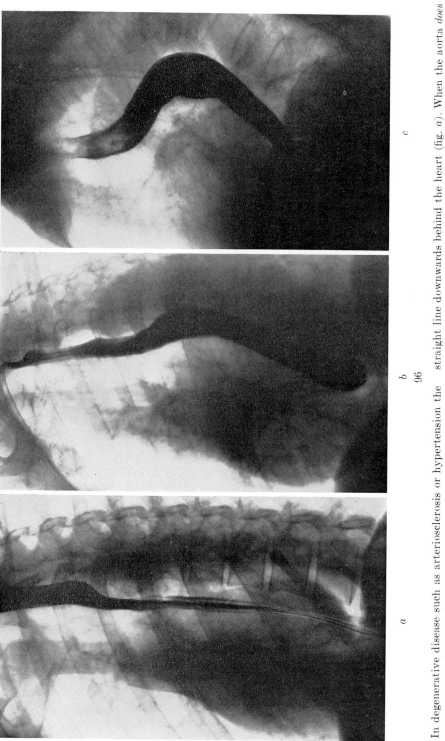

c

b

96

a

In degenerative disease such as arteriosclerosis or hypertension the aorta elongates and uncoils. The left anterior-oblique position "lays out" the aorta so that it is seen in its widest course.

Question: In the left anterior oblique position how does the *opacified esophagus* indicate the course of the aorta?

Answer: When the aorta is *not* elongated or uncoiled, the esophagus contained in the same fibrous sheath as the aorta follows a more or less straight line downwards behind the heart (fig. *a*). When the aorta *does* elongate and uncoil, the esophagus (either because it is adherent or because it is in the same fibrous sheath as the aorta) follows the aorta in its circuitous uncoiling. Figure *b* reveals some uncoiling. Figure *c* reveals a greater degree of uncoiling.

Comment: The course of the esophagus can thus be used as a clue to diagnose an unfolded or elongated aorta.

strictive pericarditis, where adhesive mediastinitis almost always exists.

In emphysema, where with *diaphramatic descent* the heart and the aortic arch tend to travel *downwards*, the aortic arch may thus be brought into closer relationship with the hook-like left main bronchus. During ordinary swallowing the pulling upwards of the left main bronchus in turn hooks under and pulls up the aortic arch.

In the normal patient, the aortic arch may normally be raised with swallowing by having the patient pull his head back and swallow. By pulling his head back he brings the left main bronchus into close association with the arch, and by swallowing, he hooks up the aortic arch.

PERICARDIAL AND VALVULAR CALCIFICATIONS

Pericardial Calcification. When present, pericardial calcification can be more easily recognized in the oblique or lateral positions of the heart. The reason for this will become evident when the examiner reflects that in the postero-anterior view the x-ray beam traveling through the calcification of the anterior or posterior walls pierces only one or two mm. of calcium, whereas in the lateral views, many cms. of this opaque material may be pierced through.

Valvular Calcification. With the eyes properly adapted and secondary radiation prevented by use of a small fluoroscopic aperture, the diagnosis of valvular calcification can frequently be made. A finding of calcification within the valves is usually made evident by their characteristic "dancing" movement within the heart shadow in the region of the mitral and aortic valves. A slight right anterior oblique view has been suggested for optimum observation.

Notes on the Visualization of Cardiac Calcifications

1. To see the calcium, especially in the valves, accommodation must be perfect, if possible taking one hour. The kilovoltage should be raised, and great care should be exercised in the search, The examiner is further aided (a) if he works with as small a fluoroscopic aperture as possible, and (b) if the patient holds his breath.

2. Calcified coronary arteries may be recognized as short parallel segments of increased density.

PERICARDIAL EFFUSION

Differentiation between cardiac dilatation and pericardial effusion, despite many clinical and roentgenological signs, is not easy, especially as the two conditions may occur simultaneously and sometimes as the result of the same cause. There are two stages particularly in which these conditions are difficult to diagnose. First, the early pericardial fluid accumulation which does not display the classic symptoms and, secondly, the extreme filling of the pericardial sac which must be differentiated from the heart enlargement such as found in rheumatic involvement, thyrotoxicosis, myxedema, etc.

Fluoroscopically or even radiographically there are certain limitations as to when or how a pericardial effusion can be diagnosed. First, it can not be diagnosed unless at least 250 or 300 cc. of fluid is present. Secondly, it is not possible to differentiate between the heart shadow and pericardial fluid shadow on the basis of difference in density.

Criteria Used to Diagnose Pericardial Effusion on the Fluoroscopic Screen

The shape of the heart has been considered characteristic, yet at least five different types have been described as pathognomonic of this condition—the triangular, the trapezoid, the spherical, the water bottle and the onion type. The common denominator of these forms of heart configuration is a loss of normal indentures (compare figure **97** with figure **98**). Whenever it is possible to identify the points of division, namely the intersection of the vascular and cardiac contours on the right or the atrio-ventricular border on the left, cardiac dilatation is indicated as opposed to pericardial effusion. Examination of these contours and search for any indentures can be done with greater accuracy on the radiographic film.

The time factor has been stressed by Friedberg,[1] who considers daily roentgen examination the most reliable method for the recognition of pericardial effusion. He considers a significant change in the size of the heart shadow during this time as the best evidence of fluid accumulation. But while this is an important sign it will also have to be revised in view of Wolf's[21] report of acute heart dilatation associated with acute pericarditis complicating respiratory infection with no fluid accumulation. Barnes and Burchell[22] have also observed many cases of pericarditis with rapid heart enlargement but without essential fluid accumulation. In these cases of pericarditis with acute dilatation recovery is complete within two or three weeks, but meantime the roentgenologist is faced with the problem of their differential diagnosis. Thus, heart size increase by itself is still not definitive.

Esophagogram. The observation of the esophagus with contrast medium holds an important place in the diagnosis of pericardial effusion as opposed to general cardiac dilatation. In this latter condition, because the left auricle is prominent, the esophagus will take on the expected variations: that is, lateral displacement may be seen in the frontal position, and with the patient in the right anterior oblique position the opacified esophagus will be displaced backwards. Brown and McCarthy[23] have confirmed this and have also demonstrated that in the presence of pericardial effusion the position of the esophagus is almost *unchanged* from the normal and presents a *normal* transmitted cardiac pulsation.

Cardiac pulsation. Diminution or absence of cardiac pulsation is an important diagnostic sign of pericardial effusion. The fluid has a damping or tamponading effect on heart movements. Often, however, as demonstrated by Stumpf, this needs kymographic proof. Stumpf[24] also demonstrated that on the fluoroscopic screen as well as on the kymograph the transmitted pulsations of a pericardial effusion frequently present the impression of true pulsation.

In the frontal projection, when fluid starts to accumulate, the pulsations in the lower borders of the cardiac silhouette may be dampened. As fluid continues to accumulate, the lateral borders of the cardiac silhouette tend to become filled out with fluid and the normal cardiac indentures chiefly on the left side tend to be straightened (figs. 97 and 98).

The accumulation of the pericardial fluid in the anterior pericardial space[39, 40] forms the basis of still another radiographic and fluoroscopic sign. The fluid accumulating in the anterior pericardial space, when present in sufficient amounts, will not only help obliterate the retrosternal clear space—as seen in the lateral chest study—but will damp the anterior cardiac pulsations as seen in the lateral chest studies. The barium-filled esophagus will, however, transmit the cardiac pulsations posteriorly.

Change of cardiac shape with change in position. With pericardial fluid, as the patient is transferred from the erect to the supine position the fluid within the pericardial sac gravitates upwards and causes a filling or bulging of the "waist" of the heart not seen in the erect position (compare figure 99 with figure 100). This change in heart shape with change of position does not occur in cardiac dilatation.

The Valsalva and Müller maneuvers to demonstrate pericardial effusion.[25] The normal heart during the Valsalva test, which consists of deep inhalation and forced expiration against the closed glottis (asking the patient to press down as if he were moving his bowels), becomes increasingly small. (See figure 67 and compare with

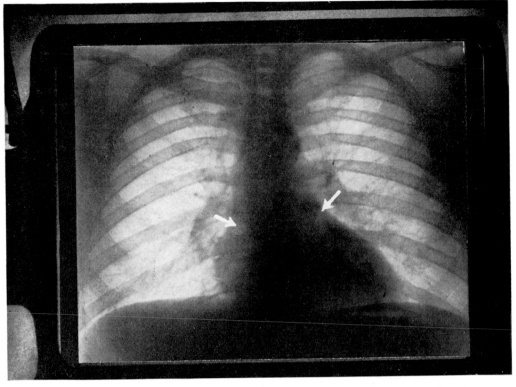

97

Normally the pericardium is closely adherent to the myocardium and the various indentures (arrows) in the normal cardiac anatomy are evident. (See fig. 98.)

68 and 69.) This is probably due to inhibition of venous inflow and increased intrapulmonary pressure compressing the heart bilaterally. Immediately after restoration of the normal respiration, the blood dammed up in the large veins rushes into the heart chambers, the original size is *rapidly* restored, and there is a temporary but marked increased rate in amplitude of pulsation.

In the reverse Valsalva, known as Müller's test, or in its modification, Pong's test—which is nothing more than a forced expiration—the normal heart shadow spreads out on the elevated diaphragm and the pulsations become freer. Their amplitude increases and the increase in cardiac size is considerable.

When a patient with pericardial effusion performs the Valsalva maneuver, the heart does not become noticeably smaller, and usually the original heart size and shape are maintained. Likewise, with relaxation of the increased pressure at the end of this test, the heart size does not increase nor do pulsatory cardiac movements become more evident. Neither does a patient with pericardial effusion, in performing the Müller or Pong test, show significant changes in heart size or shape or exaggerated pulsatory movements of the heart.

These tests can be done with the patient recumbent, and have proved helpful in differentiating pericardial effusion from cardiac dilatation. As has been stated above, a pericardial sac filled with fluid with inherent venous damming will not in spite of an increase (Valsalva) or decrease (Müller) in intrathoracic pressure vary essentially in shape or size with either maneuver. The dilated heart, on the other hand, responds

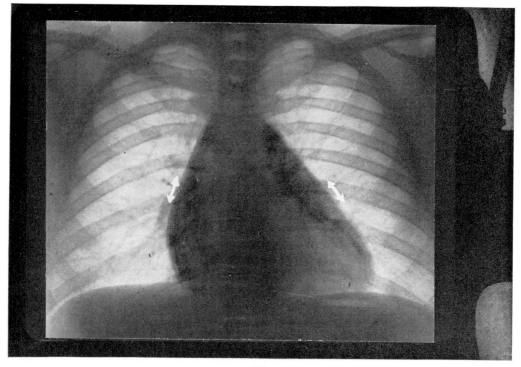

98

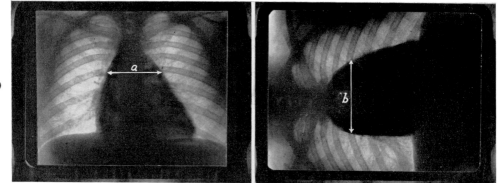

99   100

Signs of pericardial effusion.

(*Compare with fig. 97*)

98

In the presence of fluid between the pericardial sac and the myocardium, these indentures become obliterated and the entire silhouette becomes smooth.

99	100
The patient erect, fluid in the pericardium gravitates down. Diameter "a" (waist of the heart) is relatively small.	The patient lies down. Fluid gravitates upwards and diameter "b" (waist of the heart) is relatively larger.

strikingly to either test, in the same manner as described above for the normal heart.

Ungerleider[26] has recommended the intravenous injection of diodrast and observing an increase in the space between the right auricular margin and the adjacent pericardial wall. His method has been confirmed by Williams and Steinberg.[27]

Pure CO_2 injected intravenously is also used as a contrast material to diagnose the presence of a pericardial effusion.[36, 37] The patient is placed in the left lateral decubitus position. The CO_2 becomes trapped in the right auricle. Normally in the absence of a pericardial effusion, an opaque band no greater than 4 mm. in width separates the air trapped in the right auricle from the adjacent lung. Increase of this width suggests a pericardial effusion.[36, 37]

Summary of signs of pericardial effusion:

1. The Valsalva and the Müller tests are useful in the differentiation between a dilated heart and pericardial effusion. The former shows marked changes in size and shape when the patient is asked to bear down as if moving his bowels (Valsalva) whereas in pericardial effusion this does not occur. At the changeover from the Valsalva to the Müller test the weak pulsations of the dilated heart increase and become visible. In the presence of pericardial effusion such pulsatory changes do not occur in equal measure.

2. Absence of lateral and posterior displacement of the esophagus is in favor of pericardial effusion. The presence of lateral and posterior displacement or a definitely localized auricular impression are in favor of cardiac enlargement.

3. Diminution or absence of cardiac pulsation is an important diagnostic sign of pericardial effusion, often needing to be demonstrated by the kymograph. The cardiac pulsations are dampened at first inferiorly; later, with accumulation of fluid, the pulsations are dampened laterally and anteriorly.[38] Posteriorly the pulsations are present and may best be seen by opacifying the esophagus and visualizing transmitted cardiac pulsation.

4. Rapid change of heart size at repeat examinations is in favor of pericardial effusion, but is not a reliable sign.

5. Change of heart shape when changing from the erect to supine positions is a useful sign. When present it should lead to suspicion of effusion.

CHANGES IN LEFT VENTRICULAR PULSATION

Left ventricular pulsation is increased with exercise, excitement, thyrotoxicosis, valvular regurgitation (either aortic or ventricular), pneumothorax; it is diminished with enlarged heart, pericarditis (either effusive or constrictive), or with hypertrophy of the myocardium (as in hypertensive hearts). The thicker the left ventricular wall, the less apparent is its contraction. A sluggish contraction, therefore, does not always mean the heart is failing.

Although irregularity of rhythm (flutter, fibrillation, extrasystole) can be seen on the fluoroscopic screen, other procedures (e.g., electrokymography) are better for visualizing these. Apparent irregularity in rhythm may be due to diaphragmatic motion; this possibility can be excluded by having the patient hold his breath.

VENTRICULAR ANEURYSM[30]

In the diagnosis of ventricular aneurysm fluoroscopic examination probably surpasses in value the conventional roentgenogram. Since a localized bulge in the cardiac profile (fig. 101) should make one suspect such a diagnosis, the value of the fluoroscopic screen immediately becomes evident. It enables the examiner not only to search along the profile of any presenting border, but by gradually rotating the patient it enables him to observe a continuously changing cardiac profile. In the conventional roentgenogram only one profile is seen. The ideal procedure would be to make a fluoroscopic

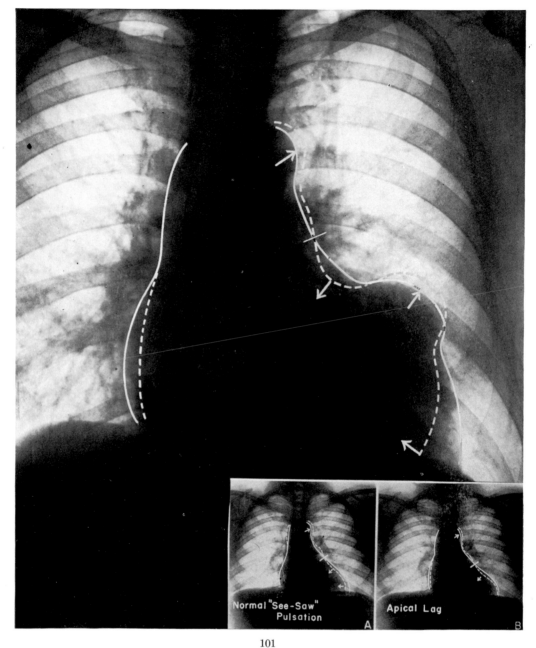

Normal "See-Saw"
Pulsation
A

Apical Lag
B

101

Contra-pulsile pulsation.

(Compare with normal inset)

Question:

What are some of the fluoroscopic signs of cardiac aneurysm?

Answer:

1. A squared appearance of the left cardiac contour.

2. With ventricular contraction during systole, the weakened portion of the myocardium (the bulge) can be seen to expand passively as a result of the raised intraventricular tension. This is called contra-pulsile pulsation.

examination first, and then follow with roentgenograms or kymographic studies in the position in which the lesion is best seen.

The most frequent site at which a cardiac aneurysm is found is at the apex and is often best seen during deep inspiration.[28]

During forced deep inspiration, the lung, overdistended with air, presses upon the heart, with the result that the cardiac shadow becomes smaller. At the same time, the intrapleural *negative* pressure is exaggerated, exerting a sucking effect upon the aneurysm, the wall of which, having lost its tonicity, is pulled out towards negative pressure, thereby becoming more prominent. In forced *expiration*, these conditions are reversed. The negative pressure has a diminished sucking effect and the aneurysmal sac tends to collapse, disappearing completely. As a matter of fact, this sign of a bulge in the cardiac silhouette produced on forced deep inspiration, which may then disappear on forced *deep expiration*, may be used as a differential feature in diagnosing cardiac aneurysm from other confusing mediastinal bulges, such as tumors and cysts of the heart and pericardium.

Using the fluoroscopic screen, one not only searches the cardiac profiles for a localized bulge, but also seeks abnormal pulsations. Abnormality in ventricular contraction, when cardiac aneurysm is present, is most evident when contrapulsile in character (fig. 101). It may manifest itself only as a localized lag of systolic inthrust or as a double systolic pulsation. Localized diminution or complete absence of pulsation is also frequently observed, but these latter are less definite and significant than the contrapulsile expansion.

Contrapulsile pulsation can be considered as a reversal of pulsation (fig. 101). It is recognized by a loss of uniformity of contraction along the left ventricular border. As the normal portion of the ventricular wall contracts synchronously with the expansion of the greater vessels during systole, the weakened portion of the myocardium (the bulge) can be seen to expand passively

as a result of the sudden rise in intraventricular tension. This reversal of pulsation is probably caused by a bulging of the weakened infarcted area; this area is thrust outward by the systolic rise of intra-ventricular pressure, while the remainder of the ventricle contracts forcibly. When the reversal of pulsation is not complete it appears as a localized lag of systolic contraction or as a double systolic pulsation. Since in normal persons the inthrust of the upper left ventricular border slightly precedes that of the apex,[5] a slight lag of the supra-apical region must be interpreted with caution. Localized diminution or absence of pulsation must be regarded as abnormal but not pathognomonic of an infarcted or aneurysmal area, and should not be confused with a normal apical pulsation which is obscured by a pericardial fat pad.

These abnormalities in contraction are observed most frequently and with greater certainty in the postero-anterior view. On rare occasions one may have to seek and find it on the posterior left ventricular wall in the left anterior oblique position.

When seen on the posterior wall these paradoxic pulsations must not be confused with the *false* paradoxic movements of the posterior wall of the left ventricle.[41] These latter are best seen with the patient in the lateral position and in full inspiration. In deep inspiration, the posterior and inferior surface of the left ventricle is sufficiently separated from the diaphragm to be well visualized. During early systole, the inferior surface moves cephalad, and simultaneously the posterior portion expands towards the spine, producing this apparent paradoxic movement. As opposed to true paradoxical pulsations these false paradoxical pulsations are transient and not seen consistently. The paradoxic bulge occurs in the early phases of contraction of the left ventricle and represents an outward bulging of a relatively amuscular area of the ventricle when the heavily muscled area of the apex initially contracts.

Although it is commonly believed that

reversal of pulsation is pathognomonic of ventricular aneurysm or myocardial infarction, Esser[29] noted impairment of apical contractions in cases of cardiac enlargement. A true reversal of pulsation has been found in certain cases of long-standing hypertensive heart disease or aortic valvular disease in which there was considerable cardiac involvement.[30]

It is interesting to note that in a recent study[30] these same phenomena were observed in myocardial infarction. A further sign of myocardial infarction has been described by Sayman. On forced inspiration, the mechanical pressure effect of the distended lung upon the heart is most apparent in the area of infarction. Here the myocardium has lost its tonicity, and the involved area, being pushed in by the distended lung, may appear flattened or depressed. With forced expiration, the pressure of the lung diminishes, the flattening tends to disappear, and the normal left ventricular border is restored.[42]

In the infarcted area, pulsations may be reversed or diminished. A comparison of kymograms obtained before and after moderate effort may reveal pulsations *above and below* the infarcted area increased in amplitude. Pulsations in the infarcted area itself were reduced or absent.[42]

Fluoroscopic examination is not likely to find wide application in the acute stage of coronary occlusion since the patients are too ill. On occasion, however, when the diagnosis is difficult, it has been used. Although the electrocardiogram is helpful in these cases, it is often inadequate and further diagnostic aids such as fluoroscopy are welcome.

HYPOTHYROID AND BERI-BERI HEART

As well as being differentiated from an enlarged heart, the roentgenographic picture of pericardial effusion must also be differentiated from the myxedema heart and beri-beri. On the fluoroscopic screen the hypothyroid heart presents marked hypoactivity, pulsation being indistinct and of small amplitude. On the other hand, Sossman describes pulsations in the beri-beri heart as hyperactive unless masked by a pericardial effusion, in which case the hyperactivity still is evident in the aorta.[31]

HYPERTHYROIDISM

In this condition there is an increase in the volume of circulation which is largely, although probably not entirely, an adaptation to the elevated metabolic rate.

Roentgenologically, the heart is often found enlarged to the left but sometimes to both left and right so that the cardiac shadow is globular. In about one fourth of the cases, the pulmonary artery segment is unusually convex and lengthened.

Fluoroscopy here gives valuable information. The pulsations of the heart are rapid, vigorous and snappy. Normal vagal slowing on holding a deep breath is likely to be absent.[31] Hyperactivity is present on both right and left contours. Kerley[32] describes the fluoroscopic appearance as that of a sponge being squeezed in and out. Increased amplitude of pulsations is obsreved in the pulmonary vessels emerging from both hilar regions.

Congenital Heart Disease

The pathologist, holding the unopened heart in his hand, attempts to diagnose the presence of lesions within by the external contours, size and shape of the heart and great vessels. In pursuance of a more accurate diagnosis, he needs additional data, and so he cuts into and opens the heart.[33] Similarly, the roentgenologist, by fluoroscopic and radiographic examination, attempts to diagnose the presence of cardiac lesions by the external contours, size and shape of the heart and great vessels and, in pursuance of a more accurate diagnosis, must rely on the additional information gleaned from the clinical picture, electrocardiography, angiocardiography and often venous catheterization and occasionally retrograde aortography[43] mainly for extracardiac lesions (e.g., aortic coarctation, patent ductus arteriosus). Malformations found by the fluoroscopist, just as those discovered by the pathologist holding the unopened heart in his hand, may be sufficiently distinctive to be characteristic of a certain defect. Yet, most often, the final diagnosis must rely on additional aids.

There are perhaps two conditions capable of diagnosis solely by the fluoroscopic and radiographic technics, and here, too, caution must be exercised to ensure that the diagnosis is compatible with the clinical appraisal of the patient.[33] One of these conditions is coarctation of the aorta, and this only after the formation of Roesler's nodes[34]

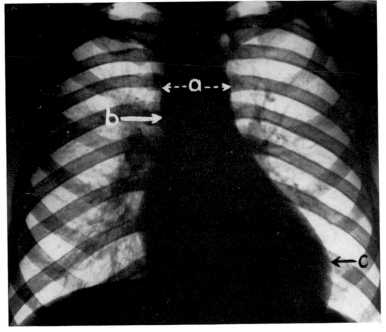

102

Question: What changes if any are present at

Answer:

Vascular pedicle (a)?.......... Vascular pedicle is small.

Ascending aorta (b)?.......... Ascending aorta is small (no bulge discernible).

Left ventricle (c)?.. .... Left ventricle is enlarged (extends beyond midclavicular line).

} These findings are consistent with subaortic stenosis.

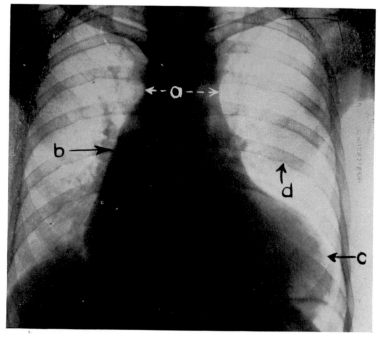

103

Question: What changes, if any, are present at	*Answer:*
Vascular pedicle (a)?.........	Vascular pedicle is small (absent aortic knob).
Ascending aorta (b)?..........	Ascending aorta is prominent. (Note bulge as compared with fig. 102).
Left ventricle (c)?.............	Left ventricle is enlarged.
Inferior rib margin (d)?........	Ribs present Roesler's nodes (notching).

These findings are consistent with coarctation of the aorta.

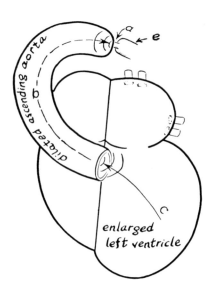

104 (Cf. fig. 103)

Coarcted aorta (a) causes more distant portion, i.e., aortic knob (e), to be diminutive.

Back pressure produced by coarctation (a) causes ascending aorta (b) to dilate.

Pressure transmitted further back causes ventricle (c) to dilate.

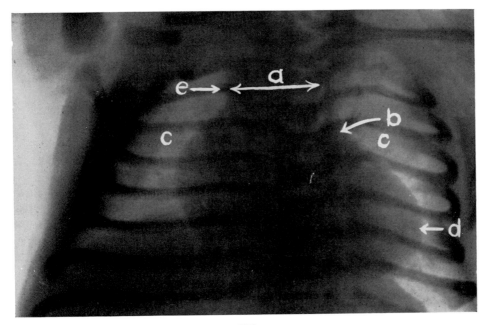

105

Question: What changes, if any, are present at

Vascular pedicle (a)?.........

Pulmonary artery segment (b)?.....................

Hila and lung fields (c)?......

Cardiac apex (d)?............

Superior vena cava (e)?........

Answer:

Vascular pedicle is small (aorta in this case is dextraposed).

Pulmonary artery segment is hollowed out (pulmonary artery is stenosed).

Hila and lung fields clear (pulmonary stenosis) (figure 107).

Cardiac apex is elevated (right ventricle enlarged).

Superior vena cava is enlarged (note small convex bulge extending into innominate artery).

These findings are consistent with tetralogy of Fallot.

Note: The rounded apex (d) simulates left ventricular enlargement. It is caused by a change in the outflow tract of the right ventricle. Right and left ventricles both pump blood into common aortic opening.

106 (Cf. figs. 105, 107)

Dextraposed aorta (a) causes smaller vascular pedicle.

Stenosed small pulmonary artery (b) causes hollowing of left cardiac contour.

Enlarged right ventricle (d) is secondary to pulmonary artery stenosis.

Enlarged superior vena cava (e) is caused by further back pressure through right ventricle, right auricle and into superior vena cava.

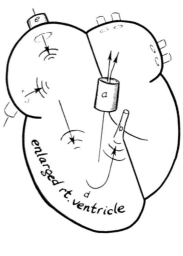

(fig. 103). The other is a fully developed case of interatrial septal defect. Both of these congenital cardiac defects will be treated more fully below.

It should be stressed that in the majority of cases, fluoroscopic and radiographic examination does not necesarily establish an exact diagnosis. This does not diminish the value of the fluoroscopic examination. The examination will detect certain facts not otherwise obtainable and these, together with other data, make a firmer diagnosis possible.

IDENTIFICATION OF DEFORMITIES

In the analysis of a given case, any existing deformities must first be recognized on the fluoroscopic screen.

The deformities listed in the questions below are basic. Complete familiarity with them is essential to the fluoroscopic examination of the congenital heart.

1. Is the right ventricle enlarged?
2. Is the left ventricle enlarged?
3. Is the right auricle enlarged?
4. Is the left auricle enlarged?
5. Are the pulmonary vessels dilated or narrowed?
6. Is the aorta or vascular pedicle hypoplastic and small? or dilated?
7. Is the superior vena cava dilated?

Before proceeding, it is important that the section on cardiac chamber enlargement be reviewed (pages **68–77**). To avoid duplication, only short summaries will be given at this time.

Each of the above seven points will now be discussed.

1. Right Ventricular Enlargement
(FIGS. 81, 82, PAGES 68, 69)

1. The point of opposite pulsations is moved down.
2. The concavity of the left border of the heart is filled in.
3. The cardiac apex is elevated.
4. The retrosternal clear space in the right anterior oblique position is filled in by the bulging anterior wall of the right ventricle.
5. There is deviation of the interventricular groove towards the left in the right anterior oblique.

2. Left Ventricular Enlargement
(FIGS. 84–86, PAGES 69–71)

1. The point of opposite pulsations is moved up.
2. The apex of the heart is displaced downwards and outwards beyond the midclavicular line.
3. In order to clear the spine in the left anterior oblique view, the rotation is usually greater than 60 degrees.
4. The interventricular groove is dislocated towards the right ventricle.

3. Right Auricular Enlargement
(FIGS. 90, 91, PAGES 76–77)

1. Enlargement of the heart takes place to the right.
2. Enlargement of the right atrial segment is seen in the left anterior oblique position.
3. The retrocardiac clear space is encroached upon, but the esophagus is neither compressed nor indented.

4. Left Auricular Enlargement
(FIGS. 81, 87, 88, PAGES 71–75)

1. Posterior deviation and compression of the esophagus occurs.
2. There is a filling in of the concavity in the left heart border.
3. A soft bulge is noted on the right side of the heart, just above the shadow of the right auricle.
4. The infrabronchial space in the left anterior oblique position is obliterated, with occasional elevation and compression of the bronchus.

5. Pulmonary Artery Dilatation and Stenosis

Dilatation and Hilar Dance. This has been discussed elsewhere (page **77**). In review, it is again stressed that the butterfly-like shadows on either side of the mediastinum, i.e., the hila, extending from the mediastinum into both lung fields, consists mainly of the pulmonary arteries and their branches. During cardiac systole, because of the ready entry of blood into the widened channels, they become widely dilated and engorged. During diastole, due to their diminished blood content, they readily collapse. The shadow of their alternate engorgement and collapse when seen on the fluoroscopic screen appears as a "blinker" light alternately turned on and off. This has been called the "hila dance" (figs. 48 and 95, pp. 41 and 81).

Stenosis and Paucity of Hilar Markings. In pulmonary artery stenosis, due to the diminished blood content of the narrowed pulmonary vessels, the markings produced in both lung fields by the pulmonary arteries (i.e., originating at the hila and extending into the lung fields) become sparse and almost absent. This paucity of markings is characteristic of pulmonary artery stenosis and renders the lung fields particularly clear. *Abnormally clear lung fields should cause the examiner to suspect pulmonary artery stenosis* (figs. 105, 107).

Further, since the left sided cardiac concavity is normally filled in, by a normal sized pulmonary artery (fig. 58, page 48, a diminutive or stenosed pulmonary artery will not completely fill the left sided concavity. Thus, a hollow, concave appearance (fig. 105) *on the left heart border should suggest a stenosed pulmonary artery.*

An important exception exists in this hollowing out of the left sided cardiac concavity. Pulmonary artery stenosis, when associated with post-stenotic *dilatation* of the pulmonary vessels, will cause the left sided cardiac concavity to be *filled in.* Because of the post-stenotic *dilatation* the region of the concavity is not only filled in, but may even appear enlarged and prominent (fig. 107).

In summary, the main fluoroscopic clue to pulmonic stenosis is the paucity of markings in the lung, i.e., abnormally clear or translucent lung fields. It is associated with an exaggerated left sided cardiac concavity. In the presence of post-stenotic dilatation, however, the expected concavity is filled in and may be replaced by a bulge.

6. NARROWING OF VASCULAR PEDICLE

Part of the routine examination of the heart should include an appraisal of the width of the vascular pedicle. For our purposes, the vascular pedicle may be considered that portion of the mediastinal shadow situated immediately above the heart and made up chiefly of the aortic arch (fig. 102). Narrowing of this shadow may be produced by any mechanism or deformity which will narrow the shadow of the transverse diameter of the aortic arch, as viewed from the front of the patient. Thus, an aorta wherein the ascending and descending limbs are brought closer together will cause the vascular pedicle to appear narrow. Ascending and descending limbs which are carried further apart will cause an apparent widening of the vascular pedicle. An aorta which is rotated, dextroposed or right sided will appear narrower when viewed from the front. An aorta wherein the knob is absent, as in coarctation, will cause the vascular pedicle to appear narrower. Subaortic stenosis, a condition wherein the full pressure or flow of blood into the aorta is inhibited, may also be associated with a hypoplastic aorta or small aortic shadow and narrow vascular pedicle.

A basic understanding of these different entities is important.

In coarctation of the aorta, the constriction and inhibited blood flow into the aortic knob causes the shadow cast by the aortic knob to *lose its prominence* and the vascular pedicle to become narrowed (figs. 103–104).

The shadow of the aortic knob may also be absent or diminutive when the aorta is rotated. During rotation, the knob may be rotated *into* the mediastinal shadow, and

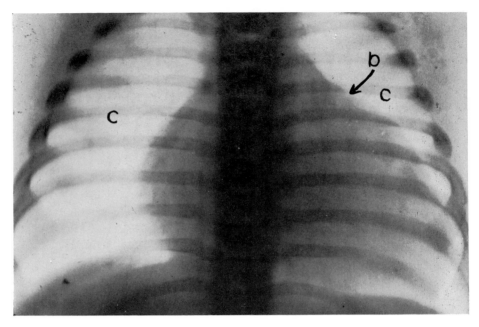

107

The heart here is also characteristic of tetralogy of Fallot.

The *prominence of the pulmonary artery* segment (*b*) is at variance with the same condition in figure 106, and is produced by poststenotic dilatation of the pulmonary artery.

Note: The fluoroscopic clue to the pulmonary artery stenosis is the *clear* lung fields (*c*) and almost absent hila (Compare with *c*, figure 108).

during frontal examination of the patient, the knob becomes hidden from view. The degree of rotation may be such as to cause the aortic knob to project from the side of the mediastinum *opposite* to which it is normally seen. In a right sided aorta, the aortic knob may be found to project from the right side of the mediastinal shadow instead of the left.

A right sided aorta should be distinguished from an aorta which is dextroposed.

A *dextroposed aorta* is one whose *origin* is shifted from the normal position (i.e., from the left ventricle) towards the right. The degree of shift is variable. In some cases, the shift is such that, instead of originating from the left ventricle, it is displaced to *overlie the interventricular septum* and arises from both right and left ventricles. This would permit venous blood from the right ventricle to enter the peripheral circu-

lation and be a cause of cyanosis. A dextroposed aorta will produce a *normal* but *shallow* indenture on the *anterior and left* aspect of the opacified esophagus.

A *right sided aorta* is one which arches to the right instead of the left, but *arises normally from the left ventricle*. It may either cross immediately to the left of the spine at the level of the arch or descend on the right and cross at the diaphragmatic level. Because of its course behind the esophagus, the characteristic indenture produced by the "normal" aorta on the *left anterior* aspect of the opacified esophagus is replaced by a *right and posterior* esophageal indenture. Also because of its course to the right, the *aortic knob* is found on the *right side* of the mediastinum instead of the left.

In Summary: The examiner seeing a narrowed vascular pedicle should suspect an abnormality in the course of the aorta.

In examining the vascular pedicle, the aortic knob must be identified. The course of the aorta anterior to the esophagus and producing an indenture into the *right and anterior* contour of the esophagus should be verified. A *left and posterior* indenture is consistent with a right sided aorta.

7. Superior Vena Cava Dilatation

Dilatation of the superior vena cava is manifested in the frontal view by a widening of the superior portion of the mediastinal shadow in the region of the aortic arch and on the right side of the mediastinum (fig. 105).

EXAMINATION FOR SPECIFIC ANOMALIES

In the discussion of the congenital heart to follow, the deformities will be pointed out as they appear on the fluoroscopic screen in the frontal position. Corroboration of the conclusions drawn from this frontal projection (i.e., the oblique studies) should be reviewed on pages 68–77).

Aortic and Subaortic Stenosis (fig. 102)

Defect. In this condition the opening from the left ventricle to the aorta is narrowed by a thickened and sclerosed aortic valve. Often, the region of stenosis may exist immediately beneath the valve.

Examination of the Heart. The routine questions, again, should always be asked:

(1) Is the right ventricle enlarged?

(2) Is the left ventricle enlarged?

(3) Is the right auricle enlarged?

(4) Is the left auricle enlarged?

(5) Are the pulmonary vessels dilated or narrowed?

(6) Is the aorta or vascular pedicle hypoplastic and small or dilated?

(7) Is the superior vena cava dilated?

Answers:

(1) The right ventricle is not enlarged.

(2) The left ventricle is enlarged (fig. 102). The stenosis at the root of the aorta,

by narrowing the outflow from the left ventricle, imposes stresses and strains on the left ventricle which cause it to hypertrophy and become dilated.

(3) The right auricle is not enlarged.

(4) The left auricle is not enlarged.

(5) No changes occur in the pulmonary vessels.

(6) The aorta and vascular pedicle: The passage of blood from the left ventricle into the aorta is interfered with because of the *narrowing at the entry into the aorta.* The aorta responds to the lessened inflow by becoming smaller than the normal. Fluoroscopically, the comparative smallness of the aorta is translated into a narrower vascular pedicle. The aortic knob is less prominent and may even be absent (fig. 102).

In certain instances the vascular pedicle may appear widened. This is produced by post-stenotic dilatation of the aorta. If the possibility of this variation is kept in mind, it can be evaluated with the other findings. It should be emphasized, however, that in aortic stenosis a narrowed vascular pedicle and a diminutive or absent aortic knob can be expected.

(7) The superior vena cava presents no characteristic dilatation.

In summary: Behind the fluoroscopic screen the important clues that should lead to a suspicion of aortic or subaortic stenosis are (a) the *diminutive vascular pedicle* and (b) the *enlarged left ventricle.*

Differential Diagnosis. 1. Behind the fluoroscopic screen an enlarged left ventricle commonly may bring to mind either hypertensive or arteriosclerotic heart disease. In these conditions, however, a prominent and unfolded aortic arch, i.e., *widened vascular pedicle*, leads to their diagnosis (fig. 94, page 80). In aortic or subaortic stenosis, on the contrary, the enlarged left ventricle is instead associated with a narrowed or small vascular pedicle.

2. Aortic stenosis of other etiology, e.g., rheumatic fever, may produce a fluoroscopic picture entirely resembling aortic or sub-

aortic stenosis. The clinical appraisal in such cases is diagnostically most important.

Coarctation of the Aorta (figs. 103, 104)

Defect. The defect in this condition is similar to the defect in aortic or subaortic stenosis but it occurs a little more distally in the course of the aorta. The narrowing exists within the arch of the aorta, distal to the origin of the left subclavian artery and in the region of the ductus arteriosus. Those cases that survive reveal a well developed collateral circulation which by-passes the coarctation.

Examination of the Heart. During the examination the examiner should ask himself the basic questions:

(1) Is the right ventricle enlarged? (2) Is the left ventricle enlarged? (3) Is the right auricle enlarged? (4) Is the left auricle enlarged? (5) Are the pulmonary vessels dilated or narrowed? (6) Is the aorta or vascular pedicle hypoplastic and small or dilated? (7) Is the superior vena cava dilated?

Answers:

(1) The right ventricle is not enlarged.

(2) The left ventricle, in an effort to pass the blood beyond the constricted portion of the aorta, becomes hypertrophied and dilated.

(3) The right auricle, (4) left auricle and (5) pulmonary vessels present no characteristic involvements.

(6) The vascular pedicle: Because of the inhibited blood flow into that portion of the aortic arch distal to the constriction, the aortic knob becomes small or absent. Due to the ready ingress of blood into that portion of the aorta proximal to the constriction, and the associated difficulty in its egress, the ascending portion of the aorta becomes prominent and causes the right side of the mediastinum to bulge (figs. 103, 104).

(7) The superior vena cava presents no characteristic involvement.

Roesler's nodes: (figs. 103, 104). Fluoroscopically and radiographically, the most important clue to the existence of coarctation of the aorta is the finding of "Roesler's nodes."

The subcostal vessels lying in the narrow subcostal grooves on the under surface of the ribs normally cause no changes in the bony contour. Because of the collateral circulation which exists in coarctation of the aorta, the subcostal vessels chiefly between the 3rd and 9th ribs become widely dilated. These widened vessels lying in the subcostal grooves gradually erode the adjacent bony margins. These erosions produce the characteristic scalloped appearance known as Roesler's nodes. Evidence of the erosion is rarely seen before 12 to 14 years of age. When present, they are practically pathognomonic of coarctation of the aorta. Similar scalloped erosions, however, can be produced by neurofibromatosis.[2]

In summary: Fluoroscopically an absent or diminutive aortic knob when associated with an enlarged left ventricle should suggest either aortic or subaortic stenosis or coarctation of the aorta. The clue to their differentiation lies in the ascending aorta. In coarctation of the aorta, the ascending aorta is prominent, whereas in aortic or subaortic stenosis the ascending aorta is small and diminutive and causes no bulge on the right side of the mediastinum. (Compare fig. 102 with fig. 103).

Roesler's nodes are present in coarctation of the aorta, but absent in aortic or subaortic stenosis.

Differential Diagnosis: Behind the fluoroscopic screen, the visualization of an enlarged left ventricle together with a dilated ascending aorta should suggest hypertensive or arteriosclerotic heart disease. In these latter conditions, however, bulging of the ascending aorta is caused by an unfolding of the aortic arch, and thus both ascending and descending portions of the aortic arch, together with the aortic knob, are prominent (fig. 94). In coarctation of the aorta, on the contrary, only the ascending portion of the arch is prominent. The aortic knob and descending portion of the aorta are diminutive or not seen. Again, Roesler's nodes will identify coarctation of the aorta.

Tetralogy of Fallot (figs. 105–107)

Defect. The defect here consists of: (a) Pulmonary artery stenosis. (b) Hypertrophy of the right ventricle. (c) Dextroposition of the aorta. (d) Interventricular septal defect.

Examination of the Heart. Again the routine questions are asked:

(1) Is the right ventricle enlarged? (2) Is the left ventricle enlarged? (3) Is the right auricle enlarged? (4) Is the left auricle enlarged? (5) Are the pulmonary vessels dilated or narrowed? (6) Is the aorta or vascular pedicle hypoplastic and small or dilated? (7) Is the superior vena cava dilated?

Answers:

We can disregard questions 2 and 4 since the left ventricle and left auricle present no significant fluoroscopic changes. Questions 1 and 5, however, play an outstanding part, and are discussed directly below after brief reference to the characteristic change:

Coeur en Sabot (Boot-shaped heart): An important clue in the identification of the Tetralogy of Fallot is the characteristic boot-shaped heart (figs. 105, 106). The question should first be asked, what deformities must the cardiac silhouette undergo to resemble the shape of a boot? In explanation, the picture of a boot should be borne in mind. Also, an appearance *resembling* left ventricular enlargement must be secured to explain the prominence of the tip of the boot. *The left side of the cardiac silhouette* which would correspond to the laced portion of the boot must be hollowed out (figs. 105, 106). The explanation of the deformity lies in understanding the changes in the right ventricle and pulmonary artery.

(1) Right ventricle: In the frontal projection of the heart, the direction in which the right ventricle enlarges, depends upon the direction of its outflow tract. Normally,

its outflow tract is upwards into the conus and pulmonary artery. Normally, the enlargement of the right ventricle is in the direction of the conus and pulmonary artery (fig. 74 page 60). In the Tetralogy of Fallot, the right ventricular outflow tract is changed. The aorta is dextroposed and the right and left ventricles, sharing a common opening into the aorta, both pump blood into the aorta. The outflow tract of the right ventricle thus resembles the outflow tract of the left ventricle. Since the outflow tracts resemble each other, the enlargement of the right ventricle in the Tetralogy of Fallot *simulates left ventricular enlargement.* Thus, simulating left ventricular enlargement, a boot shaped prominence is secured at the cardiac apex.

(5) The pulmonary artery: This left sided concavity, i.e., the laced portion of the boot, is the site of the pulmonary artery. In the normal heart the pulmonary artery succeeds in filling the concavity. In Tetralogy of Fallot, pulmonary stenosis is an important component of the congenital defect. The stenosed pulmonary artery is small, and does not fill in this concavity. This explains the hollowing out of the laced portion of the boot (figs. 105, 106; compare with fig. 107).

Another important characteristic of pulmonary stenosis is the increased clearness of both lung fields. (See pages 94–95.)

A problem confronting the examiner when appraising the paucity of lung markings is to decide whether a given degree of clarity indicates pulmonary artery stenosis. An image of the *normal* infant chest should be kept in mind. Commonly, especially in infants, if the examiner secures a clear cut clinical picture of a bronchopneumonia, the vascular markings in this *normal* chest almost appear sufficient to be consistent with a bronchopneumonia. With pulmonary artery stenosis and the concomitant paucity of lung markings characteristic thereof, even in the face of a clear cut clinical bronchopneumonia, the vascular markings are so sparse that no fluoroscopic or radiographic diagnosis could be made.

(6) Narrowed vascular pedicle: Interventricular septal defect and dextroposition of the aorta (fig. 106a) are noted. No significant fluoroscopic or radiographic characteristic arises from the septal defect. The new position assumed by the aorta causes the vascular pedicle to become narrowed.

(7) Superior vena cava (figs. 105e, 106e): The superior vena cava may be dilated; back pressure from the hypertrophied right ventricle is reflected in a retrograde direction through the right auricle and into the superior vena cava.

In summary, fluoroscopically and radiographically, the important clue that may lead the examiner to suspect the Tetralogy of Fallot is the paucity of markings in both lung fields, i.e., the abnormally translucent lung fields. This is consistent with a pulmonary artery stenosis. If, in addition, the heart is boot shaped, the diagnosis is made more certain. For final diagnosis, the clinical appraisal and other modalities discussed above should be amployed.

EISENMENGER COMPLEX (FIG. 108)

Defect: The defect here consists of:

1. Pulmonary artery dilated. It may be normal.

2. Hypertrophy of right ventricle.

3. Dextroposition of the aorta.

4. Interventricular septal defect.

Note: Except for the pulmonary artery, the defect resembles the Tetralogy of Fallot.

Examination of the Heart:

The examiner asks himself the routine questions:

(1) Is the right ventricle enlarged? (2) Is the left ventricle enlarged? (3) Is the right auricle enlarged? (4) Is the left auricle enlarged? (5) Are the pulmonary vessels dilated or narrowed? (6) Is the aorta or vascular pedicle hypoplastic and small or dilated? (7) Is the superior vena cava dilated?

Answers:

(2) The left ventricle and (3, 4) both auricles and (7) the superior vena cava present no significant fluoroscopic signs. We need deal here only with questions 1, 5 and 6.

(1) Right ventricle and (5) pulmonary artery (fig. 108): The changes described for the Tetralogy of Fallot may be applied to this anomaly. The right ventricle hypertrophies and becomes enlarged. This enlargement is secondary to the pressure increase within the chamber. This may be explained by two mechanisms. The right ventricle's pressure is raised by being associated with aortic pressure and increased pulmonary pressure. First, since the aorta is dextroposed and arises above the ventricular septal defect, the right ventricle shares with the left ventricle the function of propelling blood through the systemic circulations. Thus, the pressure in both ventricles is similar, i.e., being at systemic levels. Secondly, pressure in the pulmonary arterial system is also high. This even though the pulmonary artery appears normal or dilated. The increased pressure in the pulmonary artery depends on changes recognized morphologically within the arteries of the pulmonary vascular bed.

It is the presence of pulmonary artery dilatation that helps distinguish this complex. The pulmonary arteries, widely dilated and engorged, significantly present a "hila dance."

(6) The vascular pedicle: The dextroposed aorta is radiographically evidenced by a narrow vascular pedicle.

In summary: Although the heart may resemble the Coeur en Sabot type, it may also be normal or globular. It is the characteristic dilatation of the pulmonary arteries when present that helps direct attention that an Eisenmenger complex may be present.

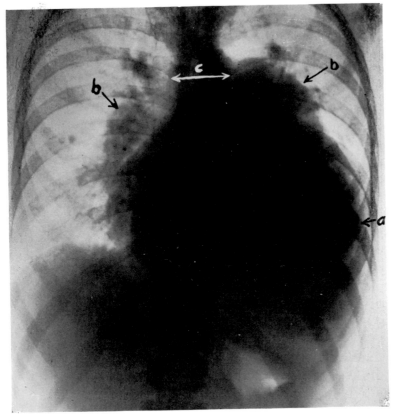

108

Apex (*a*) elevated (right ventricle enlarged). ⎫ These changes are
Dilated pulmonary arteries (*b*) (hila dance). ⎬ consistent with an
Small vascular pedicle (*c*) (dextraposed aorta). ⎭ Eisenmenger Complex

INTERATRIAL SEPTAL DEFECT
(FIGS. 109, 110)

Defect. The defect here consists of: (a) Persistent ostium primum (base of septum). (b) Persistent ostium secundum (upper posterior part of septum). (c) Patent foramen ovale.

Examination of the Heart.

(1) Is the right ventricle enlarged? (2) Is the left ventricle enlarged? (3) Is the right auricle enlarged? (4) Is the left auricle enlarged? (5) Are the pulmonary vessels dilated or narrowed? (6) Is the aorta or vascular pedicle hypoplastic and small or

dilated? (7) Is the superior vena cava dilated?

Answers (figs. 109, 110):

(1) *Right ventricle:* The dilatation and increased quantity of blood in the right auricle is soon passed on to the right ventricle, which in turn also dilates.

(2) *Left ventricle:* No significant change is noted.

(3) *Right auricle:* The configuration of the heart in this disease depends upon the direction in which the blood flows through the defect in the septum. Since the pressure on the *left* side of the heart reflects the

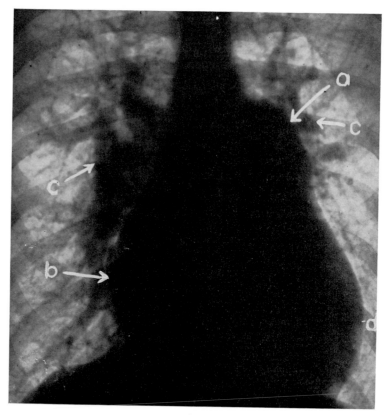

109

Question: What changes, if
  any, are present at

Answer:

Pulmonary artery
  segment (a)?

Pulmonary artery segment is prominent (pulmonary artery engorged).

Right auricle (b)? . . . .

Right auricle is prominent (its contour bulges
  due to enlargement).

Pulmonary artery
  branches (c)? . . . .

Pulmonary artery branches are dilated (hila
  dance).

Apex, right ventricle (d)? . . . . . .

Apex is elevated (right ventricle enlarged).

These changes are
consistent with an
interauricular sep-
tal defect.

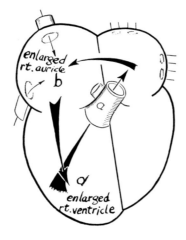

110 (Cf. fig. 109)

Right auricle (b) dilated due to increase blood
flow through the septal defect from the left auricle.

The increased amount of blood entering into
the right auricle flows into and causes an increased
amount of blood in the right ventricle (d), thus
making the right ventricle dilate.

The increased blood in the right ventricle flows
into the pulmonary artery and causes an increased
amount of blood in this vessel and its branches,
with resulting dilatation.

systemic circulation, it is higher than the pressure on the right side of the heart. For this reason the blood flow is from the *left side of the heart to the right*. Consequently, blood flowing through the defect from the left auricle to the right auricle causes the right auricle to become enlarged.

(4) *Left auricle:* No significant change is noted.

(5) *Pulmonary artery:* The increased amount of blood present in the right ventricle results in a greater inflow of blood within the pulmonary vessels. Consequently, the pulmonary artery and the hila branches

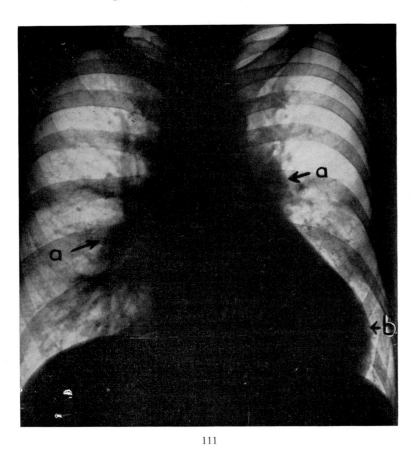

111

Question: What changes, if any, are present at

Pulmonary artery branches (*a*)?....

Apex of heart (*b*)?.................

Answer:

Pulmonary artery branches are dilated (hila dance).

Apex of heart is beyond midclavicular line and simulates *left* ventricular enlargement.

(*Note:* The electrocardiograph revealed *right axis deviation*. At post mortem, a markedly enlarged *right* ventricle was found. The left ventricle was only minimally enlarged.)

(*b*) *is really the right ventricle*. The *elevated* apex was the clue pointing toward right ventricular enlargement.

Comment: If at any time disagreement as to ventricular enlargement exists between the electrocardiographic and clinical data on the one hand, and the x-ray and fluoroscopic findings on the other, the decision should be in favor of the electrocardiogram and clinical data. This case was a Lutembacher syndrome.

become engorged. Fluoroscopically this is manifested in the "hila dance."

(6) The aorta and (7) superior vena cava present no significant changes.

In summary: The mechanism explaining the fluoroscopic image in this condition is a flow of blood from the left auricle to the right auricle and thence into the right ventricle and pulmonary artery. Enlargement, then, of the right auricle, right ventricle and pulmonary artery produces the characteristic fluoroscopic picture of this disease.

Occasionally, an atrial septal defect is associated with acquired rheumatic mitral stenosis. This complication is called "Lutembacher syndrome" (fig. 111).

PATENT DUCTUS ARTERIOSUS (FIG. 112)

Defect. The ductus arteriosus usually becomes obliterated by the third week of postnatal life. It may persist and remain patent, however forming a shunt from the aortic arch to the pulmonary artery.

Examination of the Heart

(1) Is the right ventricle enlarged? (2) Is the left ventricle enlarged? (3) Is the right auricle enlarged? (4) Is the left auricle enlarged? (5) Are the pulmonary vessels dilated or narrowed? (6) Is the aorta or vascular pedicle hypoplastic and small or dilated? (7) Is the superior vena cava dilated?

(2) The right ventricle: The right ventricle becomes enlarged. This enlargement is

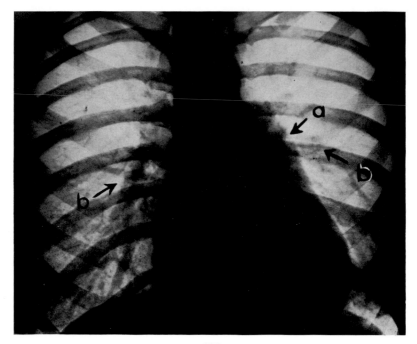

112

Question: What changes, if any, are present at	Answer:	
Pulmonary artery segment (a)?................	Pulmonary artery segment enlarged (note bulge).	These changes are consistent with patent ductus arteriosis.
Hila and pulmonary artery branches (b)?........	Hila and pulmonary artery branches dilated (hila dance).	

seen in the pulmonary artery and conus segments (fig. 112) and is produced by back pressure from the shunt and the presence of an increased amount of blood. This increased amount includes not only the blood normally circulating via the right ventricle, but also the amount added through the shunt.

(3) Left ventricle: The left ventricle has an increased load imposed upon it. It now must work not only in supplying blood to the systemic circulation, but some of it is lost to the shunt. Some enlargement of the left ventricle takes place.

(4) Right and left auricles show no significant change.

(5) Pulmonary artery and conus: These are enlarged, as discussed above under right ventricular enlargement. The increased amount of blood within the pulmonary and conus segments is also reflected into the hila and pulmonary artery branches. Some increase in prominence takes place within these structures. A "hila dance" is sometimes seen, but not as marked as in patent interatrial septal defect or Eisenmenger's complex.

(6) The vascular pedicle and (7) superior vena cava show no significant change.

In summary: Slight enlargement of the heart to the left, with a prominent conus and pulmonary artery segment and dilated hila markings, is characteristic of this defect.

DEXTROPOSITION OF THE HEART

The diagnosis of this condition is readily evident when the patient is viewed behind the fluoroscopic screen. The apex of the heart is directed toward the right instead of the left. The entire cardiac silhouette, as a matter of fact, is directed toward the right lung field.

CHAPTER IV

Examination of the Larynx, Pharynx, Hypopharynx and Esophagus

To BE EFFICIENT, the fluoroscopic examination of this region must also be me-
thodical. For the examiner to proceed with
assurance and alacrity he must first lay out
a predetermined plan of attack. With this
in mind, various fundamentals will be discussed first, and then the normal and pathological fluoroscopy of this region.

Fundamentals

NORMAL ANATOMY

Above the Thorax. As demonstrated in
figures 113–116, the hyoid bone is seen
immediately below the lower margin of the
mandible. The relationship between the
hyoid bone and the epiglottis, immediately
behind it, should be carefully noted. The
junction of the base of the tongue and the
epiglottis forms the vallecula.

To either side of the epiglottis and just
below the vallecula both pyriform sinuses
are found (fig. 113; cf. figs. 129 and 130).
The medial wall of each sinus is formed by
an aryepiglottic fold. The lateral wall is
formed by the thyroid cartilage below, and
above this the thyro-hyoid membrane connecting the hyoid bone to the thyroid cartilage.

During the act of deglutition the tongue
is raised against the palate; thus pressing
the bolus back into the pharynx. The soft
palate is raised, closing off the nasopharynx.

The larynx is raised and brought forward
towards the epiglottis. The voice box itself
is closed by the drawing together of the
true and false vocal cords.

Within the Thorax. The esophagus, which
starts at the level of the sixth cervical
vertebra (posterior to cricoid cartilage), descends into the thorax, and the first point
of normal constriction (as in fig. 117) is
found at the thoracic inlet. In a great number of cases the aorta is the only structure
that will leave its mark on the esophagus as
it travels through the thorax. Below the
aortic impression other normal indentures
will be enumerated. But it should be noted
carefully that in a great number of fluoroscopic examinations of the esophagus only
one impression may be seen, produced by
the aortic arch. In many instances, such an
impression is caused by a combination of
indentures produced by the aortic arch and
left bronchus. The esophagus finally reaches

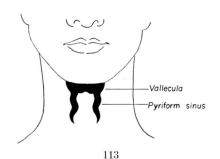

113

Barium outlining the vallecula and pyriform sinuses.

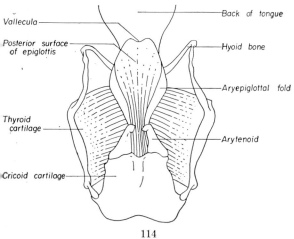

114

Normal anatomy, looking from the esophagus forward. The posterior wall of the cricoid cartilage is between the observer and the thyroid cartilage.

its spindle-shaped termination as it pierces the diaphragm to enter the stomach.

As in figures 117 and 118, other normal impressions on the esophagus are produced by the left pulmonary bronchus.[1] This impression becomes more marked when the right pulmonary artery, anterior to it, becomes dilated, thus pushing the bronchus back still more. It is possible that with pulmonary artery dilatation this latter structure itself may produce part of the impression immediately below the aorta. Below this, again, is the impression caused by the left auricle.

It would be wise to dwell for a moment on the intimate relationship between the

thoracic aorta and the esophagus. As in figure 122, the descending thoracic aorta first lies to the left of the esophagus and in this position the descending aorta normally does not cause an impression. Lower down, the descending aorta lies behind the esophagus and thus can render the esophagus broad

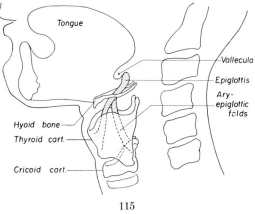

115

Normal anatomy, lateral view.

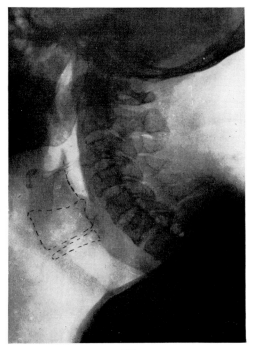

116

Normal, lateral view.

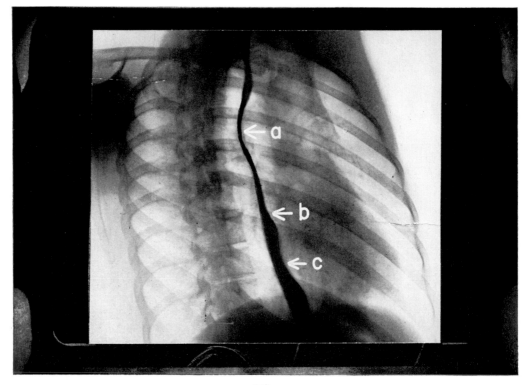

117

A. Indenture produced by the aortic arch.
B. Indenture produced by the left bronchus.
C. Indenture produced by the left auricle.

from side to side but narrow from front to back. In about its lower third and just above the diaphragm the descending aorta comes to lie to the right of and tends to compress the esophagus. This accounts for the occasional narrowing of the esophagus in this region when seen in the frontal view, and widening when seen in the right anterior oblique or lateral positions (figs. 123 and 124).

Pulsations of the Esophagus[2]

A brief review of the relationship between the esophagus and the heart and the great vessels will be helpful in understanding the esophageal pulsations. The esophagus, as has just been described, passes behind and to the right of the aortic arch, finally crossing the descending thoracic aorta anteriorly to enter into the stomach (fig. 122).

At the level of the third dorsal vertebra the aortic arch impinges on the esophagus. At the fifth dorsal vertebra the esophagus comes to lie between the upper posterior surface of the left auricle and the descending aorta, and below this it lies adjacent to the inferior posterior surface of the left auricle. Finally, as Taquine has demonstrated,[2] it comes to lie adjacent to the posterior surface of the left ventricle. These juxtapositions explain the transmission of the pulsations of each of these four portions of the circulatory system to the esophagus.

When the posterior mediastinum is narrow the various pulsations are easily transmitted. In some patients the posterior mediastinum is deeper, so that contact between the esophagus and the various pulsating structures is less close, with resultant diminution in pulsation.

In summary, it might be said that the normal esophagus pulsation varies with the level at which it is observed.

Positioning

The passage carrying the food from the mouth to the stomach is readily accessible to fluoroscopic examination.

The *pharynx and hypopharynx* are best seen fluoroscopically in anterior-posterior, postero-anterior and lateral positions (fig. 127). The first two enumerated are poor, insofar as the spine overlaps. The *esophagus* is easily seen in the right anterior oblique position (patient facing examiner and turned so that his right shoulder is closer to the examiner). The understanding of why the esophagus can be seen in this position is of prime importance. Once he understands this, the fluoroscopist not only will be able automatically to position his patient correctly but he will be able to make the necessary variations that may apply to any specific abnormalities. The burden of memorizing which position is best no longer exists.

In explanation, figures 125 and 126 should be studied. If the esophagus were to be seen with the patient rotated with the left shoulder forward (left anterior oblique position, fig. 125) the esophagus would have to travel the entire length of the heart before it would be clearly seen in its entirety without the overlapping shadow of the heart in front. On the other hand, if the patient were turned with the right shoulder towards the fluoroscopic screen, the slightest degree of obliquity would enable the esophagus to be seen without any superimposition of shadows.

When the esophageal pathology is looked for, the patient should be examined in every degree of obliquity, since lesions may be absent in one projection, yet appear consistently in another.

It is not unusual to watch the barium descend through the esophagus during a gastro-intestinal study and be lulled into a

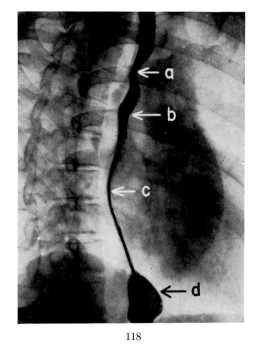

118

a—Indenture produced by the aortic arch.
b—Indenture produced by the left bronchus.
c—Indenture produced by the left auricle.
d—phrenic ampulla.

false sense of security regarding the normalcy of the esophagus. Yet, often the examiner has taken a shortcut and did not take the time to view the esophagus from every angle. Such was the case in figures 119 to 121.

Further, the esophagus can be examined in the erect, the horizontal and occasionally the Trendelenburg positions. In the latter two positions the descent of the opaque material within the esophagus is slowed and so more time is permitted for the study of the opacified esophageal contours. The slowing of the barium mixture also allows for settling out of the opaque media on the mucosa, thus bringing the various patterns and folds of the esophageal lining into relief. By using thicker barium mixtures one can slow its descent further.

Contrast Material

Fluoroscopic examination of the gastro-intestinal tract is primarily performed with

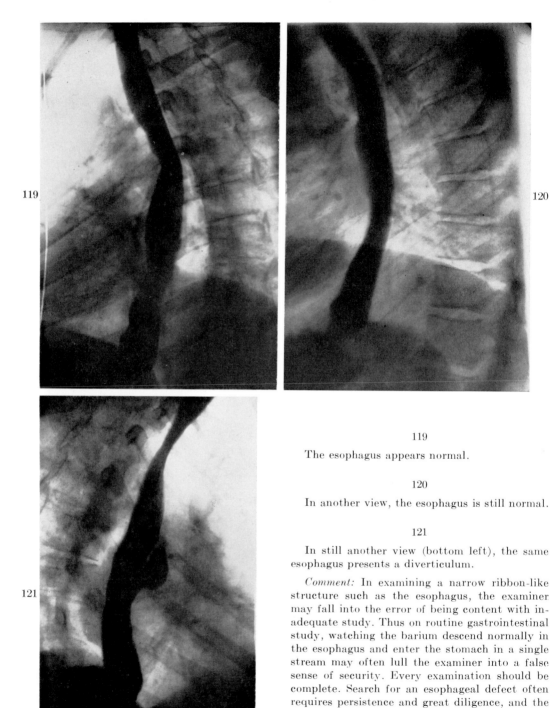

119

The esophagus appears normal.

120

In another view, the esophagus is still normal.

121

In still another view (bottom left), the same esophagus presents a diverticulum.

Comment: In examining a narrow ribbon-like structure such as the esophagus, the examiner may fall into the error of being content with inadequate study. Thus on routine gastrointestinal study, watching the barium descend normally in the esophagus and enter the stomach in a single stream may often lull the examiner into a false sense of security. Every examination should be complete. Search for an esophageal defect often requires persistence and great diligence, and the patient should be examined in all positions.

contrast material. Direct examination, i.e., without opaque material may on occasion be useful, and will be described presently.

A barium mixture is most commonly used for opaque contrast studies. These mixtures have been used flavored and unflavored.

Three concentrations of barium mixture are useful:

Thin: 1 Heaping tbsp. of barium to a glassful of water. The consistency is thin and watery.
Medium: 2 Heaping tbsp. of barium to a glassful of water.
Thick: 7 Heaping tbsp. of barium to a glassful of water. The consistency is thick and should barely run off the spoon. (Acacia may be added to achieve this end.)

The examiner should be careful in determining which mixture to use. The thicker mixtures are more advantageous when esophageal pathology is suspected, since their slower descent allows more time for detailed and careful observation. If a lesion which only partially obstructs the esophagus is so examined, the obstruction may be rendered complete by trapping some of the

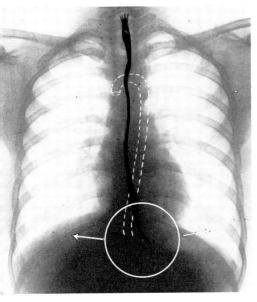

122

The lower third of the esophagus lies parallel and to the left of the aorta. In the frontal position, *since it is adjacent to the aorta it is compressed from side to side. It thus appears narrow.* But when seen from the side, i.e., right anterior oblique, the esophagus appears broader.

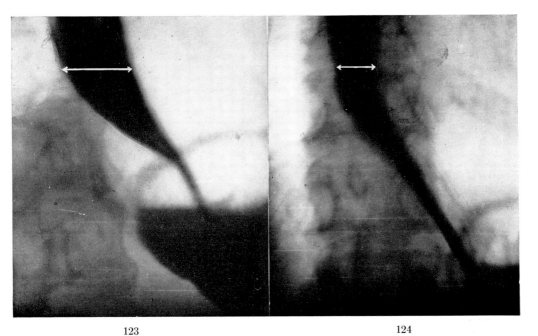

123

Lower third of esophagus appears broader in the right anterior oblique position.

124

Frontal position. The esophagus appears narrower.

mixture in the lumen. It would be wise to start with a thin mixture when such a lesion is suspected. If this passes freely the thicker mixture can then be used. A tablespoon of the latter is often sufficient.

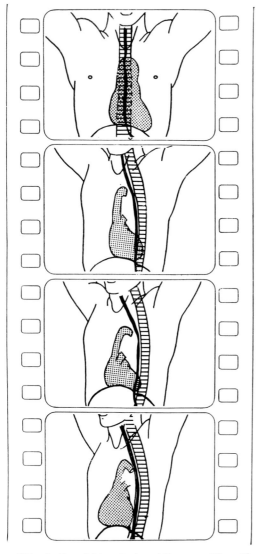

Why is the right anterior oblique position (fig. 126) superior to the left anterior oblique position (fig. 125), in the examination of the esophagus?

125

Left anterior oblique: No matter how far the patient is rotated, the heart shadow (especially the apical portion) tends to overlie the esophagus, thus not permitting adequate esophageal examination. (With extreme degree of rotation the esophagus is free of the heart.)

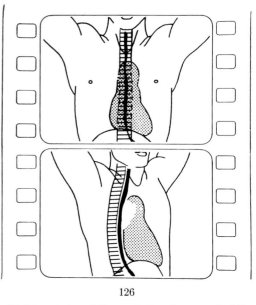

126

Right anterior oblique: A few degrees of obliquity in this position permit the esophagus to clear the cardiac shadow with no difficulty.

(*Note:* Both positions are valuable in rotating the spine free of the esophagus, although the right anterior oblique position accomplishes this with somewhat greater ease.)

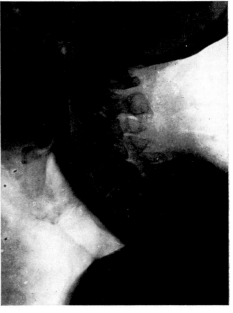

127

Barium mixture travels with great speed through the pharynx and hypo-pharynx. Note the indenture into the column produced by the epiglottis.

The thick mixture may best be given from a spoon. The patient is asked to hold the mixture in his mouth, and then, when the observer is ready to watch the barium descend, the patient is told to swallow. When thinner mixtures are administered while the patient is lying down, a glass drinking tube is used.

Halogenated oils (lipiodol) may be substituted for barium. This is done when a history is secured of violent coughing attacks associated with attempts to swallow food or liquids. Such coughing attacks may be due to the regurgitation of food or liquid particles into the trachea. When oil is substituted for the barium, it is harmless when aspirated instead of swallowed.

Barium capsules are occasionally useful to demonstrate the presence of a foreign body, such as a lump of meat, and so forth. The capsule will descend and stop at the level of obstruction.

NORMAL FLUOROSCOPIC EXAMINATION

The patient should be examined in the morning, and he must be instructed not to eat anything for eight hours prior to the examination.

The fluoroscopist, in his examination of the pharynx, hypopharynx and esophagus, should follow a definite pattern.

(1) General examination.

(2) Special examination of the pharynx, hypopharynx and esophagus. This consists, first, of a direct examination *without contrast material;* and second, an examination where *contrast material* is employed. In the *contrast* type of examination, contour, descent and position are observed.

GENERAL EXAMINATION

The patient is placed behind the fluoroscopic screen in the frontal position. The chest is first examined with the shutters wide open. The illumination of both lung fields is noted. Search is made for any abnormal shadows within the chest. The shut-

ters are next narrowed down and section after section of the chest is examined, one side compared with the other. The diaphragmatic cusps are visualized and their freedom of mobility determined. It would be wise now to move the screen downwards and study the abdomen *generally* for any opaque shadows as well as for undue air distention. This, when it becomes habit, is not a prolonged procedure.

SPECIAL EXAMINATION

Direct Examination: Without Contrast Material

The patient, standing, is turned to the right anterior oblique position (patient facing the examiner and the right shoulder brought forward) and the space behind the heart is first examined directly without contrast material. The optimum rotation is that in which the clear space representing posterior mediastinum is best seen between the cardiac shadow in front and the spine behind. Fluid levels are looked for. Any abnormal opaque shadows are noted.

The screen is next carried down and *the stomach air bubble is carefully scrutinized for any abnormal encroachment.* Absence of the air bubble should suggest either recent gas eructation or some esophageal obstruction not permitting air entry from above.

Contrast Material Employed

Due note being made of any findings, the examiner is now ready for the most important part of the examination—administration of opaque media. The patient, with the glass of barium mixture in his left hand, is asked to swallow one mouthful at a time; the opaque bolus is observed. The optimum time to observe the entrance of barium into the stomach is with the first few swallows. The entrance into the air bubble of the stomach should be carefully observed and is described in the section dealing with stomach. Acquaintance with this entry, by means of repeated study, is extremely important. Many carcinomas of

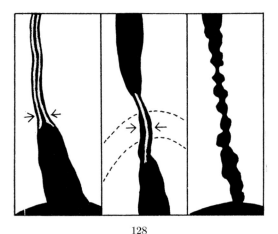

128

(*Left*) Primary peristalis
(*Middle*) Secondary peristalis
(*Right*) Tertiary peristalis

the fundus of the stomach, as well as para-esophageal hernias may be perceived only after the normal entrance of the barium into the stomach is understood and recognized (figs. 123 and 124).

At this point it should be clearly understood and emphasized that if the examiner's attention is consciously directed toward contour, descent and position, the examination will be fluoroscopically complete.

Contour. Within the pharynx the descent of barium is at such a tremendous speed that only a momentary normal pattern will be seen. The first fluoroscopic image (fig. 127) discerned as the barium enters the pharynx is an opaque bolus situated posteriorly, behind the tongue and within the oral pharynx. A tongue-like projection of the barium, although evanescent, will be seen projecting into the vallecula. As the observer watches this, he will also see the hyoid bone and larynx being raised during the act of deglutition.

From the pharynx and hypopharynx the barium quickly enters and outlines the esophagus, starting at the level of the sixth cervical vertebra. The examiner, by studying figures 117 and 118 in conjunction with the anatomical description already given,

is now well prepared to understand and recognize the various normal esophageal contours.

Barium Descent. (a) Mechanism.[4] The peristaltic action of the esophagus, although present, is not readily seen unless understood and sought for. The barium descends to the level of the diaphragm, where it remains momentarily. The cardiac sphincter soon opens and the opaque material passes into the stomach.

Three types of peristaltic activity (fig. 128) can be noted within the esophagus:

1. Primary peristalsis. Primary waves originate with the pharangeal contraction. It is seen in the esophagus as a wave-like constriction travelling downwards. The esophagus immediately in front of the wave is dilated. The esophagus behind, since it is relatively emptied, is narrowed. Training oneself to see this wave is important. As the wave descends, the examiner by observing a portion of the esophagus dilated (the portion immediately in front of the wave)— and next this same portion contracted (as the wave passes through it)—has an immediate and rapid clue helping him to prove the normalcy of the portions so examined.

2. Secondary peristalsis. Secondary peristaltic waves are attributed to local mechanical stimulation. They also occur with obstructive lesions. They are muscular contractions arising often in the mid-esophagus or in the region of the aortic arch. The wave travels both up and down the esophagus. As with primary peristalsis, observation of the dilation and constriction is valuable.

3. Tertiary peristalsis. This is more often referred to as tertiary contractions, or the "corkscrew" esophagus. It is usually only a momentary occurrence and disappears rapidly. It is not a common configuration, and the exact significance is not understood. No definite pathological entity has been described as being responsible for this pattern although esophagitis and esophageal irritability have been associated with it.

Normal descent. In upright position the most important propelling force is gravity. As the barium descends lower, or when the patient is in the horizontal or Trendelenburg positions, the primary peristaltic wave becomes important. This wave is better seen with thick mixtures. When these are swallowed the opaque material will descend to a certain point and pause. The points of temporary holdup may be at the normal esophageal constrictions, i.e., aortic level. In the region of the holdup, a narrowing or peristaltic "wave" takes place above the bolus and progresses downward following the food. Generally this narrowing is not very marked and causes no segmentation of the barium column.

Obstructive descent. When obstruction to the barium descent is present an exaggeration of the above phenomenon takes place. The barium mixture descends to the point of obstruction and stops. The esophagus above becomes dilated. Powerful peristaltic waves can next be seen attempting to push the barium through the constricted segment. A large portion of the barium mixture escapes backwards through the oncoming peristaltic ring.

(b) The descent. The fluoroscopist must understand that the descent through the pharynx and hypopharynx is so very rapid that inadequate studies are usually performed here. Because of this speed of descent even roentgenograms of this region are often unsatisfactory.

The further progress of the barium, although slower, is still rapid, and, as it descends through the esophagus, it is momentarily held up at the lower end. This holdup does not occur directly at the cardiac sphincter, but a little above, i.e. at the region where the diaphragm itself acts as a sphincter. It is normal in some individuals for a delay of several seconds to occur at this place. As the esophagus enters the stomach, it is bent backwards and to the left. This bend may vary in different indi-

viduals from an almost straight line to a marked angle. This angle is exaggerated especially when an obstruction is present at the cardiac orifice and the esophagus above is dilated (fig. 286A,B, page 214).

The entry of the barium into the stomach after the holdup in the lower esophagus is almost immediate and in a smooth single stream. This holdup and entry is noteworthy. It is important for the examiner to become thoroughly familiar with it. There is no associated esophageal dilatation. There is no retention of any significant amount of opaque media at the foot or lower end of the esophagus.

Some special procedures useful in slowing the descent in the pharynx and hypopharynx, that may be useful as well in the esophagus, are:

1. Use thick mixtures where possible.

2. Perform the examination in the prone and Trendelenburg position in addition to the erect position.

3. Valsalva maneuver[3]: after a swallow of opaque mixture the patient is asked to take a deep breath and then immediately thereafter to exhale, keeping the mouth closed and the nose pinched. This maneuver distends the pharynx with air, sharpening the contrast of the barium mixture as it lies within the various crevices. Actually, this is an attempt to achieve double contrast studies of this region.

Position. The examiner, through constant repetition, must acquaint himself with the normal position of the esophagus behind the heart, coursing downwards in a more or less straight line (fig. 77). Variations in its normal path can be caused by various mediastinal lesions such as growths, adhesions between it and an arteriosclerotic aorta (fig. 96), aneurysm, enlarged left auricle, mediastinal glands, etc. These are described elsewhere. Displacement of the esophagus may prove an important clue in the diagnosis of intrathoracic conditions. Growths in the upper thorax, when producing esophageal displacements, may cause pressure symptoms, but in the lower esophagus gross displacement may be present with no symptoms.[4a]

NORMAL VARIATIONS

Phrenic Ampulla. As the esophagus passes through the hiatus in the diaphragm it becomes spindle-shaped, being constricted by the hiatus. Immediately above this spindle-like constriction a dilatation (figs. 117 and 118) will be noted. This dilatation has been referred to as the "phrenic ampulla." The examiner may help in the formation of this normal dilatation by observing the descent of the barium, and just as the opaque media is about to pass through the esophageal opening in the diaphragm the patient is asked to take a deep breath and then press out against a closed glottis (Valsalva maneuver). As the diaphragm descends, it seems as though a sphincteric action takes place and pinches off the esophagus. The

barium collecting above this constriction forms a pouch-like distension known as the "phrenic ampulla."

This ampulla must be differentiated from hiatus hernia and epiphrenic diverticulum.

Vallecula Sign. The anatomy and normal configuration of the vallecula and pyriform sinuses has already been described. Normally, when the barium bolus is observed descending through the pharynx, the various structures can be distinguished (figs. 113–116, 127). Commonly, the barium clinging to the crevices of the vallecula and two pyriform sinuses will maintain its position for a few moments and is soon washed away. When thicker mixtures are used the temporary delay within these structures is maintained for a longer interval but nevertheless it is soon washed away also.

This must be carefully distinguished from the "vallecula sign" obtained when the barium mixture remains in the vallecula and both pyriform sinuses for an abnor-

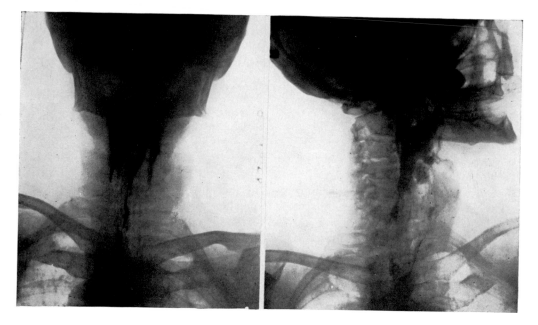

129   130

Barium, when *retained* for a prolonged period of time in the vallecula or pyriform sinuses, should be considered abnormal till proved otherwise (vallecula sign).

mally long period of time (figs. 129 and 130). Again repetition and acquaintance with the normal is requisite to the understanding of the abnormal. The presence of this sign should lead the fluoroscopist to suspect a holdup of some type in the esophagus or pharynx.

This holdup of food or barium may either be caused by organic lesions, such as carcinoma, or on the other hand may have a neurogenic etiology. This is an important sign in myasthenia gravis and various other nervous disorders. In association with the neurogenic type of obstruction, when the vallecula sign exists, fluoroscopically, in the lateral examination of the neck, the examiner will note an inability to raise the hyoid bone or larynx with deglutition.

Pathological Examination

PRELIMINARY CONSIDERATIONS

It is not within the scope of a text of this character to undertake a discussion of the various esophageal abnormalities as demonstrated on the roentgenogram. Those lesions which are of importance and require fluoroscopy for their better understanding will be described. Emphasis will be placed on those abnormalities in which the fluoroscopic study plays an important part.

When fluoroscopic procedures are used, the examiner must bear in mind that all his findings must be proved. It is not sufficient to describe an image on the screen. A radiographic film confirming his findings must follow. Perhaps the only purpose for fluoroscopy is to search for and to discover some pathological deviation. The examiner then makes note in which position the lesion is best demonstrated. For this it is wise to use a skin pencil and mark directly on the skin exactly where the suspicious shadow is best seen. This should be done in the darkened room, behind the fluoroscopic screen. The light is next turned on and the obliquity of the patient in relationship to the fluoroscopic screen noted. This knowledge is then applied in the subsequent taking of radiographic films, bearing in mind that in relationship to the patient the x-ray film must be placed in the same position as the fluoroscopic screen. If the examiner is fortunate enough to have adequate spot filming equipment the entire procedure is simplified.

FLUOROSCOPIC PROCEDURE

GENERAL SURVEY

The actual procedure in fluoroscopy of this region has already been detailed. It consists first of a general survey of the chest, mediastinal shadows, diaphragm and abdomen, and, second, of a special examination, with and without contrast material.

Direct Examination before Contrast Material

The same pattern is followed as outlined for normal fluoroscopy of the esophagus.

In the special examination, to begin with, the air bubble within the stomach is first scrutinized. Its absence is significant and if the patient has not recently eructated some gas, a pathological lesion above, causing obstruction, must be suspected. The patient is next rotated. The space behind the heart is examined for abnormal opacities or fluid levels. A fluid level recognized and proved may be significant in leading to a diagnosis of diverticulum or cardiospasm, etc. The recognition and proof of the existence of such a fluid level is demonstrated (figs. 135–137). This method of tilting the patient and observing the fluid level not changing its slope can be applied to the fluoroscopic recognition and proof of fluid levels in any other part of the body. The most common cause of a fluid level within the esophagus is cardiospasm.

Examination with Contrast Material

Special examination of the esophagus with barium mixture is next performed. The optimum position of the patient is usually prone with the left shoulder closer to the screen (left posterior oblique) (fig. 203). Supine and erect positions in various degrees of obliquity may also be necessary.

For a complete examination of the esophagus the examiner must constantly ask himself three questions:

(a) Are the esophageal *contours* normal?

(b) As the barium mixture leaves the mouth and *descends* through the pharynx, hypopharynx and esophagus is the descent normal? Are there any holdups? He must be ever watchful for the "vallecula sign." On occasion, a spill-over into the trachea may be noted.

(c) Is the barium mixture travelling from the mouth to the stomach passing through channels which are in their normal *positions*?

Contour. As the opaque media descends through the pharynx, hypopharynx and esophagus the normal curves and impressions must be looked for and identified. The patient should be observed while being rotated in various obliquities. No indenture or out-pouching must go unexplained (fig. 131–134).

As the first mouthfuls of opaque media descend through the esophagus, the patient in the erect position, the *distensibility* of the lumen and smoothness of its margins are appraised. The lumen, normally collapsed, is opened as the opaque bolus travels through it. It becomes narrowed and collapses again as the bolus passes. It is the visualization of this *dilatation and collapse* which helps indicate the normalcy of the lumen. As the bolus canalizes each portion of the esophagus, the lumen becomes dilated. The degree

of dilatation should be *commensurate with that of the segment immediately above and below*. Any segment which does not attain the width of the preceding segment can be considered *narrowed*. Narrowing of this variety is abnormal. The tapering of the esophagus at its distal end, however, must be kept in mind.

As a general rule esophageal dilatation when present and secondary to an obstructive lesion is greater the lower down the lesion exists. It is only a little widened when obstruction is high up (fig. 145). Dilatation will usually be more marked with benign conditions (fig. 143).

So, too, any abnormal narrowing must be observed and noted. Attention must be focused on the region where the normal changes to the abnormal (fig. 145). The margins of a constricting lesion separating it from the normal portion of the esophagus are often helpful in distinguishing one pathological entity from another. Is the change from the normal to the abnormal abrupt or does one fade imperceptibly into the other? Abrupt transitions should arouse suspicions of malignancy.

The observation of the region of "change" of contour is important. It is the main purpose of the fluoroscopist to discover in which position the thing he looks for is demonstrated best and next to use this position in the taking of films.

Barium Descent. Primary and secondary peristalsis has already been described. For practical purposes, as the opaque media descends it is important to note any abnormal holdups, either partial or complete. The first holdup normally should occur at the point where the esophagus is about to pass through the diaphragm. The formation at this site of the phrenic ampulla has already been described. If the descent of the barium mixture is halted at any point other than at its lower end, note must be made and explanation sought.

The type of mixture used should also be considered when the screen findings are

131–134

These studies are all of the same patient, done at various degrees of filling and emptying, during which process varying irregularities in shape can normally be expected.

Question:

Is this esophagus normal?

Answer:

The diagnosis in this case was missed. The purpose of these films is to demonstrate that an apparently insignificant abnormal configuration seen in a given position can be dismissed only if the configuration is *certain to disappear* in the *same* position. However, if that abnormal configuration is present on *two* separate studies in the *same* position, it must not be dismissed as coincidental.

The steplike irregularity on the lower left margin of the esophagus seen in figures 133 and 134 appears in two films in the *same* position (see relative position of spine, and refer to figures 197–198). When these studies were pursued with esophagoscopy, an esophageal neoplasm was found responsible.

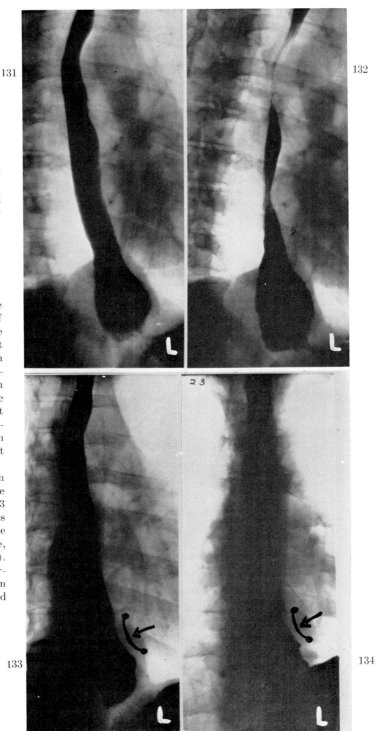

131

132

133

134

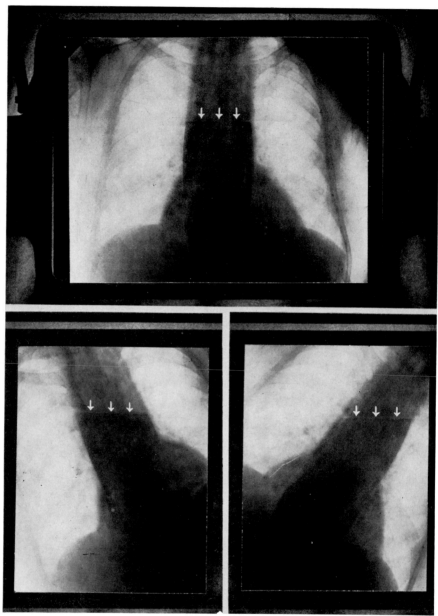

135

Proof of fluid level. Suspicious fluid level (arrows) seen in mediastinum. Proof of fluid requires tilting the patient.

136

Patient tilted to right. Only fluid would maintain its level and remain parallel to floor.

137

Patient tilted to the left. Again fluid maintains its level and remains parallel to the floor.

evaluated. Thin mixtures descend more rapidly and thick mixtures are occasionally held up—momentarily at least—in regions other than the lower end of the esophagus.

Should the examiner repeatedly fail to detect a holdup by the conventional barium swallow, Barclay[4a] recommends that the patient be fed a barium mixture containing the type of food that ordinarily induces his symptoms.

The use of a compressed barium pill[28]—the Wolf barium pill, measuring 12.5 mm. in diameter and 3 mm. thick—has also proved valuable in finding an obstructive site. The pill is flattened from side to side to permit ease in swallowing. Ater swallowing it will be halted by any obstructive mechanism. Difficulty may be encountered in elderly patients, in whom the pill may be delayed in the lower esophagus at the level of a dilated descending aorta.[25]

Reflux or regurgitation of barium is often a normal phenomenon in the lower end of the esophagus. It occurs at the momentary holdup just prior to the entry of the opaque material into the stomach. Regurgitation and reflux can, however, occur with obstructive lesions and are usually more marked the higher the lesion is located.

A normal to-and-fro motion of barium in the esophagus occasionally occurs. This is most often seen in the supine or prone positions. A condition described as *elevator esophagus* is described, which simulates this to-and-fro motion with the patient upright or in a semi-upright position. The etiology of "elevator esophagus" is believed to lie in a physiologic dysfunction.[21] A lesion in or near the lower esophagus may be the trigger mechanism which disturbs the normal neuromuscular function.[22] With this condition, a swallow of barium remains in the esophagus for a few minutes, next rises intermittently from the lower esophagus to the level of the aortic arch, and then falls back again. Occassionally it may even arise to the hypopharynx. This abnormal mobility is more likely to be seen following each of the first

few swallows and may not recur until the esophagus has been relatively inactive for some time. In cardiospasm, which may also show a to-and-fro motion, the activity is more sluggish than in "elevator esophagus." When the examiner sees this abnormal activity on the fluoroscopic screen he should suspect the possibility of an organic lesion in or near the lower esophagus or adjacent portions of the stomach.

Position (fig. 77). The position of the normal esophagus starting at C6 and coursing its way downward behind the heart must be borne in mind. Any deviations must be explained. It is interesting to note the difference (already mentioned under normal position) in descent of the normal esophagus in the presence of a normal aorta as compared to the normal esophagus in the presence of an arteriosclerotic uncoiled aorta (fig. 96).

PATHOLOGY WITHIN THE PHARYNX

The act of deglutition is usually difficult in the presence of obstructive lesions in this site. Barium mixture is often regurgitated and the "vallecula sign" is a prominent feature. After the opaque material passes the lesion, its descent within the esophagus is normal.

Diverticulum. A diverticulum within the pharynx is usually pulsion in type, i.e., due to increased pressure within the pharyngeal lumen.[5, 6]

Zenker's diverticulum is a herniation of the posterior pharyngeal mucosa through the midline of the posterior wall of the pharynx. The gap in this wall occurs just above the origin of the esophagus.

Contour: In the lateral or oblique positions as the barium mixture descends it is seen passing into a pouch-like space (fig. 138). When the pouch becomes filled the barium spills over into the esophagus. Frequently, the opaque media will pour into the pouch and esophagus simultaneously.

Holdup: A pool of barium surmounted

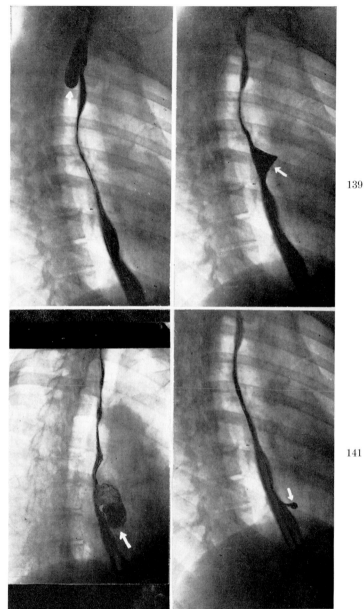

138

Zenker diverticulum, *a pulsion type diverticulum*, due to increased intraluminal pressure. It is usually situated *posteriorly*.

140

A pulsion-traction diverticulum results from increased pressure within a traction diverticulum. It too is usually situated *anteriorly*.

139

A *traction diverticulum* due to esophageal adhesions to tracheal and subaortic lymph nodes. It is usually situated *anteriorly* and is peaked in shape.

141

Epiphrenic diverticulum, a small grape-like herniation situated above the diaphragm.

by an air pocket may remain behind in the diverticulum.

Position: In the frontal position the barium column as it descends within the esophagus may be so distorted as to appear to travel to either side of the diverticulum instead of directly down in the midline.

Carcinoma. When carcinoma is discussed within this region, only post-cricoid carcinoma need be considered.

Contour: After a swallow of the barium mixture, the passage through the pharynx is so rapid that little can be seen except the absence of a smooth entry into the esophagus. Here, as elsewhere, acquaintance with the normal is of paramount importance. Regurgitation of the opaque mixture is common. Examination after the passage of the barium mixture will reveal fragments of barium entangled within the crevices of the growth. With a growth of sufficient extent, invasion of the pyriform sinuses on one or both sides may take place. In the frontal examination of the patient as the barium courses down from the mouth, the invaded space will not be visible; i.e., a persistent failure to see a pyriform space should make the fluoroscopist suspicious of an abnormality within it.

Holdup: Some holdup of the barium column occurs, the degree depending upon the size of the lesion.

Position: Some deviation of the barium column is noted. This varies with the position of the growth.

Plummer-Vinson Syndrome. Dysphagia here is probably due to spasm of the cricopharyngeal sphincter. The diagnosis is made by excluding an organic lesion and demonstrating a characteristic hematological picture. Fluoroscopically the only abnormality the examiner may see will be the "vallecula sign." The examiner may also see a smooth stricture at the level of the sixth or seventh cervical vertebra.[7]

PATHOLOGY WITHIN THE ESOPHAGUS

Congenital Atresia. From the fluoroscopic point of view, only two types need to be considered. (a) In the presence of atresia in the proximal esophagus no communication exists between the distal portion of the esophagus and respiratory passages (i.e., trachea and bronchus). A definite roentgen and fluoroscopic change is seen in this type in that the stomach air bubble is absent—since air has no way of entering from above. (b) In the presence of atresia a communication does exist between the respiratory passages and the distal esophagus.[8, 9, 10] In this type when the fundus of the stomach is examined, the normal "air bubble" will be found (fig. 142).

When esophageal atresia is suspected, Lipiodol, Diodrast, or Neoiopax should be used instead of the barium mixture, since regurgitation with a spill-over into the lungs may occur.

Contour: The barium mixture as it descends becomes arrested at the point of stricture. The portion of esophagus above become dilated (fig. 142).

Holdup: A holdup of the barium occurs at the point of stricture.

Diverticulum of the Esophagus (figs. 138–141). For practical purposes four types are described: (a) *Pulsion.* Occurring mainly on posterior wall (Zenkers). This type of diverticulum supposedly results from increased intraluminal pressure with resultant herniation of the esophageal mucosa through the posterior esophageal wall. (b) *Traction.*[11] Occurring mainly on the anterior wall, usually at the level of bifurcation of trachea or below the aortic arch, this type of diverticulum is generally triangular or tent shaped and as a rule results from adhesion of the esophagus to healed inflamed mediastinal lymph nodes. (c) *Pulsion-traction diverticula.* This is a combination of the two types above. It usually starts

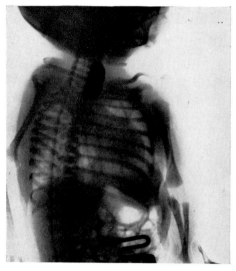

142

Question:

Child given some opaque media to swallow and the esophageal column was found to terminate abruptly in upper chest. Is there an air connection between the respiratory passages and gastrointestinal tract?

Fluoroscopic examination:

Air is seen in stomach and other loops of bowel.

Answer:

Since air from the mouth cannot enter the stomach (abrupt termination of the esophagus), it must be assumed that a fistulous connection exists between the respiratory passages and the gastrointestinal tract.

as a result of anterior adhesions. Secondary pressure of the food within the esophagus causes the diverticulum soon to balloon out and assume the roundness and sac-like contour of the pulsion type of diverticulum. (d) *Epiphrenic deverticulum* (fig. 141).

Contour: The pulsion type diverticulum (Zenkers) has already been described. The traction and pulsion-traction varieties are also visualized as out-pouchings from the normal esophageal walls. It is essential when examining for this abnormality to remember that when small it may not be detected in the erect position. Also, the patient should be turned through every degree

of obliquity, since a diverticulum not visualized at one angle may visualize at another.

Holdup: Barium may be held up in the sac.

Position: The opacified column as it courses downwards usually runs in its normal position. Its only deviation is that due to some slight displacement caused by the diverticulum itself.

Esophagospasm.[23] Spasm of the lower esophagus may occur during emotional stress. This occurs especially while eating. Symptoms include dysphagia and substernal discomfort. The pain may simulate a heart attack and a differential diagnosis must be made. Dysphagia associated with esophagospasm is an important sign-symptom complex.

Contour: This condition is not associated with any real esophageal dilatation. Fluoroscopic and radiologic examination may reveal nothing unless the patient is upset during the time of the examination. Emotional disturbance may produce a spasm or narrowing of the lower esophagus.

Holdup: The esophagus may appear normal. When the condition appears, the spasm in the lower esophagus will cause some holdup of the barium column.

Position: Unchanged.

Benign Stricture of Esophagus. Simple stricture of the esophagus usually represents the healed phase of an active ulceration following the ingestion of corrosives. These scars usually occur at the sites where the esophagus normally is narrower.

Contour: With healing of a corrosive ulcer, scar tissue develops. The change in contour when due to such abnormality is tapering, imperceptible and smooth. This is to be distinguished from the abruptness of the contour change (i.e., normal to abnormal) as found in malignancy (fig. 145). The esophagus above the narrowed segment becomes dilated.

Holdup: As the barium descends, some delay is encountered which may be partial or complete.

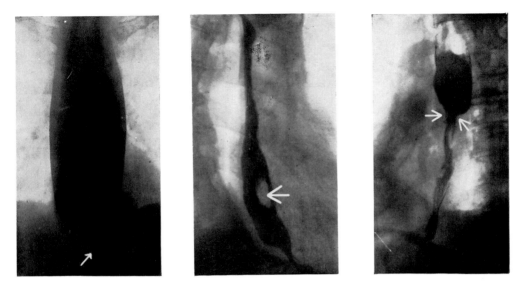

Differential diagnosis of esophageal pathology.

143	144	145
Cardiospasm	Benign neoplasm	Malignant neoplasm
1. Holdup a prominent sign.	1. Holdup of barium descent may be present, depending on the degree of obstruction.	1. Holdup is a prominent sign, but not as marked as in cardiospasm.
2. Esophagus is widely dilated.	2. Esophagus is not unduly dilated.	2. Esophagus shows some dilatation.
3. *The cardiac end of the esophagus (arrow) is sharp, tapering, and smooth.*	3. *The defect in the esophagus is smooth, round, and centrally located (arrow).*	3. *The esophageal contour changes abruptly from normal to abnormal (arrows).*
4. Amyl nitrite inhalation may open the sphincter and permit barium descent.	4. Amyl nitrite inhalation has no effect on barium holdup.	4. Amyl nitrite inhalation has no effect on barium holdup.

Cardiospasm. The multiplicity of terms describing this illness indicates the lack of uniformity of thought regarding its etiology and pathology. It is a syndrome associated with non-organic obstruction at the lower end of the esophagus and associated with marked dilatation above.

Contour: On the fluoroscopic screen during a routine chest examination, the widely dilated esophagus *may* cause a bulging of the mediastinum, mainly to the right, so that to the observer, a variety of mediastinal lesions are suggested. If the condition has not progressed to this stage of dilatation, no evidence will be seen in the routine examination unless a fluid level existed, and this would very often be missed unless specifically sought for.

The observation of a fluid level and proof thereof (figs. 135–137) are very important factors leading to a correct diagnosis. It bears repetition that *unless specifically sought as part of a routine this fluid level may be missed.*

When opaque mixture is given, the esophagus exhibits varying degrees of dilatation. Early in the disease it may be minimal, but with a long history of dysphagia dilatation may reach wide proportions (fig. 143). A marked lengthening with resulting coiling of the esophagus is present.

The peristaltic waves are generally weak and dysrhythmic. They are ineffective in propelling the barium forward. Tertiary contrations may be seen. Primary and secondary peristaltic waves are generally absent.[27]

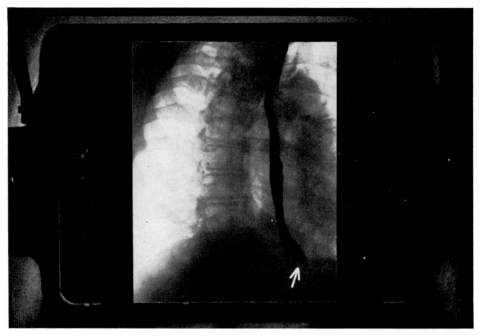

146

Cauliflower type of malignancy.

1. Holdup of barium descent.
2. Esophagus shows some dilatation.

3. *Area of invasion (arrow) is ragged.*
4. Amyl nitrite has no effect on Ba holdup.

Yet peristalsis has been described as more active in this abnormality than in any other esophageal disease.[12]

The terminal end of the esophagus is smooth and tapering vs. the raggedness of a malignancy (fig. 145). It is generally 1–3 cm. in length, most often situated below the diaphragm, presents a normal mucosa and is capable of slight changes in caliber as barium spurts through into the cardia.

Holdup: Holdup of the barium descent is always present. It varies from a temporary holdup in some cases to a marked holdup with persistent residue in others. With the patient recumbent, the opaque media may either not enter the stomach or enter only with difficulty. In the erect position, it seems as though the barium collects as in a column and when it reaches a sufficient height—generally up to the aortic arch—the weight of it appears to force the opaque media through into the stomach. Cardio-

spasm can be differentiated from carcinoma of the cardiac end of the esophagus by giving amyl nitrite inhalation. With cardiospasm, especially in early cases,[24] some relaxation may then occur and barium will pass into the stomach; with carcinoma, the cardia will not relax.

The mecholyl test will also be positive in cardiospasm. After the intramuscular injection of 1–10 mg. of mecholyl, tonic contractions will occur in the esophagus with cardiospasm. The response may include obliteration of the lumen and substernal pain.[25] The contrast material may not necessarily enter the stomach, but may be propelled backward toward the mouth.

Retention of food and barium in the esophagus is common, especially in advanced cases. Occasionally, the retained food in the esophagus may be mistaken for filling defects in the barium column and simulate a tumor. This should be borne in mind and suitable esophageal aspiration and cleansing procedures be adopted when there is a possibility that such a source of confusion may be encountered.

Position: The change in position is that due to the distortion and coiling of a lengthened esophagus.

Cardio-esophageal Relaxation.[12a] A persistent relaxation of the lower end of the esophagus is a significant, although infrequent, cause of vomiting in the newborn or young infant. The clinical picture of a persistent regurgitation or vomiting, relieved when the patient is placed in the erect position, suggests the diagnosis. Fluoroscopic examination is important in accurate determination of this condition.

Contour: Unchanged.

Holdup: Barium will be seen to descend into the stomach and next to regurgitate back up into the esophagus. This regurgitation is no more marked when the intratracheal pressure is increased, nor with deep inspiration.

Position: Unchanged.

Peptic Ulcer of the Esophagus. This abnormality of the esophagus is not commonly found. The diagnosis is made by finding an ulcer crater. The incisura when present is on the opposite wall. Hiatus hernia of the stomach may be an accompaniment. Peptic esophagitis may be present and is evidenced by a narrowing of the lower esophagus.

Contour: As the barium column descends, a little out-pouching with retention of the opaque media within it may be seen on the fluoroscopic screen.[13, 14] As the barium leaves the esophagus the black speck retained within the crater is characteristic. The esophagus in the region of the ulceration may be narrowed by secondary esophagitis or spasm (fig. 147*B*).

Holdup: There is usually no holdup in the descent of the opaque mixture except the retention within the crater. When secondary spasm is present the holdup is only temporary—if present at all. A scar sometimes forms as a result of the ulcer healing. Should the esophagus become narrowed at this point the holdup of the barium column will depend entirely on the degree of stricture.

Benign Neoplasm of the Esophagus. A benign neoplasm (fig. 144) usually produces a smooth, rounded, centrally located translucent area within the esophagus. Diagnosis is often complicated by the fact that some malignant neoplasm (sarcomas of various types) simulate this closely.[15, 16] However, a well circumscribed, translucent lesion within the lumen of the esophagus is most often benign.

Contour: When the tumor is within the lumen of the esophagus, the esophageal contours may be unchanged. Considerable dilatation of the esophagus may be present when the tumor is situated low down in the esophagus.[17]

As the opaque material passes down the esophagus and reaches the neoplasm, a splitting of the stream may be seen. It is important to note that when the tumor is small a thick barium mixture may cover over and obscure the lesion. It is therefore advisable in such cases to use a thin watery suspension.

The filling defect as seen on the fluoroscopic screen may on occasion be freely movable. This would indicate a long pedicle.

Holdup: The amount of holdup will depend entirely upon the degree of obstruction offered by the tumor.

Position: Normal.

Differential Diagnosis: A translucent area seen within the opaque mixture may be due to a trapped bubble of air. This should offer no difficulty since it is inconstant in character and not demonstrated on future examinations. Further, the swallowed air is not localized and may be noted passing through the entire course of the esophagus.

Differentiation between a benign and malignant growth should await film study where the mucosal pattern and various defects within the wall of the esophagus can better be seen.

Malignant Lesions of the Esophagus. Two important types of carcinoma found within the esophagus are:

(a) A scirrhous carcinoma which starts within the submucosa. It gradually encroaches upon the lumen and produces an angular stenosis and at still a later date the mucosa may break down and ulcerate (fig. 145).

(b) The cauliflower growth encroaches on the lumen of the esophagus and is expansive. Stenosis is produced by actual occlusion of the lumen itself (fig. 146).

Contour: The esophagus is dilated above the point of obstruction. The amount of dilatation is not usually as great as with a benign lesion such as cardiospasm. The esophageal wall is usually smooth until the actual abnormality is reached. At this point a sudden and *abrupt* change occurs. The contour becomes ragged or indented and, on occasion, irregular filling defects are seen within the esophageal lumen.

The irregularity in contour, as described, is dependent on the contour of the upper part of the growth. In the scirrhous type of neoplasm it is smoother; in the cauliflower type it is more ragged and irregular.

The most characteristic features of malignant neoplasms are their irregularity, and the constancy of such irregularities.

Holdup: As the opaque mixture passes down through the esophagus the degree of holdup depends upon the size of the growth and the occlusion of the lumen. After the opaque mixture passes, some barium may be *retained within the crevices* of the growth and *so outline the irregularity* in greater detail. Peristalsis through the invaded region is absent.

Fistula. A fistula between the esophagus and the respiratory passage can often be outlined and seen on the fluoroscopic screen. This is caused by carcinomatous connection into any of the neighboring structures, i.e.,

the trachea or bronchi. On occasion, opaque material has been seen passing into and outlining the various bronchi within the lungs. Careful fluoroscopic observation will often demonstrate that the barium did not enter *via* a fistulous tract, but instead regurgitated through the larynx.

Scleroderma of Esophagus. Scleroderma may cause sufficient mural atony to bring about obstruction, without any stenosing lesion being present.[28] Scleroderma may also be present with a constricting lesion occurring in the lower end of the esophagus associated with dilatation in the upper portion. Changes may be present within the esophagus and yet the patient may have no symptoms.[28]

Contour: The esophagus may be smooth and atonic. When a constriction is present the esophagus is dilated proximally and tapers smoothly in its distal third. A hiatus hernia may be present. The lumen characteristically remains widely patent after the passage of the opaque media and there is a tendency for a coating of suspension to cling to the walls.[29] Actual stenosis at the distal end is rare, but may be present.[30]

Holdup: Descent of barium is slowed because of the mural atony, causing peristalsis to be interfered with. It should be emphasized that, due to mural atony, considerable delay may occur in esophageal emptying, even in the absence of obstruction.[31] But since in the erect position descent may be rapid because of gravity, the *horizontal* position is preferable here as allowing more accurate observation of peristalsis and delay. In the horizontal position, the barium may pass quickly through the proximal part and be held up in the distal esophagus. Hoesli[32] noted a delay here of 40 minutes, as compared with a normal control of eight seconds.

Position: Esophageal position is normal.

SPECIAL PROCEDURES

In the course of the routine observations of contour, holdup and position it may become necessary to perform additional examinations to help delineate a lesion or some abnormality. Only special maneuvers will be described in the following.

Foreign Body. If the foreign body is a fishbone or some other opaque material it may occasionally be seen on direct examination, i.e., without the aid of contrast material. If, on the other hand, it is radiolucent it may make itself evident by various deviations appearing in the barium mixture as it descends through the pharynx, hypopharynx and esophagus. These will be described presently. On the other hand, no help may be secured by observing the barium mixture descend and so special examinatons may be necessary.

Deviations in the Descending Barium Column: As the barium descends a small amount of opaque media may become trapped either on the foreign body or in some crevice between the foreign body and the esophageal mucosa. The opaque media, unable to move out of this crevice in which it has become lodged, will tend to remain in this position even after several swallows have washed the rest of the barium down into the stomach. In the presence of a suitable history, a persistent barium residue after the main bolus descends is important evidence of a foreign body. A clump of barium may be retained within the folds of the esophageal mucosa at any point. Therefore, the observation of a holdup is not con-

147A

Because of the short esophagus, hiatus hernia (A) and ulcer crater (arrow), a diagnosis was made of peptic ulcer of the esophagus. The defect remained persistent over a three-week period in spite of treatment. Esophagoscopy was not helpful.

At operation a carcinoma was found. In retrospect, the *asymmetry* of the defect should have led to the correct diagnosis. Spasm from peptic esophagitis is more symmetrical and not one-sided.

A differential diagnosis for this type of defect would include peptic esophagitis, carcinoma of the esophagus, cardiospasm, and scleroderma (cf. figs. 147B–E).

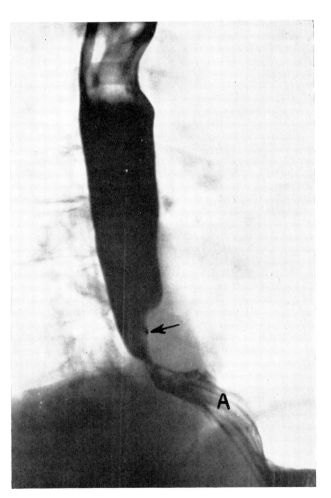

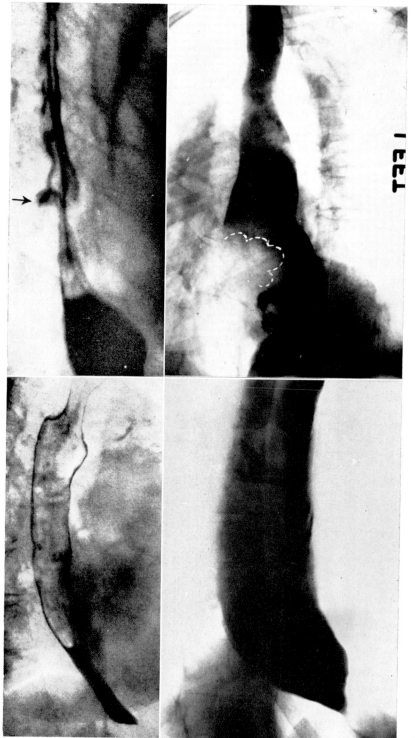

147B

147C

147D

147E

147B–E (see facing page)

clusive unless it appears consistently with repeated examinations.[3]

When a thick suspension of barium is given, a forking of the opaque media may in some cases indicate the presence of a foreign body.

Scott and Moore[18] recommended the use of a very thin suspension of barium in water. Thus the opacity of the esophagus after it is filled with the opaque material is considerably diminished. The translucent filling defect caused by a foreign body is often best seen through this thin layer.

It has been recommended that a piece of cotton be soaked in a barium mixture and this given to the patient to swallow. Theoretically, the cotton attaches itself to the foreign body and so delineates it. Practi-

cally, this is often confusing and not successful. Small pellets or capsules of barium have been used and their descent observed fluoroscopically. At the site where the foreign body is lodged it may obstruct the esophagus and so cause the pellet to stop, or else the examiner may visualize a tumbling effect when the pellet passes the foreign body protruding from the wall of the esophagus.

When a foreign body, such as a coin, lodges within the esophagus (as opposed to the larynx), its location is easily discernible. Since the esophagus is flattened from front to back, the coin will be seen in the frontal plane (fig. 148). In the larynx, because the space created by the vocal cords is narrowed from side to side, the coin is seen on end.

147B

Reflux Peptic Esophagitis

Symmetrical narrowing at the lower portion of the esophagus, except for projecting ulcer (arrow), when present.

Mucosa thickened but generally intact.

No great dilatation above.

Often associated with hiatus hernia (permitting reflux of gastric contents).

(Figures B and D reproduced, respectively, from figures 3819 and 3817 of Schinz, H. R., et al.: Roentgen-Diagnostics, Vol. IV. New York, Grune & Stratton, Inc., 1954; courtesy of Georg Thieme Verlag, Stuttgart, Germany.)

147C

Carcinoma

Narrowing irregular and asymmetrical (scirrhous may be symmetrical).

Mucosa destroyed.

Dilatation above lesion not great, since with malignancy not sufficient time is given for it to develop. Holdup generally not marked and barium will enter stomach.

Stomach (fundus or cardia) invasion common.

147D

Scleroderma

Mural atony, peristalsis reduced or absent.

Mucosa tends to become smooth.

Esophageal lumen tends to remain patent after the barium has passed.

Delay in esophageal emptying mainly in lower portion even in absence of narrowing. The delay best demonstrated in decubitous position when the barium mixture just appears to "lie there." In the erect position, with the aid of gravity, barium tends to fall through.

Scleroderma affecting the cardia allows gastric regurgitation which in turn may produce secondary peptic esophagitis with resultant narrowing of the distal third of the esophagus. Hiatus hernia may be associated.

147E

Cardiospasm

Symmetrical, smooth, tapered segment at cardio-esophageal junction of esophagus (below diaphragm).

Mucosa intact.

Benignancy of lesion allows adequate time for wide dilatation of esophagus to take place above.

Amyl nitrite and Mecholyl tests valuable (see text).

Holdup of barium prominent; in the erect position, when barium in the column is high enough, the weight of the column sooner or later overcomes the resistance and the barium squirts into the stomach. The stomach is not involved.

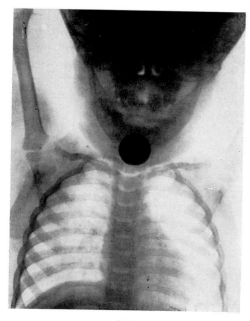

148

Question:

Assuming the child has swallowed a coin, and this is the picture seen on the fluoroscopic screen. With no further investigation, where is the coin?

Answer:

A coin held up in the respiratory passage in the neck lodges between the vocal cords and is seen on end.

A coin held up in the neck and within the esophagus, fills the space formed by the esophagus, i.e., flattened from before backwards, and is seen as above, "en face."

Visualizing a Lesion from Below. The inexperienced observer is often confused when an obstructive lesion is found within the esophagus. The barium column is well outlined above, but almost in its entire extent, from the point of obstruction to the stomach, it appears narrowed. In his inexperience the examiner may fail to recognize that this narrowing of the esophageal contour is not entirely due to the pathological process but rather to inadequate filling with resultant narrowing of the entire esophagus *below* the lesion. In actuality, although the narrowing may extend for many inches, the lesion itself may occupy only 2 or 3 cm. of the esophagus.

After due experience it becomes unnecessary to view a lesion from below in order to recognize its full extent.

When it is desirable to observe a pathological process on its inferior aspect, this can be accomplished by (a) double swallow or "fooling" the cardiac sphincter, and (b) utilization of phrenic ampulla.

(a) Double Swallow: The patient first drinks a glassful of barium, thus filling his stomach with opaque media. He is then placed on the fluoroscopic table in Trendelenburg position (preferably supine). The opaque media will now gravitate towards the fundus. Our method now aims at opening up the cardiac sphincter and allowing the escape of barium up the esophagus. The patient in Trendelenburg position with the fundus full of barium mixture is now given a second swallow of barium. The cardiac sphincter will open to receive the new supply of opaque media. In the process of opening, the barium from the fundus will find its way back through the cardiac sphincter and up the lower end of the esophagus. In truth, the sphincter was opened to receive the new barium from above but the barium trapped in the fundus got out instead.

(b) Utilization of Phrenic Ampulla: The formation of the phrenic ampulla has already been described. When this latter dilatation is noted in Trendelenburg position and the patient asked to breath out against the closed glottis (Valsalva maneuver), the opaque media (as in fig. 150) may, on occasion, be seen to gravitate upwards in the esophagus and so delineate a lesion from below.

Hiatus Hernia. During any fluoroscopic examination of the esophagus a dilatation may be seen immediatly above the diaphragm. This may be due to a hiatus hernia. An attempt will be made in the following section to present a practical differential diagnosis for this condition. Maneuvers necessary to make a hiatus hernia evident when the entire stomach is below the diaphragm will be described in the chapter on "Stomach."

Hiatus hernia and its differential diagnosis (figs. 149–152). Hiatus hernia must be differentiated from: (1) Phrenic ampulla; (2) short esophagus; (3) epiphrenic diverticulum, and (4) eventration of the diaphragm.

1. Phrenic ampulla.

The diagnosis of hiatus hernia is often confused by the presence of the normal dilatation of the esophagus above the diaphgram—that is, the phrenic ampulla. A valuable clue may be secured by observing the esophageal entry into the questionably dilated shadow situated immediately above the diaphragm. This entry is outlined by giving the patient a swallow of barium and observing its descent down the esophagus into this shadow. In the presence of a phrenic ampulla, the esophagus—in an uncoiled and more or less straight line—will be seen to enter the apex or top of the ampulla. On the other hand, in the presence of a hiatus hernia the esophagus in a twisted and coiled condition enters into the side of that portion of the stomach situated above the diaphragm. In order to see this twisted, coiled esophagus entering into the side of, and often below, the herniated stomach, the patient often must be rotated through various degrees of obliquity.

Indeed, if the herniated portion is full of opaque material, and the patient is so positioned that the barium as it descends down the esophagus travels *behind* the herniated portion, the lower portion of the esophagus—even though outlined by barium—will be hidden behind the herniated stomach. As a result, the examiner will see the descent only to the apex of the herniated portion, its further course being hidden by the barium-filled herniated portion of stomach which is an effective barrier to observation of the true point of entry. This apparent, but actually false, finding may well lead to the erroneous diagnosis of phrenic ampulla. To overcome this difficulty, the patient should

be rotated through various degrees of obliquity until the examiner, observing the barium-outlined esophagus, can determine whether the point of entry he had previously observed was true or whether the esophagus was hidden behind the herniated stomach.

Further differential features between phrenic ampulla and hiatus hernia may be secured by a study of the mucosal pattern as seen in the dilated portion in question. Thus, the examiner should further try to observe the mucosal pattern of the region involved, and note the characteristic considerable increase of thickness of the gastric mucosa as compared with that of the esophagus (cf. fig. 149 with figs. 151, 152). When the confusing dilatation above the diaphragm is due to phrenic ampulla, the esophageal folds as seen within the ampulla are fine, slender and easily differentiated from the wider gastric folds seen when a hiatus hernia is present. However, since it is difficult fluoroscopically to identify with certainty the type of mucosa involved, for verification this finding must be checked with radiographic films.

Finally, the normal esophagus (with or without presence of a phrenic ampulla) as it passes through the diaphragm is about one cm. or less in diameter, whereas the stomach when herniated and passing into the thorax is about twice as wide. In the presence of a hernia the diameter of the stomach shadow passing through the diaphragm is usually 3 to 5 cm. and may be wider.[19]

2. Short esophagus.

Partial thoracic stomach associated with a short esophagus is generally thought to be congenital.[20] If this theory is correct, the condition is not a true hernia. Some observers believe, however, that the etiology and pathogenesis is the same as other varieties of hiatus hernia, but that the esophagus in these cases of partial thoracic stomach shortens after the hernia develops.

Having established the existence of part of the stomach above the diaphragm, it is important to differentiate the short esopha-

149   150

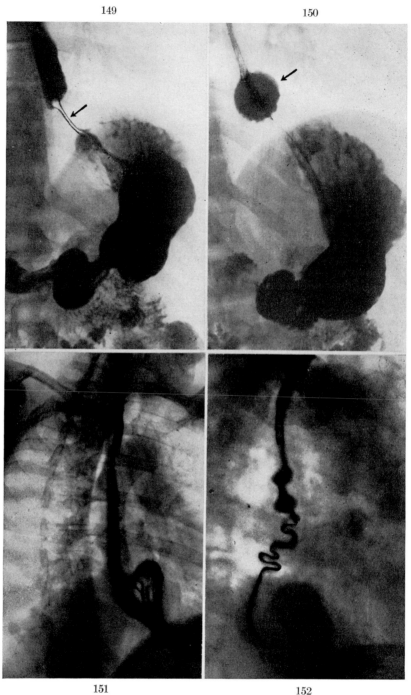

151   152

The differential diagnosis of hiatus hernia.

(See opposite page)

gus from a true hiatus hernia. For this diagnosis the length of the esophagus becomes important. If this structure is not coiled or obviously too long, we are dealing with the short esophagus type of hiatus hernia (fig. 151). On the other hand, when it appears elongated and coiled, and apparently enters into the side of the herniated portion above the diaphragm, it is a true hiatus hernia (fig. 152).

A short esophagus is a little more difficult to differentiate from the phrenic ampulla, since in both these conditions the esophagus will be seen to enter into the apex or roof of the dilated shadow. Perhaps the best way to differentiate the one from the other is to observe the constany of the dilatation above the diaphragm when due to stomach. This is especially true in the Trendelenburg position. The phrenic ampulla, on the other hand, will not be as constant, and as it is observed fluoroscopically it will disappear and reappear later, only to disappear again. *The wide gastric folds passing through the diaphragmatic hiatus are pathognomonic of stomach;* i.e., the observer, seeing this type of mucosa within the abnormal dilation, will know that the latter must be of gastric origin.

3. Epiphrenic diverticulum.

The hiatus hernia must be differentiated from the epiphrenic diverticulum. An epiphrenic diverticulum (fig. 141) will be noted to have a thin pedicle and a small marble-like contour. Once observed and proved on the radiographic film it presents no problem.

4. Eventration (see p. 33).

For a diagnosis of diaphragmatic eventration, the superior margin of the dilated and questionable shadow should be observed. Here the examiner's eys should be fixed on what he believes to be the diaphragm. *If it does prove to be the diaphragm, a diagnosis of eventration is made.* To verify whether he has actually found the diaphragm, the examiner observes the various diaphragmatic movements (as outlined in the chapter on "Chest"), including diaphragmatic paralysis (Kienbock's sign).

Deformities of the Esophagus due to Cardiac Abnormalities. (This is discussed in Chapter III, which deals with cardiac fluoroscopy.)

Esophageal Varices. The cobblestone appearance of the esophageal mucosa or the scalloping of the esophageal contours will

---

The differential diagnosis of hiatus hernia (*see opposite page*).

149

Normal esophagus (*upper left*).
1. No dilatation above diaphragm.

3. Esophagus normally straight.
4. Two to three fine mucosal folds present in part of esophagus visualized.
5. Changes in contour due to normal passage of media.

151

Short esophagus (*lower left*).
1. Dilatation above diaphragm.
2. Esophagus enters dilatation at apex.
3. Esophagus above dilatation normally straight.
4. Many thick, *coarse mucosal folds* present within dilatation.
5. Dilatation persistent.

150

Phrenic ampulla (*upper right*).
1. Dilatation above diaphragm.
2. Esophagus enters dilatation at apex.
3. Esophagus above dilatation normally straight.
4. Two to three fine mucosal folds present when ampulla contracts and empties, and permits visualization of mucosal folds.
5. Dilatation not persistent, i.e., comes and goes.

152

Hiatus hernia (*lower right*).
1. Dilatation above diaphragm.
2. Esophagus enters dilatation at side and below.
3. Esophagus curled and tortuous.
4. Many thick, *coarse mucosal folds* present within dilatation.
5. Dilatation persistent.

*need confirmation with radiographic exam-
ination.* A helpful procedure for this study
is to have the patient in the prone position
(left posterior oblique, fig. 203). With the
patient thus positioned, the typical pattern
may best be seen during deep inspiration.
Thick media should be employed. During
the passage of the barium, all of these markings will be covered over. The mucosal
markings should be studied after most of the
opaque mixture has passed and only a small
amount is left behind to outline the various
crevices and markings necessary to make
the diagnosis. When difficulty is encountered
in outlining the mucosal contours with

opaque material, the Valsalva maneuver is
useful in that it often may hold up the barium in the phrenic ampulla and may allow
retrograde flow of the barium thus outlining
the varices when they become distended.
Several swallows of barium each followed by
the performance of a Valsalva test are often
necessary before the veins fill. In some
cases they may not distend at all.[4]

Ulcer in Hiatus Hernia. Ulcer craters may
form within the sac of a hiatus hernia. They
are seen as barium trapped in a crater. This
is described more fully in the discussion of
gastric ulcer. Ulcers in a hiatal sac may be

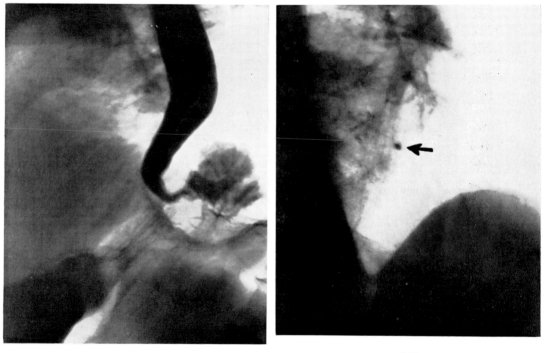

153

The patient presents a history of tarry stools.
A hiatus hernia is found. No lesion is seen within
the herniated portion of the stomach.

154

This is the same patient 5 hours later. The
barium mixture has passed on its way. The stomach and its herniated portion have emptied. A
"fleck" (arrow) of barium is present above the
diaphragm. This might be a "fleck" of barium
retained either within the region of the esophagus
or in the herniated portion of the stomach.

Question:

How can you determine what and where this
"fleck" is? (See fig. 155, facing page.)

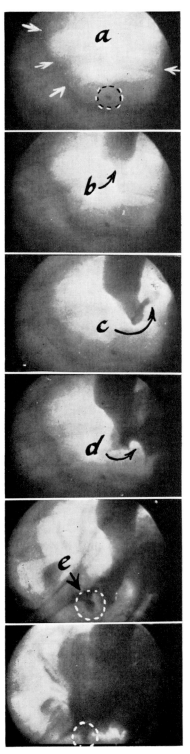

155

missed during conventional studies. A procedure here recommended is to study the involved region *after* the opaque media has passed out of the sac. A *persistent* barium "fleck" left behind after the bulk of the barium has passed may be caused by barium trapped in an ulcer. See figures 153–155 for a demonstration of the method of confirming such a case.

Summary

By way of summary it should be pointed out that in order to be able to cope with the abnormal, the normal must first be clearly understood. When an abnormal process appears it would be wise to secure a radiographic film for a clearer and more sharply delineated study of the image. Again, it should be noted that the information derived from the fluoroscopic screen should be looked upon as only one of the links of the chain leading to a correct diagnosis.

LARYNX

The vocal cords and the supraglottic areas are usually examined through the mouth by mirror. The subglottic region is not seen by mirror, but may be clearly outlined on spot films during fluoroscopy. It is also seen on tomographic study (fig. 156). It should,

155

Answer:

This is a re-examination to determine both the nature and the exact position of the "fleck" of barium, which has already served as a suspicious lead. With greater persistence and with careful examination in all positions, the examiner can trace sequentially—as in this series—the entry of barium down the esophagus (b), into the hiatus hernia (c and d) and into the "fleck" (e). Thus, the presence of an ulcer in the herniated portion of the stomach is confirmed.

Comment: A valuable aid in the barium study of any hollow viscus is the examination of the region in question *after* the barium mixture has passed. In searching for an ulcer which may have been missed, a residual "fleck" in the region would be highly suggestive. Persistent study in various positions would next confirm it (fig. 155).

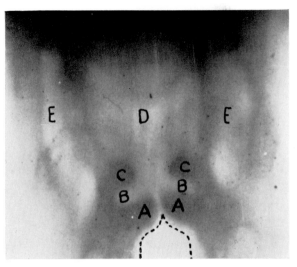

156

A. Vocal cords. B. Ventricles. C. False vocal cords. D. Vestibule. E. Pyriform sinuses.

Note the top of the tracheal air space and the glottic opening above it (dotted line) as the patient says "E." It appears as the dome of a building with a central spire.

however, be stressed that roentgen examinations employing the spot film during fluoroscopy can yield valuable information as to the site of origin and also the extent of a lesion. The roentgen examination is not intended to compete with the clinical examination. It is meant to fortify, confirm or complement the findings. Thus, findings on the spot film may demonstrate the extent of a lesion not seen clinically. This is particularly true of subglottic lesions or lesions of the hypopharynx.[26] Fluoroscopy and spot filming may also enable the examiner to interpret minor variations seen on the laminograph.

In order to examine the larynx, the

Figs. 157–160 (see facing page)

157

The patient is saying "E" and the vocal cords are normally approximated. The space between the cords (glottis) is centered over the tracheal air column. The tracheal air column appears as a tall building and the centered space between the cords as a spire (dotted line).

158

The patient is breathing in and the vocal cords are symmetrically abducted. The vocal cord region is seen patent, with symmetrical soft bulges (arrow) on either side where the vocal cords are abducted. This is normal.

159

Question:

When the left vocal cord is paralyzed and the patient attempts to say "E," what does the right vocal cord do?

Answer:

Since the paralyzed left vocal cord cannot do its part in approximation (see fig. 157), the right vocal cord *reaches across* the midline to compensate for its weak partner. Thus, the space between the vocal cords is asymmetrical. The glottis is shifted toward the paralyzed cord. The "spire of the building" is shifted toward the paralyzed cord.

160

When a vocal cord is paralyzed, it cannot abduct during inspiration. Thus, whereas the normal cord is retracted and disappears, the paralyzed cord (arrow) remains projecting into the air column. This exposure was made during deep inspiration.

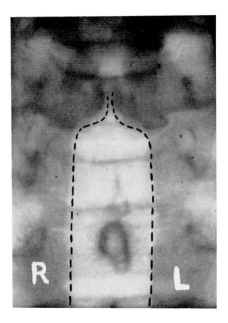

157

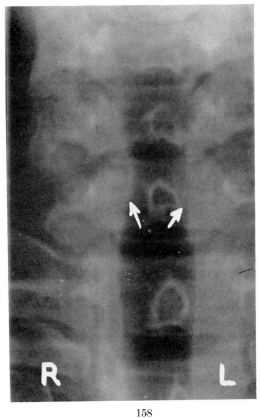

158

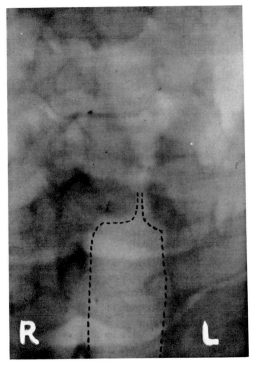

159

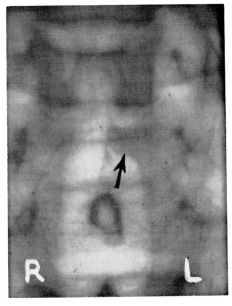

160

patient is placed behind the fluoroscopic screen, facing the examiner. The chin and occiput are so positioned that they do not obstruct visualization of the larynx. Films are exposed as the patient first phonates the letter "E" and then inspires slowly and deeply.

Phonating the letter "E" *closes* the glottis. With the glottis closed, the fluoroscopic spot film should reveal symmetry of the vocal cords. The glottis should be in the center of the tracheal air column. The tracheal air column, surmounted by a central sitting glottis, has been likened to a tall building with a spire sitting on the top[1] (fig. 157).

Films are next exposed during a slow,

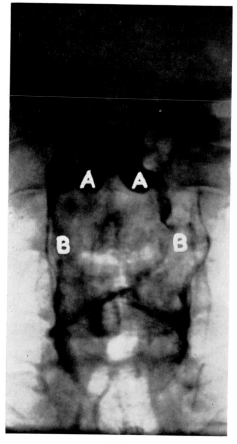

161

The vallecula (A) and pyriform sinuses (B).

deep inspiration. The glottis at this time *opens*. When normal, the vocal cords are symmetrically abducted. With symmetrical complete abduction, both vocal cords almost disappear. They are seen as soft bulges on either side of the air column (fig. 158). When a cord is paralyzed it fails to abduct and will project into the tracheal air column (fig. 160). It is recommended[26] that, in order to secure complete vocal cord abduction, the patient during deep inspiration be completely relaxed. Incomplete abduction due to incomplete relaxation may simulate vocal cord paralysis to an examiner not familiar with normal variations.

Symmetry of the vocal cords on phonation of the letter "E" (fig. 157) and symmetry of abduction on deep inspiration (fig. 158) indicate normalcy; asymmetry in either phonation of the letter "E" or deep inspiration indicates abnormalcy.

To explain further: With paralysis of one vocal cord during the patient's phonation of "E," the other (normal) vocal cord in the attempt to make the sound finds it necessary to reach across the midline to approach the paralyzed cord. The paralyzed cord is unable to fully partake in the closure,[27] and cannot reach the midline during the phonation of "E." Thus, the normal cord compensates by "over-reaching" across the midline to approach the paralyzed cord. Thus, finding asymmetry would indicate that the "tall building" has had its "spire" shifted to one side, thus implying that the side towards which the spire has shifted is paralyzed (fig. 159). These changes are subtle but may be seen with awareness of the possibility.

With deep inspiration, a paralyzed vocal cord will *not* abduct and thus remains projecting into the tracheal air column (fig. 160). A vocal cord fixed by tumor will also remain projecting into the tracheal air column. On the other hand, during deep inspiration, the normal vocal cord will seem to have disappeared since it became abducted (fig. 160). A small soft bulge may be seen at the site of abduction of a normal vocal cord (figs. 158 and 160).

For an efficient examination, the finding on the spot film should be considered in conjunction with clinical findings and tomographs employing the same maneuvers, i.e., exposure when sounding "E" and during deep inspiration.

With the patient behind the fluoroscopic screen and in position for the examiner to visualize the larynx, the pyriform sinuses may also be outlined. The patient ingests some thick barium paste. After the major bolus is swallowed, the pyriform sinuses (fig. 161) and lateral pharyngeal walls may be well outlined. Encroachment of a mass into this region may be seen as invasion of the normal outline with resultant asymmetry of the pyriform spaces.

The patient placed in the lateral position would also enable valuable findings to be made of the cervical esophagus and pharynx (figs. 115 and 116).

In the lateral fluoroscopic spot film examination of the larynx, the same maneuvers (i.e., phonating the letter "E" and deep inspiration) are followed. It is recommended[26] that for best visualization of the lateral laryngeal structures, the central ray be placed at the level of the superior notch of the thyroid cartilage. The spot film will now disclose the laryngeal ventricles. Motion of the arytenoid cartilage can also be appraised, as can the mechanism of swallowing. The upward motion of the larynx with posterior tilting of the epiglottis during swallowing is seen. Motion of the tongue in swallowing can also be appraised.

CHAPTER V

Examination of the Stomach

Fundamentals

ANATOMY OF THE STOMACH

FOR DESCRIPTIVE PURPOSES, the stomach can be divided into three sections: the fundus or cardiac end of the stomach, the pars media or body, and the antrum (fig. 162). The incisura angularis divides the body from the antrum. The cardiac incisura is the superior angle formed by the junction of the esophagus with the cardiac end of the stomach. The greater curvature can be considered as starting at this angle and continuing upwards and around over the fundus and down on the lower border of the stomach to end at the pyloric sphincter. The sulcus intermedius is an impression on the greater curvature not often found, but nevertheless occasionally present to the confusion of the novice. Other normal impressions found on the greater curvature may often be produced by either the spleen, the splenic flexure of the colon or the ribs

(fig. 163). It is important to know these normal impressions in order to avoid the error (frequent among beginners) of interpreting such apparent defects as abnormalities. The pyloric canal separates the duodenum from the antrum.

The duodenum is divided into four portions: superior, descending, transverse and ascending. The first half of the superior portion is considered as the "cap." The reader should be aware that the Kerkring folds start at about the apex of the cap and the parallel duodenal folds (to be described below) become lost at this point (fig. 175).

MUCOSAL PATTERN

Understanding the normal mucosal pattern will prove of great value, since changes in these folds are valuable clues leading to a diagnosis of organic disease.[1, 2]

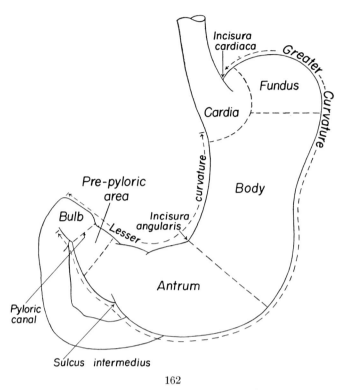

Incisura
cardiaca

Greater

Fundus

Cardia

Curvature

curvature

Pre-pyloric
area

Body

Bulb

Incisura
angularis

Lesser

Pyloric
canal

Antrum

Sulcus intermedius

162

Anatomy of the stomach and duodenum.

For practical purposes the stomach can be considered as a hollow tube lined with a mucous membrane, the lining being much larger than its outer covering. In order for it to fit into its small tube, much "crinkling" of this lining must occur. The patterns formed by the wrinkled folds in the stomach are many, but in spite of these many variations one can identify a basic pattern. As shown in figures 164 and 165, it is noted that the mucosal pattern along the lesser curvature is smooth, striated and consists of parallel folds. In the antrum the folds are also parallel and disposed in a horizontal fashion. Occasionally, the antral folds may be vertical or even variegated. The basic pattern of the folds on the greater curvature side are oblique and occasionally transverse. Thus the lesser curvature contour is smooth, whereas the greater curvature is serrated or tooth-like.

The folds within the fundus are variable (figs. 166–168).

Understanding the formation of mucosal folds will aid in understanding normal appearance. A passive effect is secured from the stomach muscle wall. Thus, when the circular muscles contract, the mucosa arranges itself in folds parallel to the gastric lumen. Longitudinal muscle contracting wrinkles the mucosa vertically (perpendicular to the lumen). A variegated pattern is caused by different groups of muscles contracting. Practically, the observer will note that the wrinkled mucosa is in *groups* of parallel folds. Seeing a bizarre pattern, the examiner should try to break this maze down into small *groups* of parallel folds.

The muscularis mucosa is active in the formation of folds, and often accounts for visualization of folds where gastric distention is greatest, their absence where gastric contraction is marked.

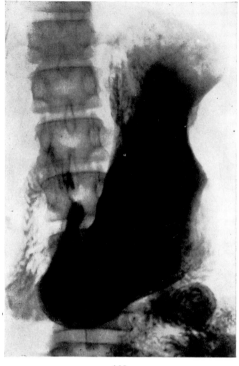

163

A notch high up on the greater curvature may be normal and produced by pressure from the spleen.

Question:

When accessible to the palpating hand how may this deformity be determined as normal?

Answer:

See figures 177 and 178, page 151.

The mucosal pattern of the duodenum is also quite variable but as it will be seen (fig. 175) the basic pattern can be considered as a group of parallel folds.

FLUOROSCOPIC PALPATION

For satisfactory palpation and manipulation it is first important to place the patient so that the fluoroscopist can easily observe the parts investigated. The patient stands on an elevated platform, so that his stomach is just above the fluoroscopist's eye level, while the examiner sits comfortably on a small stool. It is next important to secure complete relaxation of the patient's ab-

dominal wall. For this, he should be instructed to "slouch"—lean back against the backboard, drop his chin, droop his shoulders, let the abdomen sag and breathe naturally.

Generally palpation is performed with one hand while the other controls the tube and screen. By immobilizing the tube and screen both hands may be used.

In fluoroscopic palpation the observer does not press directly inwards. Pressure is applied "below" the part examined.[3] It is thus possible to keep the hands out of the fluoroscopic field, outside the field of illumination. The fluoroscopist, in his effort to protect himself further, will as far as possible attempt to hide the palpating hand behind the opaque barium meal; the latter acts as a barrier against the x-rays emanating from the tube behind.

Radioscopic palpation is not quite the same as the clinical, that is, done by touch alone. In fluoroscopy, a combination of touch and sight is required. For example, to see the mucosal pattern, the touch must be firm enough to press away excess barium and still be sufficiently gentle so that just the right amount is left behind to permit the mucosal folds to become opacified. In addition, the examiner must be able to estimate the force needed to move any part considered mobile. The relationship of movement to the degree of pressure exerted will permit the observer to appraise the relative "freedom of mobility" of the various parts examined.

GRADED COMPRESSION

An extremely important part of the fluoroscopic examination of the gastrointestinal tract is the study of the barium-filled lumen by means of graded compression. The barium suspension within the stomach may innundate and obscure important underlying pathology. It is the purpose of the examiner to thin the overlying media. He does this by means of careful pressure,

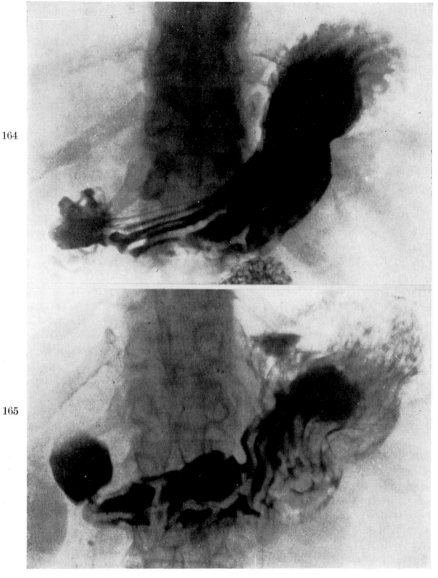

164

165

164

Normal gastric rugae.

165

Normal gastric rugae. Note the variegated pattern of the antrum.

i.e., by pressing away some of the overlying barium and visualizing the relief pattern of the underlying structures. *Too much pressure* may rid the region under investigation of *too much* of the opaque media, not leaving enough to outline the structures.

Too little pressure applied to the region under investigation may not sufficiently thin the overlying media to cause the underlying pathology to become visible. It is important to train oneself to judge the correct amount of pressure that must be applied in order to

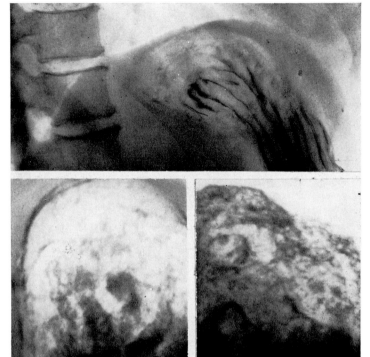

166-168
Varying mucosal patterns of the fundus.

visualize the underlying structures. Graded compression may be performed with the palpating hand, pressure cone, or other devices (figs. 172–174).

MOBILITY

The stomach can be considered as a hammock hanging suspended from the esophagus on the left, and from the juncture of the first and second portion of the duodenum on the right. The actual displacement that this hammock can undergo is considered the mobility of the stomach.

Behind the fluoroscopic screen (fig. 176), with the patient erect, the palpating hand can move the greater curvature and actually lift it up from a level in the region of the pelvis to above the umbilicus. Mobility may also be demonstrated by changing the position of the patient. When the position is changed from erect to supine, the normal stomach may exhibit a wide range of movement. Barclay[3] places the normal pylorus between L3 and L4 when the patient is in the erect position, but displaced to L1 with the patient horizontal.

This characteristic of the stomach is extremely important in arriving at various diagnoses. Adhesive processes such as fibrosis following operation or actual invasion of neighboring organs by pathological processes arising in the stomach, or vice versa, may not allow this mobility.

FLEXIBILITY

Gastric Contour. Flexibility or pliability can be considered as the softness of any portion of the stomach. This is determined, as in figure 176, by indenting different accessible portions of the gastric contour. Although the whole hand may be used, the examiner may find it advisable to use as

169

170

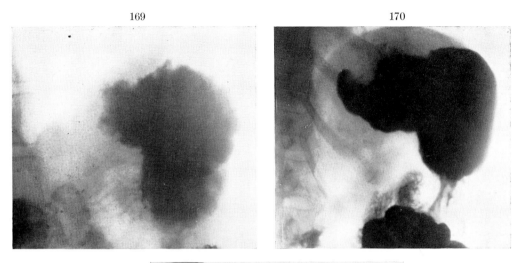

171

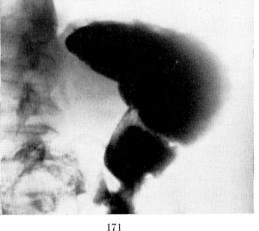

169–171

These figures demonstrate the barium filled fundus in the supine Trendelenberg position. Note that the roof of the fundus in figs. 169 and 170 are irregular. The roof of the fundus in fig. 171 is smooth. Figs. 169 and 171, when distended with air, were found normal. Fig. 170, when distended with air, revealed a tumor mass.

Comment: Placing the patient with the barium-filled stomach in the Trendelenberg position should reveal a smooth fundal roof. Irregularity of the roof is suggestive of tumor; since it is evident that an occasional *normal fundus* may appear *deformed* (fig. 169), a tumor must always be confirmed by suitable air distention of the fundus. (See fig. 287A, B page 215.)

small a pressure point as possible, since this allows smaller portions of the gastric wall to be studied at a time. This maneuver presents a method of actually determining and differentiating the rigid infiltrated parts of the stomach from the normal soft and flexible parts.

The normal soft gastric contours when indented by the hand will yield and assume an indenture corresponding to the pressure point. The rigid pathological wall may be mobile and allow itself to be raised by the pressure upwards of the fingers, but will not yield and thus become indented. With a loss

172

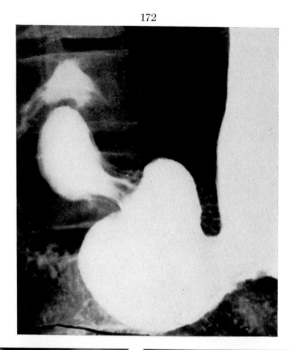

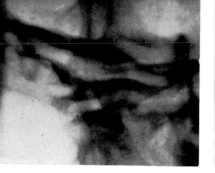

173

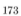

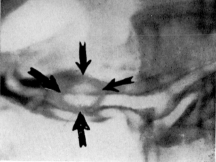

174

172

Conventional filming without the benefit of
compression study during fluoroscopy reveals a
normal stomach antrum (see fig. 148–149, same
patient).

173

Same patient next viewed with benefit of compression behind fluoroscopic screen. *Excessive
compression*, however, did not leave enough barium behind to coat and *properly* outline the mucosa or any pathology.

174

Same patient. *Correct graded compression* re-
moves excessive barium but sufficient residue remains to coat and outline an underlying polyp.

of flexibility, that portion of the gastric contour involved refuses to be indented by the
palpating finger, nor will it display normal
elasticity by springing back after the pressure is removed.

Unfortunately, portions of the gastric
outline and duodenum which are high and
beneath the ribs can not always be reached
by the examiner and thus other methods of
determining the softness of these gastric

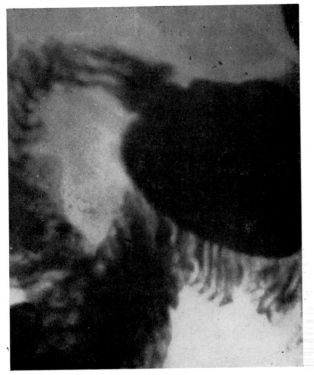

175

The normal rugal pattern of the duodenal bulb is usually a group of parallel folds.

Question:

Where difficulty is encountered in determining which of the structures present on the screen is duodenal bulb, what are some useful aids?

Answer:

1. Finding the point at which barium descends locates the descending duodenum. The part immediately proximal to this must be the first portion of duodenum and bulb.

2. The folds within the bulb are parallel. The folds immediately distal, starting at the apex of the bulb, are herring bone in appearance, i.e., Kerkring folds. Finding the origin of the Kerkring folds locates the apex of the cap.

3. The pyloric sphincter is a constant space of separation between bulb and stomach. A peristaltic wave which may simulate the pyloric sphincter moves and keeps changing position.

contours must be looked for. The pliability of the fundal end of the stomach, may be gaged with the patient in the supine position. The experienced examiner will look for fine undulations on the greater and lesser curvature which will suggest softness. Also, the change of contour which takes place in the fundus with deep inspiration and expiration, when once learned, helps to determine the pliability of this inaccessible region.[4] At its best, the determination of flexibility and pliability in these inaccessible parts is not too easy and when a pathological process is suspected, repeated examinations and careful film studies must be performed.

Mucosal Patterns. The flexibility and pliability of the stomach is also determined by observing the mucosal patterns and again with the palpating fingers distorting them. A pattern which can be changed and molded by pressure and which assumes contours corresponding to this pressure, proves to be free of abnormalities (figs. 177, 178).

A mucosal pattern also demonstrates its

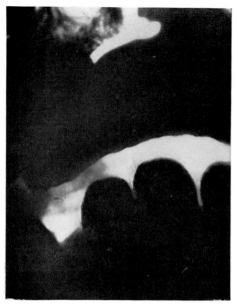

176

1. The palpating hand determining the *mobility* of the stomach by actually *lifting it up*. This would tend to rule out an adhesive process binding the stomach down.

2. The palpating hand by *indenting* the stomach wall demonstrates the *flexibility* of the stomach wall.

pliability by permitting the normal parallelism of the folds to occur when a peristaltic wave passes through it (fig. 181). Often this may not be seen on the fluoroscopic screen but instead on the radiographic film.

Flexibility and pliability are fundamental and important. When the examiner sees an abnormal mucosal pattern he should immediately try to distort it with the palpating hand. When this pattern refuses to distort itself and persistently maintains the same abnormal configuration, a pathological process must be suspected (fig. 284).

DISTENSIBILITY

Still another method of determining softness or ability of the gastric wall and duodenum to "stretch" is by observing its distensibility. An area which at any one time appears narrow and later becomes wider and ballooned is probably not rigid (contrast with fig. 285).

The rugal folds in the normal stomach assume important changes when the stomach is distended. In the empty state, much wrinkling of the mucosa is permitted; on the other hand, with the stomach full, the mucosa is stretched and the toothlike indentures due to the wrinkled mucosa become more shallow and may even disappear. These mucosal changes (i.e., exaggeration of the folds when the stomach is empty, and their tendency to disappear when the stomach is full) can be taken as evidence of pliability of the mucosa. Such knowledge is of value when the stomach contour shows an assumedly abnormal indenture which is actually caused by a rugal fold. One of the maneuvers the examiner can use as a test in this situation is to overdistend the stomach. This overdistention can be done with barium or air. Especially in the fundus is air valuable (figs. 227–230). If the mucosa is normal and caused the indenture, the indenture will tend to disappear; if the deformity had no such normal cause, it will tend *not* to disappear (figs. 227–230, pages 175, 176).

It should be noted that the gastric wall can be so stretched by the palpating hand that the mucosal pattern may be completely obliterated. This too is suggestive of a normal mucosa.

PERISTALSIS

The observation of the peristaltic wave is another method useful in appraising the rigidity of the stomach wall. Peristalsis may be considered as a rhythmical muscular contraction encircling the stomach and traveling smooth and wave-like towards the pyloric tip. By means of this movement the contents within the stomach are carried towards the pyloric opening. Peristalsis is initiated by taking food into the stomach. There is often some delay between the entry of barium mixture into the gastric lumen and the formation of these waves. This may depend on the psyche of the patient or emotional factors.

In the erect position the waves usually

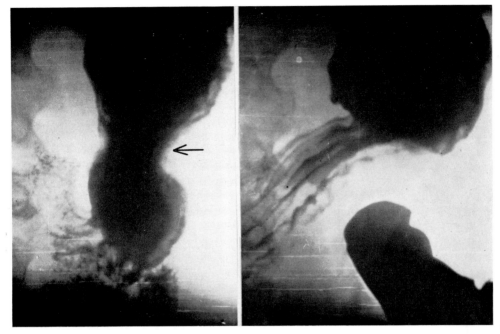

177   178

Question:

Is the concavity in the gastric outline (arrow) due to a stomach lesion?

Fluoroscopic Findings:

1. Palpating hand indents involved region. The gastric outline *changes* and the change corresponds to the pressure (gastric wall proved flexible).

2. Enough barium is pressed out of the region so that the rugal pattern is seen. The pattern is normal and also distorted (draped over finger) corresponding to the applied pressure (mucosa thus proved soft and flexible).

Answer:

The above findings are characteristically normal. The concavity in figure 177 is not due to a gastric lesion.

start at the incisura angularis or perhaps a little above this point. They are, however, best studied with the patient prone.[4] In this position the waves start a little higher up near the cardia. They are initiated as shallow ripples and become deeper and stronger as they advance towards the pyloric sphincter. Peristalsis is usually not prominent in the upper third of the stomach and is thus of little help in the study of this region.

The wave, as a band encircling the stomach wall, travels at a regular rate towards the pyloric sphincter. The closer the wave gets to the sphincter, the deeper does it become. This encircling band or peristal-

tic wave pushes some of the stomach contents forward. As the wave approaches the pyloric sphincter, the space containing food, between the sphincter and the oncoming wave, becomes progressively smaller until obliterated. If the sphincter does not open, the food contents trapped between the wave and sphincter must of necessity fall back past the wave into the stomach. But after a few such abortive waves the pylorus should open and a mass of stomach contents be expelled into the duodenal bulb.

In the normal individual, only two or three such peristaltic waves or bands are present in the stomach at any one time.

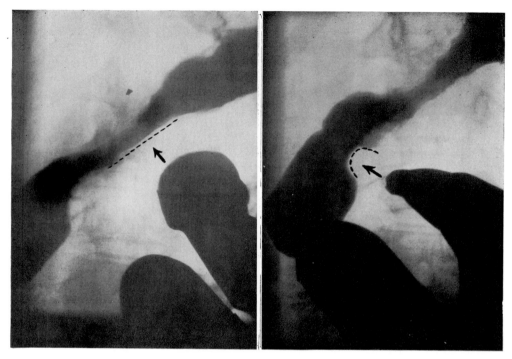

179

Palpating hand discovers rigid section on greater curvature of the stomach (dotted line), which will not bend on applied pressure.

180

Palpating finger delineates extent of pathologic rigidity by indenting normal soft tissue at distal termination of lesion. (Cf. normal, figs. 177, 178.)

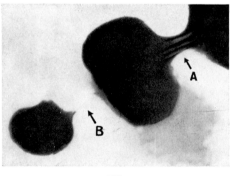

181

1. A deep peristaltic wave may press away sufficient barium so that parallel mucosal folds (A) become evident. Often this is a valuable finding in concluding that the *mucosa in the region is normal.*

2. A normal peristaltic wave may succeed in pressing all of the barium out of the region (B). The more distal part of the stomach, to the inexperienced observer, may then be mistaken for the duodenal bulb. (See fig. 175.)

Hyperperistalsis (fig. 182) is characterized by the presence of more waves, and usually these make deeper impressions into the gastric contours.

Occasionally, the opposing walls of the peristaltic contraction can become so deep as to press all barium out from between them, and therefore on the fluoroscopic screen the stomach may appear as though one portion were separated from the other (fig. 181 B). Actually, however, some mucosa coated with barium is separating the one portion from the other, but because of the deep peristaltic waves the folds become so fine that they can be seen only on radiographic films—not on the fluoroscopic screen.

When any portion of the wall is rigid, the peristaltic wave will not pass through it. Under these circumstances, the wave may be seen as a constricting band approaching the invaded segment, but once the lesion is reached the wave is no longer evident. On the opposite wall, however, the wave as a contraction ring continues on its course. At the distal end of the infiltrated area the wave again appears on both curvatures. In other words, the wave only disappears in that part of the wall where the rigid process exists. When rigidity of a wall is confined to a small segment it may be difficult or impossible to recognize lack of peristalsis through it.

Peristalsis as seen within the antrum is slightly different from peristalsis in the rest of the stomach. Although a peristaltic wave may be deep enough for the opposing walls to meet, this is generally not the case except as seen during antral contraction, better termed antral systole.[4a] On the fluoro-scopic screen, during this phase of gastric activity, the contracting antrum expelling its contents is replaced by barium-coated thin mucosal folds. The examiner *must learn* to look for this antral systole with resultant momentary obliteration and prompt relaxation to normal width. Once seen during an examination, it can be accepted as a valuable clue in helping establish the normalcy of the antrum.

It should be understood that the observation of peristalsis and the absence of it in the presence of an infiltrative process does not, of necessity, signify malignancy since either a malignant process or a benign process may produce a lack of peristalsis in a given area. However, when the benign process heals, peristalsis again becomes evident.

Reverse persistalsis occasionally occurs with obstructive lesions. Here the course of the wave is reversed and it passes in a retrograde fashion from the pylorus towards the cardia. Reverse peristalsis may occasionally be functional in origin, occurring with nauseousness as a result of the unpalatable barium mixture. It may also occur with inflammatory lesions.[20]

FILLING DEFECT

The examiner should understand that radiographically the gastric wall is not actually seen. What he sees is a cast of the interior formed by the barium. A *positive defect* can be defined as an abnormality wherein the cast reveals a protrusion. A benign gastric ulcer projecting from the lesser curvature represents such a defect. A *negative defect* is an abnormality wherein a portion of the cast appears to be lacking or cut off. This type of defect is produced by spasm or an intrinsic lesion. *An intraluminal defect* is a variety of negative defect (figs. 183–186). In this type of defect the contours of the cast remain intact. The portion that is lacking is situated between the greater and lesser curvatures of the stomach. This is demonstrated in the presence of an intraluminal polyp.

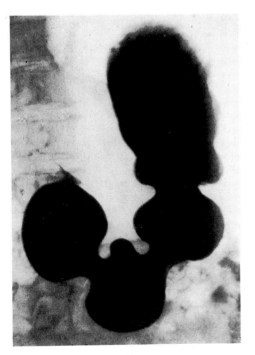

182

Question:

What characterizes hyperperistalsis?

Answer:

The waves (above) are deeper and more numerous than the normal.

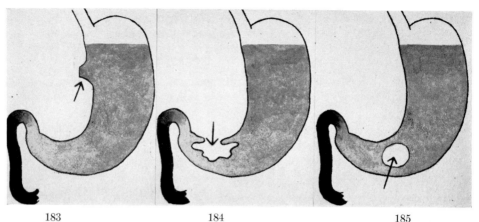

183   184   185

Positive defect.   Negative defect.   Central negative defect.

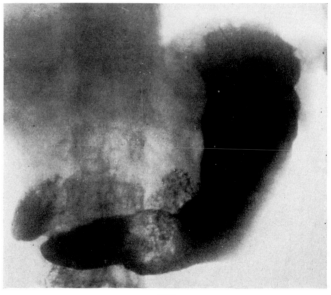

186

A central negative defect produced by a large polyp. Note that the lesser and greater curvatures remain intact.

Question:

Explain the absence in this case of mucosal folds in the region of the polyp.

Answer:

The mucosa may be stretched over the polyp to such an extent as to obliterate the wrinkling, or folds.

The importance of using a small quantity of barium during the first part of the fluoroscopic examination becomes evident. An excessive amount of barium may cover or obscure the intraluminal defect.

Normal intraluminal defects may occasionally occur in the barium-filled stomach and it is important that they be understood. As in figure 190, with the patient in the supine position the spine may bulge upwards and divide the stomach into two compartments, one each appearing on either

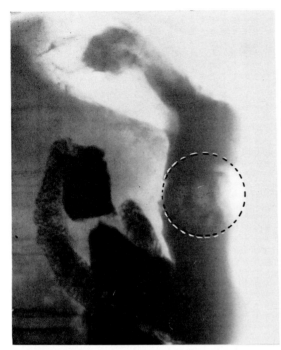

187

Right lateral view of the stomach. The examiner is viewing the stomach from the side of the lesser curvature.

Question:

What may produce the defect encircled?

Answer:

1. A space-occupying lesion within the stomach would thin the barium at the site and produce such a defect.

2. Any factor which would bring the walls of the stomach together within the region, i.e., extrinsic pressure or a normal incisura, would result in poor filling at the site and produce such a defect. (Cf. figs. 188–189.)

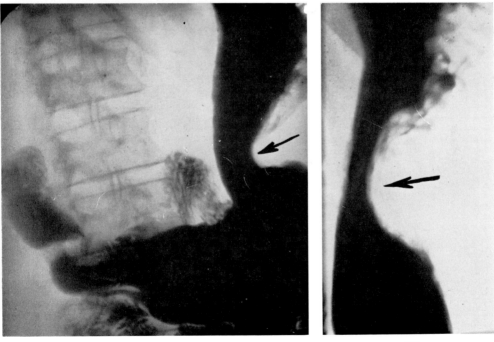

188   189

The stomach is here seen in the *frontal* projection. The defect in figure 187 is seen to be produced by an incisura, bringing the greater curvature close to the lesser curvature. (NOTE: The greater curvature of the stomach is not seen in figure 187, since in the right lateral projection the greater curvature is behind.)

Comment: A normal greater curvature incisura may sometimes be deep enough to produce a defect as here demonstrated (fig. 189).

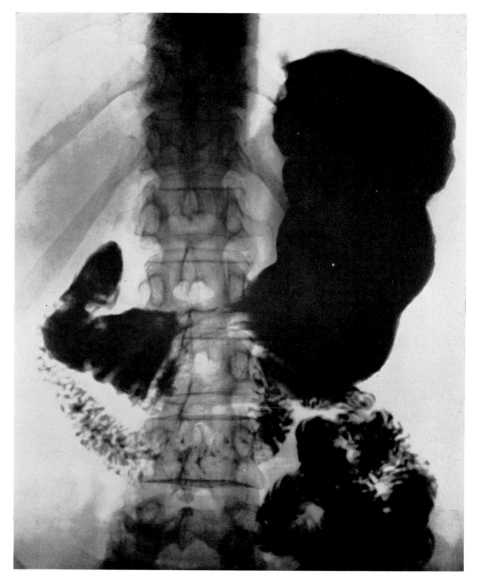

190

Question:

How does this defect in gastric contour come about?

Answer:

Pressure from the spine. This pressure can come about when the patient is *prone*, without pillow support, and the spine sags, pressing on the stomach. This defect may also come about when the patient is *supine* and the stomach drapes itself on either side of the spine.

side of the spine. This same defect may sometimes occur when the patient is in the prone position when the spine sags. Understanding the cause of these defects may help in avoiding them. Thus, in the prone position, pillows under the chest and pelvis are used to lift the spine away (fig. 203).

Another defect which may appear in the body of the barium filled stomach may be produced by approximation (drawing to-

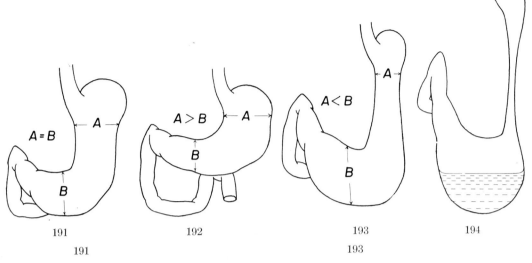

191

191

192

192

193

193

194

194

Orthotonic stomach, A = B

Hypotonic stomach A < B

Hypertonic stomach, A > B (In this type of stomach particularly, the cap and distal antrum, since they are directed from before backward, can not be satisfactorily examined in the frontal position.)

Atonic stomach, A < B (Vertical walls touch each other. Third part of the duodenum crosses the cap at its base.)

gether) of the walls in the region of normal extrinsic pressure (fig. 190). The walls may be approximated from the extrinsic pressure from a normal spleen or normal ribs (figs. 187–189). The approximation of the walls thins out the barium in the narrowed region and this may have the appearance of an intraluminal defect. Putting the patient in different positions will clear the dilemma.

TONE OF THE STOMACH

The stomach can be considered either orthotonic, hypertonic or hypotonic. This estimation is made, with the stomach filled with opaque media, by comparison (as in figures 191–194) of the relative widths of upper and lower parts of the gastric lumen.[5] In *hypertonic* or "steer horn stomach" the lumen is widest above and narrower at the antrum. There is practically no incisura angularis and the stomach more or less lies

distributed obliquely across the spine. The division into horizontal and vertical portions is not evident.

In the *orthotonic* stomach the incisura angularis is well marked. The lumen above in the fundus of the stomach is approximately equal in diameter to the lumen within the antrum. The vertical portion is seen to the left of the spine, ending at the incisura angularis. The horizontal portion or antral region crosses the spine. The greater curvature usually extends down to about the intercristal level.

In the *hypotonic* stomach the diameter of the fundus is less than the antral region. The most dependent portion of the greater curvature often lies close to the symphysis pubis. The *atonic* stomach is an exaggeration of the hypotonic stomach. It hangs with its vertical walls approximated and touching with the foot of the stomach dilated and pouch-like. The normal relation-

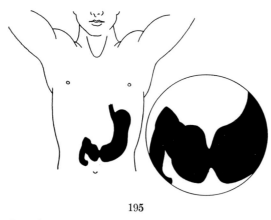

195

Question:

The antrum and bulb appear persistently normal in this position. Why must the examiner not be content with his findings?

Answer:

Because often in this position the distal antrum and bulb are directed from before backwards, and therefore there is a superimposition of shadows concealing existing defects.

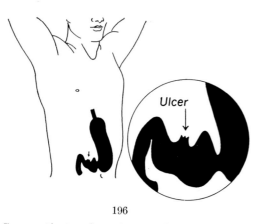

196

Same patient as figure 195 examined in the right anterior oblique position reveals a constant and persistent deformity, as of an ulcer.

ship of the transverse or third portion of the duodenum to the cap is characteristic (cf. figs. 193, 194). It should be noted that in the atonic stomach this third portion of the duodenum lies at the same level as the base of the duodenal cap. This arrangement prevails because the base of the duodenal cap is pulled down by the atonic stomach, but the third portion of the duodenum is held up in position by the ligament of Trietz.

POSITIONING DURING FLUOROSCOPY

The beginner in radiology may wonder why a defect is called constant, yet does not appear on all films taken during the examination. A stomach may be the seat of a serious abnormality although it may appear entirely normal when viewed in the frontal (i.e., postero-anterior) position. Thus a gastric ulcer, usually distinguished as a projection from the posterior wall,[5a] may not be seen if the patient is examined in the frontal position (cf. figs. 195 and 196). This is because in this latter position the lesser and greater curvatures are seen in profile, and any projections from these will become clearly evident, but a projection from the back wall of the stomach will not be seen since it is not in profile. It thus becomes important to know how to position the patient in order that the posterior gastric wall can be seen in profile by the fluoroscopist. Following the same reasoning, the understanding of exactly which walls are seen in profile with the patient in each position must be achieved. With this in mind, the following section is presented.

In the several different types of stomach as described above, the antral region, pyloric sphincter and duodenal cap are disposed not only from left to right but also backwards. In the hypertonic type of stomach this region turns slowly backwards, starting at a variable point in the distal portion of the antrum so that by the time the cap is reached, this first portion of the duodenum is directed backwards and upwards and slightly to the right. In the orthotonic type of stomach the distal antral region is directed upwards and when the first portion of the duodenum is reached, this latter structure points backwards and upwards. In the hypotonic type the distal antrum is so directed that the duodenal cap is directed upward and slightly to the left.[5]

The importance of the various stomach and duodenal directions will make itself evident upon a moment's reflection. In al-

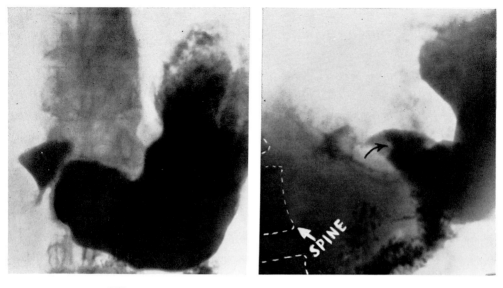

197   198

In the anterior-posterior projection (fig. 197), this stomach appears normal. See figure 198: The stomach viewed in another angle reveals a defect (arrow).

In the fluoroscopic examination, since the patient in front of the examining physician is positioned at will, the position of the organ is obvious to the examiner. When the examiner is confronted with a *film*, however, he must use other means to determine the *position* in which the organ is seen. In figure 198, for example, the stomach shown in figure 197 is now viewed from a different angle and reveals a defect (arrow). To determine the angle used, the *position* of the spine as seen in *relation to the stomach* will provide the clue. Note in 197 the spine is behind the stomach and in 198 the patient is seen from the side, since the spine is now rotated to the side of the stomach.

most any one of these types of stomach, wherever the antrum is bent and directed from before backwards, if one observes this region only in the frontal plane (patient facing the examiner) it will be analogous to looking through the open end of a tube. To see the profile of the side walls of such a tube, one would turn it so that it is seen from the side. Likewise, to see the profile of the side walls of the stomach the patient should be turned to one side, i.e., right anterior oblique position (previously defined) (figs. 195, 196). If the distal portion of the antrum and pyloric sphincter as well as the duodenal cap lies directly behind the stomach, as with a stout individual, only a true lateral position will demonstrate these contours.

The physician need not necessarily memorize all these positions. What *is* important

to remember is that behind the fluoroscopic screen the patient is to be rotated until the portion of stomach in question is seen in its *greatest length*. In this position the examiner can consider he is getting the best side view of the part under study. This procedure is called "laying out" the part, and this same principle can be applied to colonic examination.

It is important for the examiner to understand the exact lateral position of the stomach within the body. As in figure 199 B a side view of the patient reveals the stomach is distributed more or less obliquely, with the fundus or upper portion being posterior, the antral or lower end being anterior. This knowledge is important since when the patient is placed in the supine position the opaque media will fall posteriorly into the fundus and the air within the stomach will

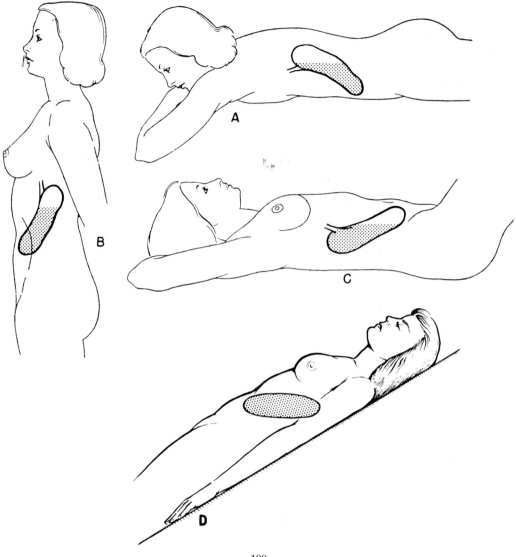

199

Because of the oblique disposition of the stomach in the body, note how *air contrast studies* of different portions of the stomach may be accomplished by *changing the patient's position.* (Similarly, note how barium may be directed by the examiner into different parts of the stomach.)

A. Patient prone: Air in the fundus, barium within the antrum and the body of the stomach.

B. Patient erect: Same as A.

C. Patient supine: This examination lends itself to air contrast studies of the antrum. The air in this position *rises* to the antrum; if a barium mixture is present within the stomach, it will gravitate towards the fundus. With the patient in the Trendelenberg position, and the stomach so "tipped" that its contents tend to pour into the esophagus (left side off the table), a hiatus hernia may best be made evident.

D. Patient supine at 45 degree angle. This position allows complete filling of the stomach.

Table 1.—*The Six Positions for Proper Examination of Stomach and Duodenum*

1. Erect Frontal. (fig. 200)
   a. Gastric walls in profile. Lesser and greater curvature
   b. Duodenal walls in profile. Lesser and greater curvature
   c. Miscellaneous
      (1) Antrum may overlie first portion of duodenum
      (2) Descending duodenum may overlie first portion of duodenum
      (3) Distal portion of antrum and duodenum often directed from before backwards and to the right

2. Erect Right Anterior Oblique. (fig. 201)
   a. Gastric walls in profile. Posterior and anterior
   b. Duodenal walls in profile. Lesser and greater curvatures
   c. Miscellaneous
      (1) Duodenal cap free from overlying antrum and descending portion of duodenum

3. Erect Left Anterior Oblique. (fig. 202)
   a. Gastric walls in profile. Anterior and posterior
   b. Duodenal walls in profile. Anterior and posterior
   c. Miscellaneous
      (1) Posterior wall of duodenum may not be seen unless the palpating hand pushes the stomach back towards the spine

4. Supine Frontal. These profiles are essentially the same as for the erect frontal
   a. Miscellaneous
      (1) Barium gravitates upwards and distends fundus (fig. 199)
      (2) Air contrast study of antrum and cap (fig. 199)

5. Supine Right Anterior Oblique. The profiles are essentially the same as for the right anterior oblique
   a. Miscellaneous
      (1) Barium gravitates as in section 4 above; similar air contrast studies (fig. 199)
      Note: With the palpating hand the fluoroscopist can lift the greater curvature upwards towards the epigastrium and so best see the duodenal jejunal flexure

6. Prone Left Posterior Oblique. (fig. 203)
   a. Gastric walls in profile. Posterior and anterior
   b. Duodenal walls in profile. Lesser and greater curvature
   c. Miscellaneous
      (1) Barium mixture is now within the pars media and antrum
      (2) Peristalsis best visualized
      (3) Cap free from overlying shadows of antrum and descending loops of duodenum

rise into the antrum. Thus air-contrast studies of the antral region can be secured. On the other hand, with the patient placed in the prone position, the gastric contents can be expected to travel downwards into the antral region and air-contrast studies of the fundus can thus be secured (fig. 199).

For a proper examination of the stomach and duodenum, the examiner should view each patient in at least six different positions. Table 1 and the illustrations indicated therein should be understood carefully, and applied methodically.

FLUOROSCOPIC FIELDS

The proper usage of the fluoroscopic shutters is extremely important for protection of examiner as well as patient; also, through correct application secondary radiation is diminished and finer detail is secured on the fluoroscopic screen. Throughout this discussion no specific directions will be given as to where to employ a small or large fluoroscopic field. But knowledge of this is of primary importance, and the rationale has been discussed in another chapter. The rule in handling of the shutters is first to view the entire field through as large a fluoroscopic opening as the screen permits, remembering, as described under "Protection," to have the shutters arranged so that a shutter or lead frame is seen on each side of the field. Having oriented himself, the examiner then selects and "cones down" on specific regions. The aperture through the diaphragmatic shutters is reduced and as small a field as possible secured. With repetition and experience, the handling of this mechanism becomes automatic.

BARIUM MIXTURE

A watery unflavored barium mixture is usually used for this study. This consists of a half glass of barium powder to which sufficient water is added to fill the glass. The mixture should be prepared with a mechanical mixer since an emulsion not allowing barium globs or large air bubbles is desirable. The preparation should be at room temperature. Cold solutions may cause gastric spasm.

The contrast medium to be used is important only in that it should be fluid enough to flow easily, and at the same time be sufficiently dense to obscure on the screen all bone and soft tissue detail, even in fairly thin layers. Flavored suspending agents usually produce too fluid a mixture and are still ineffective in disguising the taste of the barium sulfate.[6] A drop of peppermint oil to a glass results in fewer objections to the mixture.[3]

Fluoroscopic Procedure

The actual fluoroscopic examination of the stomach may be divided into five stages. Each of these stages will be considered with the following questions in mind: What is the position of the patient? How much barium should the stomach contain? What is the purpose for this stage? What is the method employed? This section should be read with constant reference to figures 200–203.

STAGE I

Position. Erect frontal (fig. 200).
Gastric Contents. Fasting stomach.
Purpose. Gross pathological deviations in the chest, mediastinum and diaphragm as well as abdomen are sought.
Method of Examination. The examination is performed on the fasting stomach. The patient, standing on a small platform with his stomach just above the examiner's eye-level, is placed behind the fluoroscopic screen facing the examiner (frontal position). The chest is first studied in its entirely. The cardiac contours and mediastinum are observed. Next, starting at the apices and traveling down toward the diaphragm, the chest is studied segmentally. The mobility of the diaphragm is determined. The screen is next carried downwards and the entire abdomen is surveyed. Any abnormal calcifications are sought for and noted. Occasionally opaque gallstones or renal calculi as well as calcified mesenteric nodes may be found.

Any abnormal air distention of the bowel should be noted. The examiner then focuses his attention on the cardiac end of the stomach or magenblase. Normally, a small bubble of air should be present. If this is not visible, and if the patient has not recently eructated some gas, an obstruction higher up (in the esophagus or pharynx) must be suspected. The presence or absence of a fluid level within the stomach air bubble indicating secretion is then determined. Any encroachment into the normal round air bubble is searched for, the examiner being ever mindful of the normal impressions occasionally made by either the heart, liver or spleen (figs. 204, 205, 206). The thin narrow space between the diaphragm and the su-

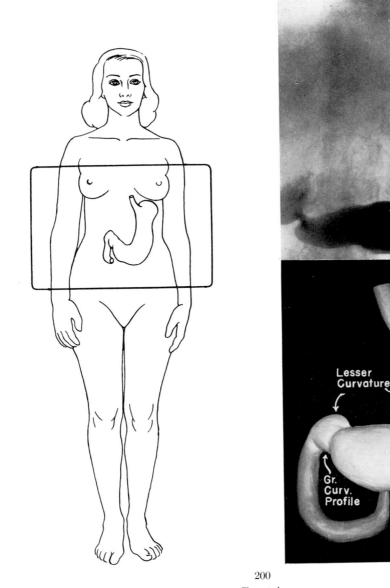

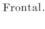

200

Frontal.

Question:

What are the important advantages of the frontal position?

Answer:

Ulcers projecting from the lesser and greater curvatures may be seen in profile.

Question:

What are the important disadvantages of this position?

Answer:

1. Posterior wall ulcers cannot be seen. Only with the stomach in a relatively empty state or by using compression may a posterior wall ulcer be seen "en face" in this position.

2. Examining the distal antrum and duodenal cap in this position is often analogous to examining a tube by looking through its open end, i.e., no completely satisfactory examination of the antrum and duodenum may be performed in this position.

Comment: The right anterior oblique position (fig. 201) corrects the disadvantages of this position.

163

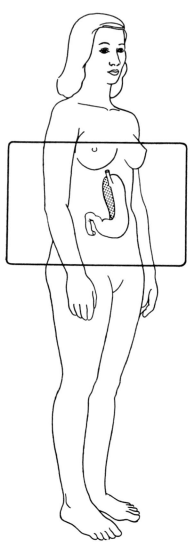

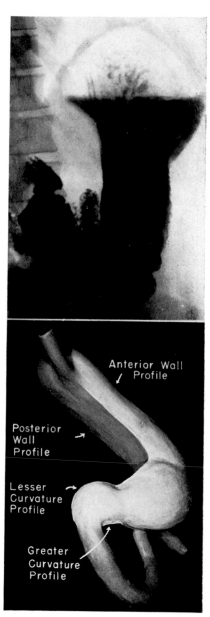

201

Right anterior oblique.

Question:

What are the advantages of this position?

Answer:

1. The posterior *gastric wall* is examined in profile, and an ulcer frequently found here may be seen as a projection.

2. Note that the distal antrum and cap is "laid out" and examined in profile. (Compared with fig. 200.)

Comment: This position corrects the deficiencies of the frontal position (fig. 200).

Question:

What are the disadvantages of this position?

Answer:

1. The anterior and posterior walls of the *cap* are not seen in profile; thus an ulcer projecting from the posterior surface will not be seen except "en face." (See fig. 202; cf. figs. 231, 232.)

2. The lesser and greater gastric curvatures cannot be adequately examined in profile.

164

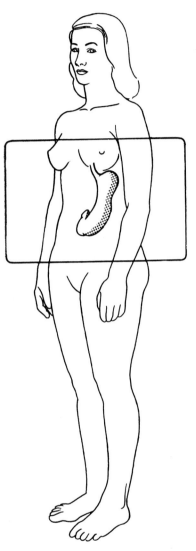

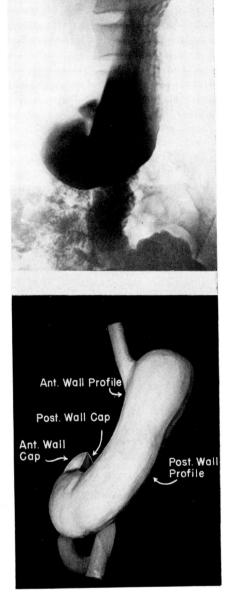

202

Left anterior oblique.

Question:

   What are the important advantages of this position?

Answer:

   The anterior and posterior walls of the cap can be examined in profile. (See figs. 231 and 232.)

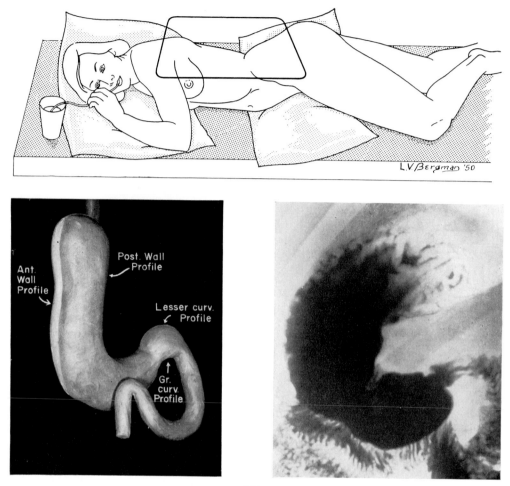

Ant.
Wall
Profile

Post. Wall
Profile

Lesser curv.
Profile

Gr.
curv.
Profile

203

This is the strategic position.

1. Since ulcers are common on the posterior gastric wall, it is this wall which is in profile in this position.

2. The duodenal bulb is "laid out" in profile.

3. With the patient prone, peristalsis is more pronounced and thus easier to study.

Comment: This has all the advantages of the right anterior oblique position, but in addition peristalsis can be more easily observed.

Barium normally enters the stomach air bubble as a single stream.

perior margin of the fundus is next sought for and observed (fig. 26). Any undue thickening or widening of this space in the *erect* position should be considered pathological until proved otherwise. On rare occasions only can the normal diaphragm, liver or spleen cause such a widening.

STAGE II

Position. Erect: frontal, right anterior oblique, left anterior oblique (figs. 200–202).

Gastric Contents. One to two swallows of barium mixture.

Purpose. The examiner seeks to determine

first whether the passage of the opaque material into the stomach is normal. Unless a lesion of the esophagus is suspected, the examination of the esophagus is ignored at this stage and the entrance into the cardia is observed. He will bear in mind that the barium mixture should enter the stomach through the cardiac sphincter as a single stream (figs. 207, 208). If the stream is split, it is probably pathological (fig. 209).

Next the stomach proper is studied. With the first few swallows of barium, sufficient opaque material will enter to coat the stomach walls and permit study of the gastric mucosal pattern. The examiner knows the basic pattern and will seek it. Deviations in rugal pattern must be proved normal by being flexible and mobile. The examiner is ever mindful that the normal mucosal pattern can be distorted by applied pressure (fig. 178) and may even become obliterated if the pressure is too great. He will at this time try also to wash the opaque material into every nook and crevice in an effort to uncover any craters in and between the gastric rugae. When opaque mixture lodges in an ulcer, he must determine whether this is a true ulcer crater or a glob of barium accidentally caught up between two adjacent mucosal folds (figs. 211, 212), producing an ulcer-like shadow, i.e., a "persistent fleck."

If after repeated attempts he can not dislodge the "persistent fleck" he will suspect an ulcer. A further manifestation of a true ulcer niche will be its oval contours (fig. 212). The examiner's suspicions must be further confirmed as described in the next stages.

Pain and tenderness is also sought for and its relationship to the part palpated noted.

Method of Examination. The patient is placed in the right anterior oblique position and asked to take one or two swallows of the barium mixture. At this time the esophagus is ignored and the entry into the stom-

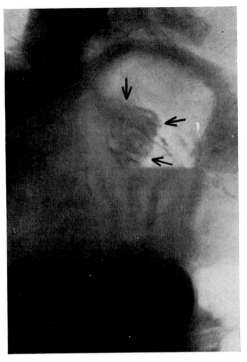

204

A tumor mass (arrows) is seen projecting into the stomach air bubble. The normal gastric air bubble should be round. Normal deformities within the bubble must first be ruled out before any finding is determined as abnormal. (Cf. fig. 26B.)

ach is carefully studied. Normally, this should be in a single stream (figs. 207, 208).

In the hypertonic type stomach a wedge is soon formed (fig. 213) by the opaque media which slowly travels down and fills out the entire gastric lumen. In the hypotonic type stomach the barium mixture without wedge formation will quickly sink down to the greater curvature or lower pole of the stomach.

The patient is next rotated into the true frontal position and the barium within the stomach is spread or washed over the mucosa. The gastric walls and mucosal pattern are studied and for this they must be opacified with a thin layer of barium. This is accomplished in a very simple manner when the opaque material is already dif-

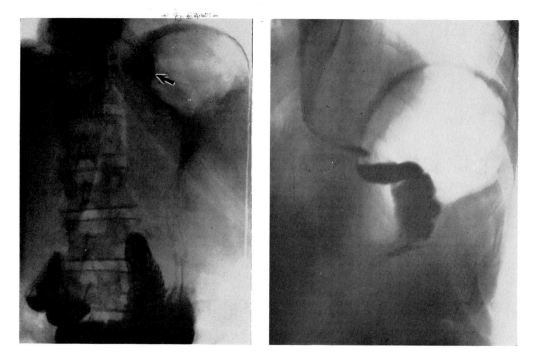

205   206

Question:

    The arrow (fig. 205) demonstrates the normal indenture of the liver onto the stomach fundus; in cases of doubt, how may the normalcy of this shadow be determined?

Answer:

    With further distention of the stomach fundus (fig. 206), the distended mobile fundus may push itself away from the liver. Often, with some rotation into the left anterior oblique position, the stomach fundus can be separated from the liver shadow. Normalcy is further confirmed by seeing a normal entry of barium through the esophagus into the stomach.

fusely spread through the stomach. Pressure is applied with the fingertips and the gastric mucosa "pressed" upon in an effort to spread the folds apart. Pressing too deeply may obliterate the rugae completely. A method of studying the mucosal pattern recommended by Barclay[3] is for the examiner to press with his hand on the stomach as as to halt the entry of barium just as it enters, then gradually to allow the hand to move down so that the opaque material follows slowly, outlining the mucosal pattern. In cases where the entire barium mixture has already gravitated to the lower pole of the stomach, the mucosa may be studied by placing the hand directly below the stomach so that the opaque material rests immediately above the fingertips.[5] The opaque media is now slowly pushed upwards as high as possible within the stomach. This is called "washing" the gastric mucosa and provides adequate observation of the gastric relief pattern[4] (fig. 214).

The study of the gastric rugae is performed methodically. With the first sweep of the examiner's hand upwards, it is suggested that the lesser curvature be observed and defects in this region sought for. As the hand moves down and the folds slip out from beneath the fingers, it is suggested that the middle of the gastric lumen be observed. Finally, when the hand is carried up again, the greater curvature should be studied. The same procedure is carried out for all acces-

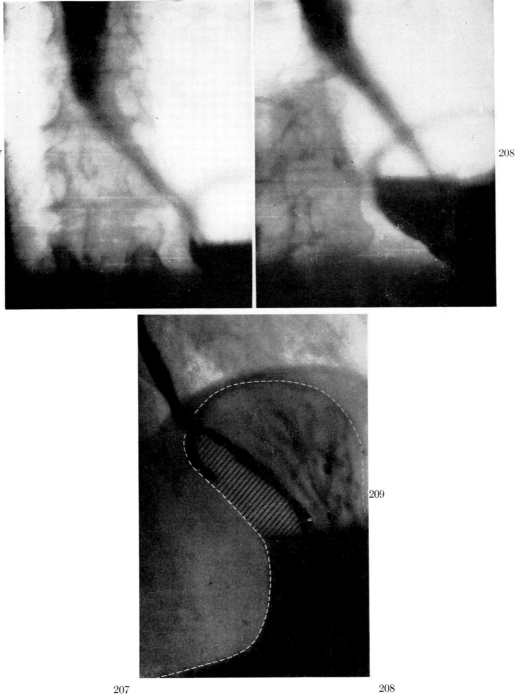

207

Normal entry of barium into stomach. Frontal view.

208

Normal entry of barium. Right anterior oblique view.

209

The flow of barium is split abnormally by a tumor, as the barium enters the stomach.

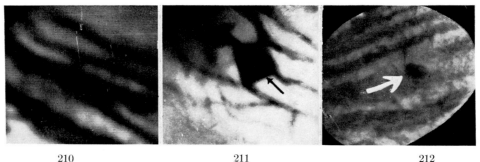

210

Normal gastric rugae.

211

212

Question: Which of these barium flecks is a true ulcer crater?

1. This barium fleck washes away with the massaging hand.

2. This barium fleck has "square" margins.

3. This barium fleck is not apt to appear in the same place with repeat examinations.

A fleck with the above characteristics is a false crater.

1. This barium fleck does not wash away easily with the massaging hand.

2. This barium fleck has oval margins.

3. This barium fleck should reappear with repeat examinations.

A fleck with the above characteristics is a true crater.

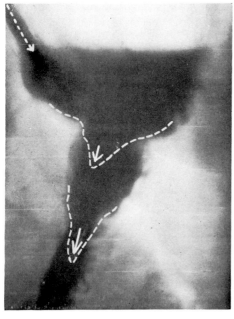

213

Barium normally enters the stomach in a single stream. In the hypersthenic stomach it next descends in wedgelike fashion.

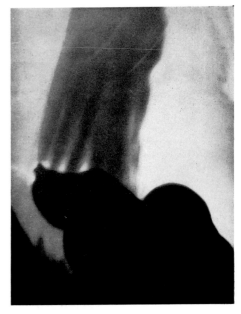

214

The palpating fingers press on the stomach with sufficient pressure to push most of the barium out of the way. The pressure must not be great enough to remove *all* the barium *nor to obliterate the mucosal folds.* The mucosal pattern is studied immediately above the fingertips.

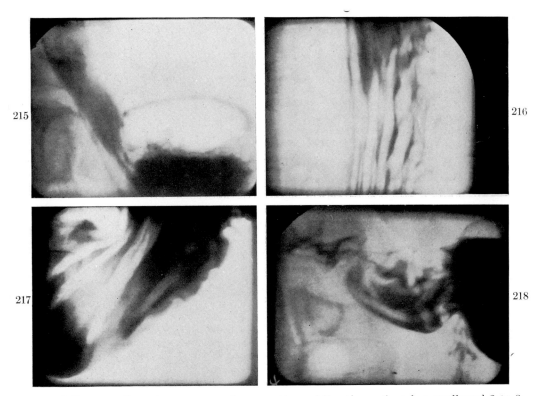

Rapid film recording of mucous membrane pattern. After the patient has swallowed 2 to 3 mouthfuls of barium, the fluoroscopic screen with the attached compression device is carried down and successive films taken of:

215	216
Esophageal entry into stomach normal.	Verticle portion of the stomach normal.

217	218
Region of incisura angularis normal.	Antrum normal.

sible portions of the stomach. The duodenal cap, if it appears at this time, may be studied in the same manner. When the hand is washing the stomach like a brush, it is also attempting to spread the barium mixture into all crevices and nooks.

Flexibility as well as mobility of the various accessible mucosal patterns is determined. The duodenal cap may appear at this time but filling will probably be inadequate and thus not permit ample study. No special effort should be made to fill this first portion of the duodenum during this stage, since barium within the duodenal loop and jejunum may obstruct further study of the stomach.

The mucosal pattern as seen fluoroscopically should next be visualized on the radiographic film. A simple method of doing this is to move the fluoroscopic screen and take consecutive spot films, first of a single mouthful of barium entering the stomach. Next the screen, together with the spot filming device, is carried over the opacified gastric contour, and, by means of graded compression, spot films are taken of the pars media (vertical portion of the stomach), the region of the incisura angularis (junction of the vertical and horizontal portions) and finally, the antrum (figs. 215–222).

If peristalsis is now present the relation-

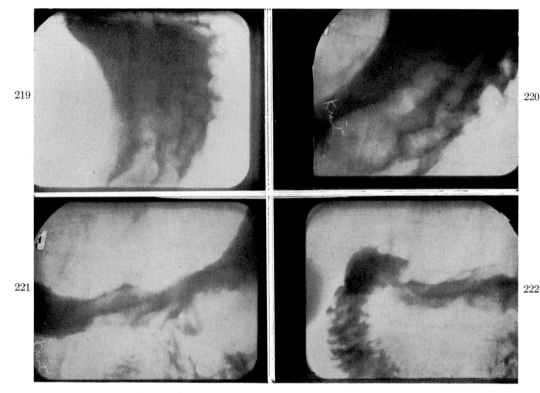

Abnormal mucous membrane pattern (cf. figs. 215–218).

219

Verticle portion of stomach reveals thick folds (lower portion of spot film). (Cf. fig. 216.)

220

Region of incisura angularis reveals thick folds. (Cf. lower portion of folds, fig. 217.)

221

Antrum reveals destruction and distortion of mucosa. (Cf. fig. 218.)

222

Antrum reveals destruction and distortion of mucosa. (Cf. fig. 218.)

ship and distortion of the mucosal pattern by the various waves is also noted (fig. 181A).

STAGE III

Position. Erect: frontal (fig. 200), right anterior oblique (fig. 201), and left anterior oblique (fig. 202).

Gastric Contents. Glass full of barium mixture in stomach. This entire stage may be delayed until Stage IV or V.

Purpose. The examiner now wishes to examine *the full stomach.* The stomach in a contracted, more or less empty state, may be suitable for gastric rugal studies, but this

has its disadvantages. The fluoroscopist is aware that large craters with heaped-up edges which are more or less approximated when the stomach is not fully distended, may not fill with opaque media (figs. 267–272). This will be only the more true if the ulcer lies hidden between several closely approximated gastric rugae. The examiner knows that by filling the stomach the rugae will be spread apart, allowing barium mixture to enter the formerly inaccessible crater. The observer also knows that if the stomach contains only enough barium to spread out on the foot of the stomach, he may occasionally miss a crater high up behind the ribs where the palpating hand

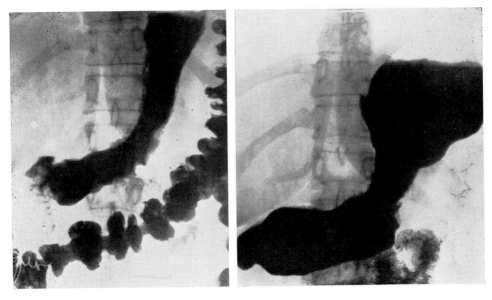

223   224

The stomach seen in figure 223 appears well filled. Yet, the same stomach with further filling seen in figure 224 reveals a constricting lesion in its midsection, with dilatations above and below.

Comment: Although the stomach may appear full, at least once during an examination the stomach should be filled and seen when it contains the full complement of barium to be given (16 ounces).

cannot wash the barium mixture. This, too, will prompt him to give the full quota of opaque media. The inadequate filling, so valuable for mucosal studies, also may not permit efficient study of the gastric contours (figs. 267–272).

The true position of the stomach as it hands in the abdomen cannot be properly appraised in this comparatively empty state. Pressure defects from extra-gastric masses may not make themselves evident unless the various gastric and duodenal contours are ballooned out.

The magenblase holding only one or two swallows of opaque media (i.e., the empty stomach), will not permit as efficient a study as when many swallows follow one another (i.e., the full stomach), since with each swallow a little air is carried down to rise into the fundus. This air trapped within the fundus will distend it, and better air-

contrast studies of this region are thus permitted (figs. 204 and 227–230).

Another important reason for having the stomach filled at this time is to permit more adequate study of the duodenal cap. Furthermore, with increased distention of the walls, peristalsis makes itself more evident.

Last but not least, up to this time the pharynx and esophagus have as yet not been adequately examined. During the additional filling of the stomach the examiner may study these. Because of the advantage secured in the slowing of the opaque media in the horizontal position, this part of the examination could be profitably delayed until this latter position has been reached.

Method of Examination. The screen is centered over the pharynx and the patient is asked to swallow. The passage of the barium mixture through this region is observed. Each bolus is followed throughout

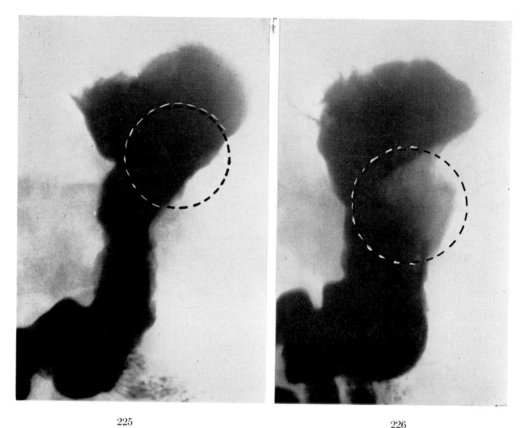

225

The stomach here appears filled.

226

The same stomach as in figure 225, with further increments of opaque media, reveals a defect (encircled) not seen in figure 225.

Comment: The stomach in figure 225 appears full. Some portions of it were not completely distended. The examiner must make certain that during any examination the stomach must be seen at least once with its full complement of opaque media (16 ounces).

its entire course until it enters the stomach. The various normal esophageal contours are observed, and, as the barium bolus descends, the normal distensibility of the esophagus as well as any defects are noted.

With the patient in the frontal position, the position of the stomach is noted (fig. 200). Its relationship to surrounding organs is observed. The fundus is examined next and the air bubble will now appear more distended and distinct than formerly, since air has been swallowed with each swallow of barium mixture. The gastric lumen distended by the additional barium, the rugal folds more widely separated, the examiner

continues his search for craters and other mucosal abnormalities. The palpating hand will push aside sufficient barium mixture so that the mucosal pattern and gastric contour can be observed. This observation is performed methodically, first the lesser curvature, then the mid-portion of the stomach and finally the greater curvature. Flexibility and mobility are determined. Any defects are noted and barium mixture is washed over these in an effort either to fill them out or perhaps obliterate them.

It is important in studying the gastric and duodenal contours to use only just enough pressure to force excess barium aside

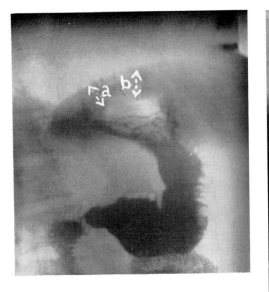

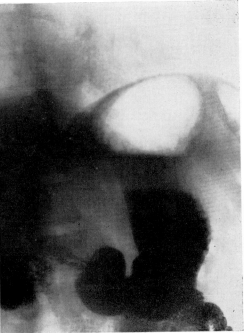

227   228

Question:

The distance between the superior margin of the fundus and the lung above (arrows A and B) is increased beyond the normal. The roof of the fundus is also deformed. Is an abnormalcy present?

Answer:

The same stomach fundus is now fully distended with air. The roof of the fundus is smooth and the space between the roof of the fundus and the lung above is now normal.

Comment: Incomplete air distention of the *normal* fundus may cause the apparent abnormal changes in figure 227. The distance between the roof of the fundus and the lung above should normally measure from 5 to 15 mm. This, however, must be appraised only when the fundus is properly distended with air. Similarly, the smoothness of the fundal roof can be appraised only when the fundus is properly distended with air (see fig. 228).

so that the folds are seen. Too much pressure will obliterate them entirely. Peristalsis, if it is present, may now be observed also, although this phenomenon can be better appraised in the prone position.

For the examination to be complete at this stage, the patient must be examined in both oblique positions. The fluoroscopist utilizes the right anterior oblique position for optimum study of the antrum, pyloric sphincter and duodenal bulb (fig. 201). If the "cap" or bulb is not seen, maneuvers to fill it as described below should be performed. The bulb being completely filled, its various contours are examined in the

right anterior oblique position. The searching hand will smooth out and examine the mucosal pattern and try to determine the presence of any deformity. An attempt will be made, if the first portion of the duodenum is accessible, to wash or massage the opaque media into any craters. The patient is next turned to the left anterior oblique position. The contour of the anterior gastric wall may now be studied, any defects being noted. The *anterior* and occasionally the *posterior walls* of the duodenum are also brought into profile and defects noted (figs. 231 and 232).

The entire duodenal sweep is next ob-

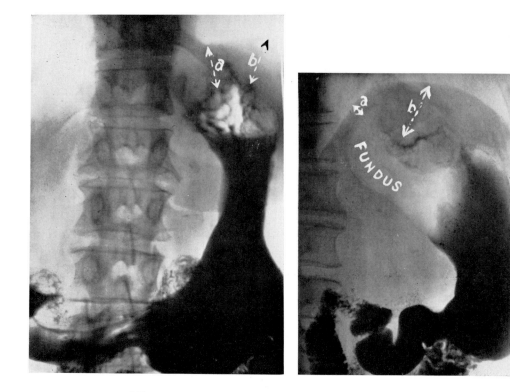

229

230

The space as indicated by arrows a and b, separating the roof of the fundus from the lung above, is increased beyond the normal. The roof of the fundus itself is grossly deformed as it projects into the stomach air bubble (see fig. 230).

The same stomach as figure 229, with the fundus now properly distended with air, reveals the region of arrow a to be normal. The region of arrow b reveals a tumor projecting into the stomach air bubble, and the tumor itself causes an increase in the distance from the base of the lung to the roof of the stomach (arrow b).

served. The duodenum forms a loop which is more or less fixed to the posterior abdominal wall. The duodenal arc curves like the letter "C." Variations in the curves of the duodenum have been recognized (figs. 233–236). The mucosal pattern within the bulb has been described as basically parallel (fig. 175). At the apex of the bulb the feathery appearance produced by the valvulae conniventes (or Kerkring's folds) starts and is continued through the entire loop and into the jejunum.

Motility within the sweep starts with a contraction of the bulb and is visualized as a sudden overflow of the first portion into the second or descending portions. Peristaltic waves propel the food through the de-

scending, transverse and ascending portion of the duodenum. Another type of movement other than a peristaltic wave which may be seen in this region is a rhythmic segmentation which produces a to-and-fro movement. Antiperistalsis is commonly seen in both normal and abnormal conditions and is found in the second and third portions of the duodenum. It is seen as a localized contraction forcing the opaque material backwards. These movements have been described by Bolton and Salmond.[8]

STAGE IV

Position. Horizontal supine, and right anterior oblique (gastric profiles similar to figs. 200, 201). With the patient still supine.

he is next slowly rotated with the left shoulder up, i.e., slowly onto his right side.

Gastric Contents. One glass of barium mixture.

Purpose. Barium which in the erect position could not reach and enter all of the various nooks and crevices, as well as ulcer craters within the stomach and duodenum, even though the stomach was filled, may do so in the horizontal position. The examiner knows that with barium gravitating into the fundus in the supine position (fig. 199 C), a defect here may become evident (figs. 169–171). In this position, also, since the barium gravitates upward toward the diaphragm, a hiatus hernia may possibly be discovered. Air contrast studies of the antral region may also be secured, because in this position air from the cardia travels down to the pyloric end of the stomach (fig. 199 C). Finally, with the patient supine and the right shoulder brought a little forward, the duodenal sweep is best seen. If, now, with the patient in this position the palpating hand of the examiner pushes the greater curvature of the stomach up towards the diaphragm, the duodenal-jejunal flexure may be brought into view. Next the examiner should attempt to demonstrate lesser curvature ulcers high up in the stomach near the cardia. This is described below under Method of Examination and gone into more fully in the section on DIFFICULTIES AND VARIATIONS (Schatzki maneuver).

Method of Examination. The patient is next placed in the supine position with his right side closer to the screen. (Note that the gastric profiles are similar to figures 200 and 201.) Air-contrast and mucosal studies of the antrum are obtained as the barium in the body of the stomach exchanges position with the air in the fundus. The duodenal bulb may also be seen in air-contrast if the duodenal mucosa is coated with the opaque media, and air from the antrum passes through the pyloric opening.

After examining the bulb and antrum, the fundus is studied next. The various

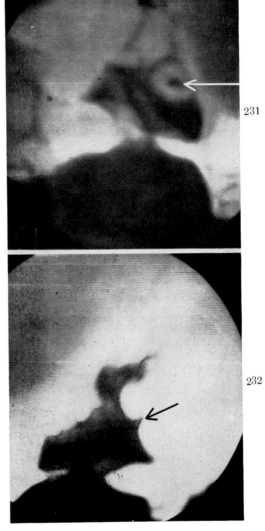

231

232

231

The duodenal cap examined in the right anterior oblique (fig. 178) reveals with compression studies an ulcer (arrow) "en face."

232

The same patient examined in the left anterior oblique (fig. 179) reveals the ulcer as a projection from the posterior profile of the cap.

folds may be obliterated by overdistention with barium mixture. With deep inspiration and expiration, some change in this region may occur (narrowing with inspiration).[4] These respiratory changes may not be readily seen, but nevertheless once learned, they

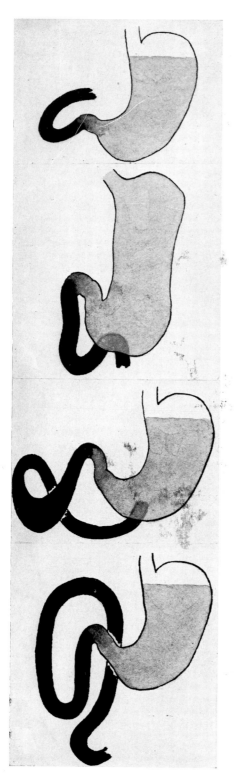

Variations in the course of the duodenal sweep.

Figures 233 and 236 are examples of mobile duodenum.

233
Demonstrates the patient in the erect position.

234
Demonstrates the same patient as in figure 167 in the prone position.

235
A variation in the duodenal sweep.

236
A variation in the duodenal sweep.

can be useful in determining flexibility of this part of the stomach. Finally, the duodenal sweep and duodenal-jejunal flexures are observed. For the latter, the supine position with the right shoulder brought slightly forward is useful. The palpating hand lifts the greater curvature of the stomach upwards, thus uncovering the duodenal-jejunal flexure behind.

This being completed, the patient is again placed in the supine position. The left shoulder is slowly raised, i.e., the fundus is raised, and the patient is slowly moved onto his right side. With this maneuver the barium in the fundus is made to pour as from a cup down along the path of the lesser curvature into the stomach below. This is done slowly and under direct visual control. The examiner should note that with the left shoulder raised the fundus and the left side of the stomach—the greater curvature—become higher and the lesser curvature lower. Barium is thus, by aid of gravity, permitted to enter into any ulcer craters of the lesser curvature which may have previously been missed. This is described more fully in the section on special variations (page 187 and figs. 247, 248).

STAGE V

Position. Prone left posterior oblique (fig. 203).

Gastric Contents. (As in Stage IV.)

Purpose. The observer not only wishes to see more of the posterior gastric wall, but also wants to observe gastric peristalsis more adequately. In this position, both can be accomplished. As a matter of fact, it is often the best position in which to watch peristalsis. The cap and duodenal sweep are also clearly visible. This has been called the "strategic" position.

In this position, too, the esophagus is clear of the spine. Many prefer this position for viewing the esophagus and therefore delay filling of the stomach until this stage. When this is done, Stage V precedes Stage IV.

Method of Examination. With the table still in the horizontal position and the patient lying supine, he is now asked to turn and lie on his stomach with his left shoulder closer to the screen (fig. 203). It is wise to direct the patient to turn with his right side down. In this manner it is obvious that the barium from the fundus will be tipped into the antrum and duodenum (fig. 199 A). Gastric peristalsis and filling of the duodenal bulb are noted. Occasionally it may be necessary to achieve a greater degree of left posterior oblique to free the duodenum from the overlying spine and gastric antrum.

DIFFICULTIES AND VARIATIONS

The course of the duodenal sweep may be varied (figs. 233–236). The various loops, however, may be easily detected by watching the barium flow. It is often a matter of trial and error to find the position in which the duodenal cap is best visualized in such cases.

An interesting anomaly is the mobile duodenum. This is illustrated in figures 233 and 234. It will be noted that the position of the sweep will depend upon the position of the patient, i.e., whether standing or recumbent.

In the prone position, *the antral region of the stomach may be compressed between the table below and spine above.* This does not permit adequate antral study. This difficulty can be overcome by supporting the chest and hips on pillows, thus raising the spine off the table (fig. 203).

Cascade Stomach. The cascade or "cup and spill" type of stomach can be considered for practical purposes as caused by a draping of the stomach over the gas filled colon below so that the fundus or upper end is posterior and the antrum or lower end is anterior. The middle of the stomach, as in figure 256 is constricted by pressure from structures beneath.

Barium entering this type of stomach will enter into the fundal "cup" above and become trapped. When sufficient opaque media accumulates, the "cup" or fundus becomes filled to the brim. With additional barium mixture a spilling-over occurs into the antrum below (figs. 289, 290). The spilling is usually in an anterior direction, but may on occasion go to either side.

Until the examiner is thoroughly acquainted with the mode of barium entry into a cascade stomach, this may cause him confusion. The first puzzle he encounters is seeing the barium come down, enter into the cardia and fundus, but not make further descent. With further increments of barium and with the patient so positioned that the examiner can see the barium travel out of the fundus and into the body of the stomach, it may appear to the inexperienced observer that the barium is travelling over a mass (fig. 287). The difficulty may be overcome by remembering that in the cascade stomach the formation of two fluid levels—one within the fundal region of the stomach and the other at the foot of the stomach—is an important clue to the diagnosing of the type of stomach seen. A fuller understanding of this can be secured by comparing figures 289, 290 with figure 288.

The examiner may have difficulty in properly filling such a stomach. In this event, he will try to "tip" the contents of the fundus above into the antrum below. To accomplish this he may have to place the patient in various positions, testing the ingenuity of the examiner. Often, by asking the patient to bend forward as far as possible and lean from one side to the next, he may achieve the same end. Upon entering the foot of this type of stomach, the weight of the barium mixture, if sufficient in amount, may pull it straight. Should this fail, emptying the colon of its gas by an enema or cathartic may often cause the cascade to disappear. Other suggested causes for this type of stomach are a localized spasm or a contraction of some epigastric adhesions.

Finding the Duodenal Bulb (fig. 175).

The inexperienced examiner occasionally has difficulty in determining which exactly of the opaque structures on the screen is the duodenal bulb. A portion of the antrum separated from the rest of the stomach by a deep peristaltic wave may often deceive him (fig. 181 B). The duodenal bulb may be identified in these ways: (1) Barium, upon leaving the bulb, spills over and travels *downwards* into the second portion of the duodenum. On the other hand, barium within the gastric antrum usually will travel in a horizontal or upward direction and no "spill over" takes place. *A method useful in finding the bulb would be to observe at which point the barium makes its descent, and that portion immediately proximal to this must be the bulb.* (2) The Kerkring folds starting at the apex of the bulb can be used as a landmark (fig. 175). (3) The pyloric sphincter is a useful landmark in finding the bulb. This may often have to be differentiated from a peristaltic wave. The former is a constant space which separates the bulb from the antrum, whereas the latter is a moving contraction which travels towards the distal end of the stomach and finally obliterates itself. Careful observation behind the fluoroscopic screen should obviate any error.

Filling the Bulb. The experienced observer is familiar with the fact that often the duodenal bulb will appear after only one or two swallows of barium mixture. It seems as though in the resting state the pyloric sphincter remains open, and soon after food or barium mixture enters the stomach the sphincter closes, only to be opened subsequently by the mechanism of peristalsis. Where the examination is restricted to the first portion of the duodenum alone a useful method to fill this part of the bowel rapidly is to ask the patient to drink down the entire glass of barium mixture at once.

During routine gastrointestinal fluoroscopy the examiner may encounter difficulty in filling the first portion of the duodenum. The following maneuvers may prove useful in accomplishing this aim.

If peristalsis is slow in starting, this may be stimulated either by some palpatory manipulation (smooth and simulating peristalsis) of the stomach, or by asking the patient to take a few deep breaths. The examiner then attempts to push some barium through into the bulb. Pressure should be applied behind a wave when it is still a considerable distance from the pyloric sphincter. The pressure should be smooth following the wave, and directed toward the sphincter, *not* upwards toward the liver.

The patient, finding himself in a dark room with unusual surroundings, may be upset. Pleasant conversation or perhaps discussing some of the food that he usually enjoys may release the pyloric sphincter and allow passage of the barium into the duodenum. It may be necessary, in order to overcome this emotional factor, to ask the patient to sit outside and then recall him in five or ten minutes. Now, accustomed to his surroundings, the duodenal cap may be readily observable. It may be wise while he is waiting to have him lie on his right side, thus gravitating the barium towards the duodenum.

Especially to be emphasized is the necessity of having the patient in a thoroughly relaxed state, mentally as well as physically. This was emphasized by Kirklin.[7] He observed that nervous tension from any cause commonly gave rise to rigidity of the abdominal muscles, upward retraction of the stomach and spasticity of the pyloric sphincter. Accordingly, all his efforts were directed toward achieving complete relaxation of the patient.

The following manipulation has been employed by Kirklin[7] with success: After advising the patient to relax, the examiner applies manual pressure at a point in the stomach just above the incisura angularis. The cupped right hand is placed obliquely across the stomach so that pressure is exerted by the palmar and ulnar sides of the fingertips and the ulnar side of the hand. The fingers are slightly flexed and approximated. The index finger is applied just mesial to the lesser curvature and the little finger and ulnar side of the hand at the greater curvature. The thumb is parallel to and below the greater curvature of the antrum (fig. 237). The hand in this position assumes the form of a scoop, and although the gastric contents can be driven forward, the backward escape of these contents may also be prevented. With the hand held this way, pressure is applied at the moment when the disappearance of a peristaltic wave at the pylorus is succeeded by full antral dilatation. The examiner exerts sufficient pressure to produce a more or less visible division of the barium suspension and then pulls his hand downward and at the same time rotates it slightly clockwise without permitting his fingers to slip from their position on the skin. The effect of the entire maneuver is to drive the suspension toward the pyloric sphincter by indirectly increasing the intra-gastric pressure in the antrum. If necessary, simultaneous upward pressure against the antrum can also be made with the thumb. The pyloric sphincter may open after one or two such manipulations.

It is highly important that the entire manipulation be executed at the precise moment when the antrum has relaxed and a peristaltic wave is in progress toward it. Pressure should not be applied when the prepyloric region of the antrum is contracted.[7]

The manipulation of the gastric walls in an effort to open the pylorus also bears emphasis. Pressing upwards on the antrum in an attempt to pass the opaque media through the pylorus results in compressing the cap against the liver and thus prevents the cap from filling.

A massaging movement from the pyloric sphincter directly downwards for some unexplained reason is successful in occa-

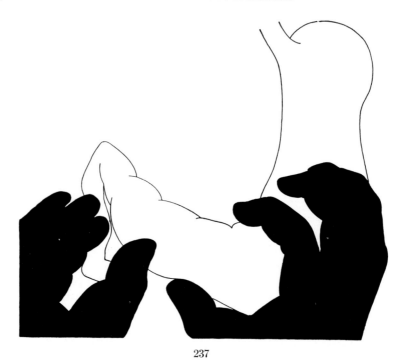

237

Proper position for right hand and fingers in order to fill the duodenal bulb. Note the left hand may compress the descending duodenum, thus helping prevent rapid emptying of the bulb.

sionally opening the pylorus and allowing the barium to fill the cap.

Employing the help of gravity may also prove useful. The patient is asked to lie so that the cap and antral portion of the stomach are below with the pars media and fundus above. This is accomplished when the patient is lying directly on his right side. Once the cap is filled in this position, the patient can be turned to any other suitable position for study of the cap. It is occasionally advisable when this maneuver is employed to give the patient the barium in an outer room and ask him to lie on his right side. After five minutes (during which time the physician can proceed with another patient), the patient is recalled for examination.

A useful method is to only *partially* fill the stomach and have the patient lie on his right side. In this position, again, gravity helps fill the bulb. The patient lying on his right side places the bulb closer to the table top. The fluoroscopic screen and *spot film*

device is on the *top side or left side* of the patient. The bulb located adjacent to the table is in a suitable location for conventional radiography, i.e., being close to the film beneath. Where spot filming is employed, the greater distance from the spot film device, however, will cause the image of the bulb to be blurred.

The examiner employing a spot film device must thus bring the filled bulb closer to the fluoroscopic screen, i.e., to the spot film device. He is ever mindful that in gradually rotating the right side of the patient towards the screen, i.e., in bringing the bulb up, the bulb may empty. The patient, then, lying with his right side down, must *gradually* be rolled so that his left side is pushed away from the examiner and his abdomen tends to face upwards towards the fluoroscopic screen. This is done under constant direct fluoroscopic visualization.

The importance of performing this maneuver when the stomach is only *partially* filled with opaque media lies in the fact

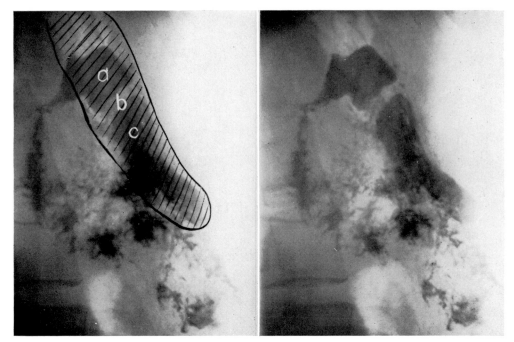

Another method of filling and filming duodenal bulb.

238   239

a. Duodenal bulb.
b. Pyloric sphincter.
c. Stomach antrum.
Cross-hatched lines represent the empty stomach behind.

Comment: If the stomach were filled with barium, the shadow of the *filled* body of the stomach (cross hatching) would blot the shadow of the bulb.

Empty, or *partially* filled, body of the stomach (see text, page 182) permits visualization of the duodenal bulb.

that the amount of rotation necessary to visualize the *"filled bulb"* is such that if the stomach were filled, its shadow would overlie the duodenal bulb and prevent its visualization. (See figs. 238, 239.)

A bulb which contracts rapidly, not allowing for adequate study, may be visualized to greater advantage by compressing the second or descending portion of the duodenum (fig. 237). This when successful acts as an obstruction, preventing emptying of the duodenal contents above.

Occasionally, the patient may help fill his own bulb, especially when the examiner has both his hands occupied. For example, the examiner may attempt to obstruct the descending portion of the duodenum with one hand and with the other operate the spot film device. He would also like to help the stomach empty and so fill the bulb. The patient's hand may be brought into the fluoroscopic field and strategically placed on his own abdomen with the exact position and the *direction and degree of pressure* determined by the examiner as the situation requires (fig. 246).

Complete Filling of the Bulb. The importance of fully distending the bulb cannot be overstressed. In the absence of a previous surgical procedure in this region, and a suggestive clinical history, any persistent deformity in the bulb represents a scar of duodenal ulcer.[9] One of the most common causes for an *apparently deformed* bulb is incom-

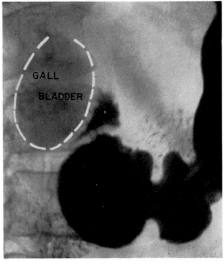

240

The gallbladder may produce a concave or hollowed out deformity of the duodenal bulb.

plete filling. With its lumen collapsed on itself and its mucosa wrinkled, it may simulate duodenitis or ulcer.

Normal Deformities of the Bulb. The cap may normally be deformed by the overlying gallbladder. This can be seen in both the right anterior oblique and left anterior oblique positions (fig. 240).

Fluid Levels in the Bulb. The fluorocopist often encounters an air bubble in the duodenal cap when the patient is in the erect position, the barium forming a horizontal fluid level (fig. 241). In this circumstance, the various contours and mucosal patterns of the duodenal bulb cannot be adequately studied, especially if they are inaccessible to the palpating hand.

Incomplete filling may cause an ulcerated bulb to appear normal. For example, in figures 242–244 the duodenal bulb appears normal because the pathology in the bulb exists above the level of the opaque media. This portion of the bulb, not being opacified, cannot be seen. It is thus important to eliminate this fluid level—*or air bubble.*

In the prone position the cap is filled and deformities not seen when the fluid level was present may now appear.

In the erect position, the examiner should attempt to force a large quantity of barium through the sphincter, thus filling the bulb and displacing the air.

Placing the patient in the prone position will "press" the air out of the duodenum. The patient can next be examined in the erect position. It is important in going from the prone to the erect position to make certain that the patient is not first turned into the supine, since air rising into the antrum may escape into the duodenum (fig. 199 C).

The Technique of Air Contrast Studies of the Bulb (see occasions for such studies, p. 205). Air contrast studies of the duodenal bulb are performed *after* the bulb has been filled with barium. It is advisable to have the patient lie on his right side, since, as already noted, the bulb is thus filled with the help of gravity. After the bulb has been filled with the barium suspension, the patient is placed in the supine position. In this position, the air normally passes to the gastric antrum, i.e., the highest portion of the stomach when the patient is supine (fig. 199C, p. 160). The bulb will fill with air when it is elevated *above* the level of the stomach. *This is accomplished by raising the patient's right side off the table.* The degree of obliquity in which the patient is placed varies with the position of the bulb. A high oblique or sometimes lateral position may be necessary to demonstrate a bulb directed posteriorly. A slight oblique is sufficient to demonstrate a bulb which lies in the transverse plane.

Generally, air from the antrum rushes in and fills the bulb in a few seconds. When the bulb is not properly filled with air, gentle pressure on the antrum or having the patient lie on the left side for a minute can be helpful. The air causes the barium suspension to leave, but a thin coating of the opaque media is left behind to outline the mucosa. Barium trapped in a crater, especially on the posterior wall, is also left behind and can be seen in air contrast. *Spot films are routinely made, since fluoroscopic visualization of the air-filled bulb is poor.*

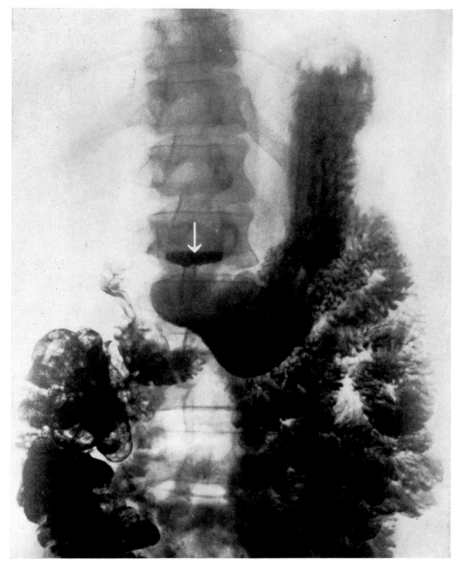

241

A common difficulty the novice encounters is a fluid level within the cap not permitting proper examination of this part. (See figs. 242–244 and 245B.)

Because the air-filled bulb may be difficult to see on the screen, and hence difficult to position for filming, a useful method in helping to locate the bulb is to opacify the gallbladder and use it as a landmark. The air-filled bulb is expected to lie immediately medial to the gallbladder. Another useful landmark in like fashion is the opacified descending portion of the duodenal sweep. The bulb can be located and spot filmed by remembering that it is situated at the top of the descending duodenum and leads into it.

Fluid Levels in the Stomach. The fasting stomach may present a fluid level within the fundus. This can be taken as evidence of hypersecretion. It is possible for a large amount of secretion to be present in some stomachs and yet not be evident as a fluid level. This may occur when excess fluid col-

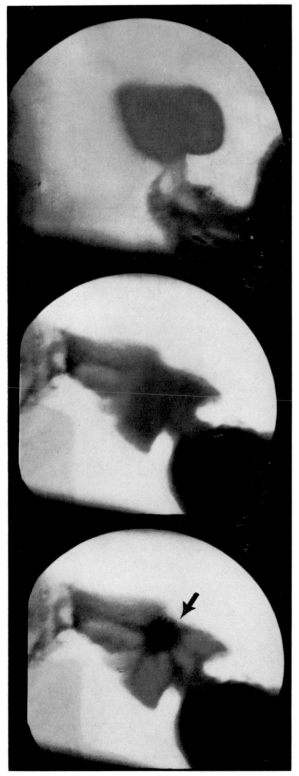

242

Is this smooth, triangular bulb normal? (See f
243.)

243

Bulb in figure 201, filled only in its lower ha
appears normal. By *completely* filling the bu
the indented deformity (arrow) on the superi
margin is seen. This deformity indicates the pro
able presence of an ulcer. (See fig. 244.)

244

Air contrast study of the same bulb reveals
crater underlying the deformity confirming
active ulcer.

lects in the sac-like lower portion of an atonic stomach, the gastric walls above being drawn together (fig. 194). The barium mixture as it descends into and through the excess fluid forms globs and can be seen cascading down. The fasting fluid subsequently settles out as a layer above the barium mixture.

With the patient in the erect position, a barium fluid level at the foot of the stomach, i.e., in the region of the antrum, must be critically appraised. It should be borne in mind that defects in the lesser curvature of the stomach—above the fluid level—may be present and not seen. Either barium may have gravitated out of an ulcer above the fluid level or a lesion may not be properly outlined because the barium has not come in contact with it (fig. 245B).

Abnormal Entry of Improperly Prepared Barium Mixture into the Stomach. Masses lying along the course of flow of contrast media may separate the stream into two or more components. This splitting is not normal but may on occasion appear in a normal stomach when very thick mixtures or pastes are used, since these break into globules and fail to spread evenly into the stomach. Confused patterns may thus occur at the site of entry of the barium into the gastric lumen. This can be overcome by being sure that the mixture is properly prepared.

Aids in Examining the Cardia. The following manipulation has been employed successfully by Kirklin.[7] The patient is advised to "push out" his "stomach" against the hand of the examiner. Although the phrase is not precise the patient understands what is meant and responds properly by lowering his diaphragm, cramping his abdomen and causing the stomach to descend. At the moment of greatest descent the fluoroscopist applies sufficient pressure directly below the left costal arch so that the walls of the stomach are approximated. The patient is then told to relax his efforts slowly. During the relaxing period, while the stomach is ascending to its normal position, the ex-

aminer applies this constant pressure. By this procedure a great part of the cardia is brought down into the field of manipulation and the mucosal relief can be examined more adequately.

A method of detecting ulcers in the upper portion of the stomach, i.e., the lesser curvature, is described by Schatzki.[21] An ulcer in these regions may be missed because it is so situated that either barium cannot enter into it or, if the barium does enter, the filled opaque stomach may be so situated in relation to the ulcer that it is difficult to view the ulcer in profile or through the opaque, filled stomach. This method attacks both problems. It attempts not only to fill the ulcer with barium, but, next, to so position the patient that the ulcer is either thrown into profile or seen en face with the overlying barium sufficiently removed so that the ulcer crater is visible.

The principle employed is to place the patient so that the suspected ulcer site is in a *dependent* position, and next filling it with barium (figs. 247, 248).

Since the majority of ulcers appear at or near the lesser curvature, the examiner should arrange this region of the stomach so that it becomes the most dependent portion. Thus, when the patient lies on his back, barium collects in the fundus and the balance of the stomach is relatively empty. In this, the supine position, the patient can next be rotated with the left side up. By lifting the left side, the fundus becomes elevated and barium will pour out into the stomach beneath. The degree of elevation of the left side will determine how much barium leaves the fundus and how far down the lesser curvature it will travel. Note that the lesser curvature, with the left shoulder lifted, becomes the dependent portion of the stomach. The barium mixture can now more easily enter into ulcer craters situated in this region. If too much barium runs out, part or all of it can be made to run back into the fundus by lowering the left side.

With this method it can be seen that by

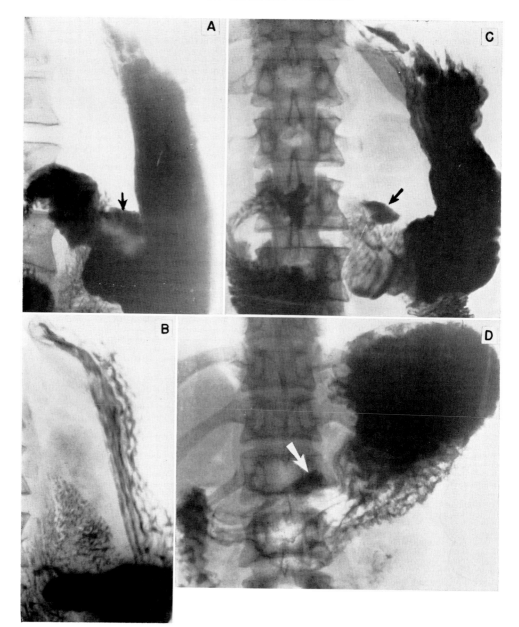

245 A–D

Interpretation made by a new resident.

A. Stomach appears normal. Arrow points to what appears to be a loop of intestine behind.

B. Normalcy seems to be confirmed by upright study.

C. Normalcy seems further confirmed by apparently normal stomach and barium seen entering apparently normal triangular duodenal bulb (arrow).

D. Air contrast study of antrum obtained with patient supine appears normal. Barium (arrow) appears trapped between normal (?) folds.

(*See comment, bottom of page 189.*)

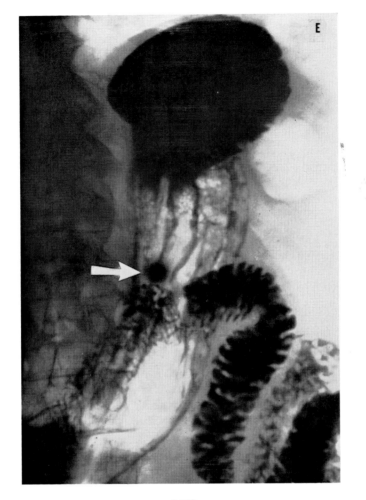

245E

Further value of air contrast study of stomach

E. With patient supine, air contrast study of the stomach (not fundus) may be secured. To obtain this type of air contrast, patient, with barium in his stomach, first lies on his left side. This clears the antrum and a large part of the body of the stomach by "dumping" the opaque media into the left side of the stomach. The barium is next made to gravitate into the fundus by placing the patient in the supine position (see fig. 199C, page 160). This view may on occasion show a *posterior wall* crater too shallow to be seen in other projections and positions. Such was true in fig. 245E.

---

245 A–D (continued)

Fig. 245A–D as interpreted by a new resident serves to illustrate the care that must be taken to be sure that the anatomic parts are properly labeled and the affect positioning and air have on a gastric study. Actually, the following is the correct interpretation:

A. An ulcer is seen on the lesser curvature (arrow) antral portion of stomach. Note thick mucosal collar beneath, i.e., lesser density.

B. In the *erect* position, the ulcer cavity empties itself of barium and the stomach appears normal.

C. In the *prone* position, the antrum is compressed between spine and the table top. Antrum empties, but ulcer on lesser curvature retains barium and is again visualized. Duodenal bulb is ill-defined and poorly filled, seen overlying spine.

D. Patient *supine*, air contrast study of the antrum is obtained, barium is seen trapped in lesser curvature crater (arrow).

Now note fig. 245E above.

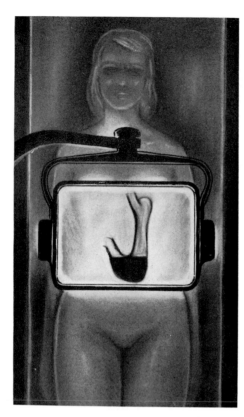

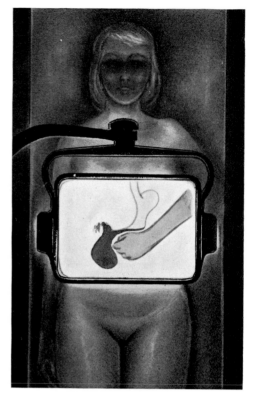

246 A

246 B

Patient in erect position. Barium settled to foot of stomach. Bulb difficult to fill without manipulation.

The patient may help fill his own bulb by strategic positioning and pressure of own hand.

elevating the patient's left side, ulcer craters on the lesser curvature and adjacent portions of the anterior and posterior walls of the stomach can be made dependent and so filled (figs. 247, 248). Simultaneously, by lowering the left shoulder, barium flowing back into the fundus may thin the overlying barium sufficiently so that the ulcer can be seen en face. The examiner's ingenuity may also be successful in bringing the ulcer into profile.

As in fig. 199 D, it is seen that the stomach lies more horizontal when the table is *tilted*. Tilting the table instead of holding it horizontal during this maneuver is also of value in those patients where the stomach tends to fall backwards upon the fundus when they are supine. With the stomach in one horizontal plane, the examiner can more easily shift barium about in the stomach with lesser degrees of rotation of the patient.

The optimal degree of table tilt varies with each patient. With repetition of this maneuver, however, the examiner may soon acquire the feeling of the proper tilt for each patient. His own ingenuity and imagination may occasionally lead him to examine patients in Trendelenburg and other positions, utilizing this same maneuver.

In practice, this procedure can become routine. After fluoroscoping the patient in the erect position, the table is tilted backward. If barium has not run into the fundus. it will if the patient is turned to his left side.

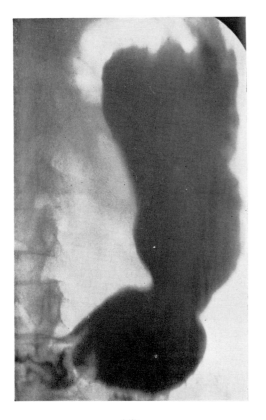

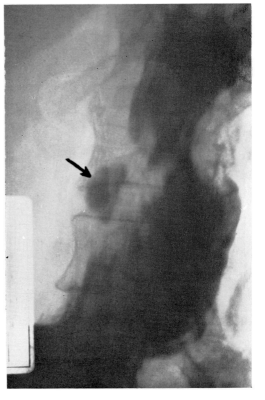

247

248

No ulcer is seen, although one is suspected. What further maneuver can be performed to delineate an ulcer crater high up on the lesser curvature? It is assumed that the palpating hand cannot reach the involved region to press barium into the possible crater. (see fig. 248.)

The lesser curvature must be put into such a position so that barium can pour directly onto it; i.e., the lesser curvature becomes the floor of the stomach and not the side wall. The greater curvature thus becomes the roof of the stomach.

For this to occur, the barium is first trapped in the fundus, i.e., the patient is placed in the supine position (fig. 199C). Barium is then poured from the fundus onto the lesser curvature by raising the left side of the patient, i.e., rolling him onto his right side. By rolling the patient with the left side up and the right side down, the greater curvature becomes the roof of the stomach, and the lesser curvature the floor. Barium now pouring from the fundus onto the floor (lesser curvature) enters and fills the crater (arrow).

The maneuver next starts when the patient is turned gradually on to his right side and the flow of barium from the fundus is observed.

False Craters. The examiner must be aware of the possibilty of diagnosing an

ulcer crater when in truth none exists. A small clump of barium from an improperly prepared, or occasionally even a properly prepared mixture, may be trapped between two mucosal folds and appear as though a crater existed (figs. 211, 212). With suffi-

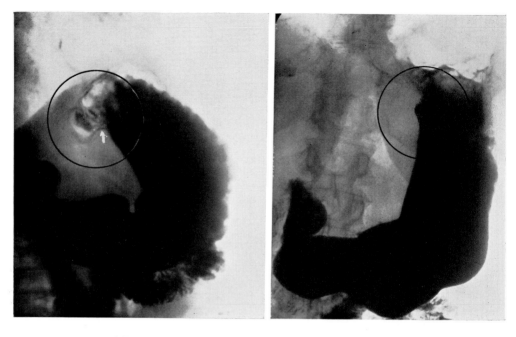

249   250

Question:

What common irregularities may occur in the profile of the cardia of the stomach?

Answer:

(1) A gastric diverticulum (fig. 249).

(2) A regional ulcer (fig. 250).

(3) The normal "star shaped" folds when seen on end (figs. 251 and 252).

Comment: As in figures 247 and 248, positioning the patient supine and next performing the Schatzki maneuver would place the questionable region so that barium can be poured on to it. A diverticulum is made evident by its smooth grapelike appearance and pedicle (fig. 249). An ulcer would not be as smooth and would have no pedicle (fig. 250). The normal "star shaped" folds would be confirmed first by the inability to prove an ulcer as present and, second, by demonstrating folds radiating from a point as in figure 252.

cient washing of the involved region by the palpating hand the glob of barium should be easily displaced. If doubt exists, the examination must be repeated. It is unlikely that barium will be trapped in the same position twice.

Barium within a gastric diverticulum may appear as though it were a crater. To avoid such an error the examiner must attempt to position any defect so that it is seen in profile. In the profile projection, the true diagnosis becomes evident. The sac-like contours and pedicle of a diverticulum, hanging like a grape, together with its typical location on the upper and posterior wall near the lesser curvature are the signs looked for in arriving at a diagnosis (figs. 249, 250). Also, an ulcer crater is likely to be associated with some rigidity of the walls, whereas a diverticulum will leave the walls uninvolved. Further, an ulcer crater in the region of the cardia large enough to be confused with a diverticulum will be readily seen as such by the Schatzki maneuver described above. Spot films will often be necessary for final confirmation.

Normal Variation in Lesser Curvature at Cardia.

The lesser curvature of the stomach is

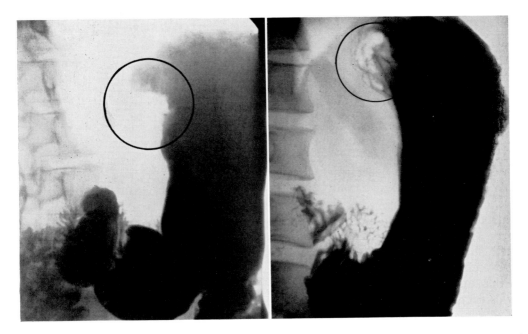

251   252

Question:

The lesser curvature of the stomach should normally be smooth. What normally may produce an irregularity within the region (encircled)?

Answer:

The normal "star shaped" folds of the fundus, when seen in profile, may sometimes produce the irregularity seen in figure 251.

described as characteristically smooth. The only deformities are the soft undulations of the peristaltic waves. Yet, a deformity may occur within the cardiac region which may be normal and yet cause confusion: When the normal star-like folds radiating from the esophageal entry into the stomach are seen in profile, a defect may be produced which might simulate an ulcer (figs. 251, 252). Differentiation from an ulcer can be obtained by discovering radiating folds responsible for the deformity. Further, if a question of ulcer arose in fig. 251, it should be pointed out that an ulcer large enough to be seen in profile as in figure 251 would be picked up and further confirmed as ulcer

by the Schatzki maneuver (see page 187).

Negative Defects. Any food or mucus in the stomach, when present to a considerable extent, may produce a negative defect, either within the mucosal relief pattern or in the gastric contours. To differentiate these from true pathological processes the examiner must, upon observing these defects, move them about with the palpating hand. The freedom of mobility without apparent deformity of the gastric walls is diagnostic (fig. 300).

A patient properly prepared will not present this difficulty. Occasionally it may be necessary to re-examine the patient after preliminary gastric lavage.

The Pathological Stomach

Although there are examiners who consider fluoroscopy the best basis for making a diagnosis of gastric or duodenal disease, the consensus is opposed to this. Because of the greater detail secured on the radiographic film and the greater time permitted for study, a diagnosis should properly await film examination. The fluoroscopic findings as detailed below should be considered as clues, each to be proven on the subsequent roentgenogram. When any pathological process is noted, spot films should be taken. Whether or not this is possible, it is wise for the examiner to make careful note of the position and method used to demonstrate any defect and to reproduce these when later taking conventional films.

SPASMS EXISTING IN THE STOMACH

The following paragraphs review the various types of spasm found in the stomach.

Pylorospasm. Pylorospasm may be functional or organic in origin. A diagnosis of pylorospasm may be accepted as justifiable if, after the various procedures recommended for filling the duodenal cap have been employed, the pyloric sphincter persistently fails to open.

In this condition the peristalic waves are active and deep. They may start higher up than the incisura angularis and their depth increases as the distal end of the stomach is approached. None of them are successful in pushing the opaque mixture into the bulb. In the presence of pylorospasm, the spastic sphincter remains closed for approximately fifteen minutes.

Circumscribed Spasm. A circumscribed type of spasm may be such as the incisura opposite an ulcer. This latter type of defect can be caused by either a malignant or a benign ulceration. When a malignant ulcer is present, the spasm is usually broader but shallower and often does not reach the lesser curvature. With a benign ulcer the defect caused by the spasm is narrower and deeper and often reaches the lesser curvature (fig. 253).

Antral Spasm. The antrum may become markedly narrowed and at times almost completely obliterated. This will closely simulate an antral carcinoma. However, when this narrowing or obliteration is due to spasm as the opaque mixture passes from the pars media of the stomach to the antrum, the antral profile will be smooth. Should a small amount of barium remain behind to coat the mucosa, it will be found intact. The contour may, moreover, show variation of outline at different times. These phenomena (namely, smooth profile, intact mucosa, and change of contour), especially the intact mucosa, are important in differentiating the spasm from antral carcinoma.

The examiner must bear in mind that this diagnosis often can not be determined on the fluoroscopic screen and requires the full clinical acumen and adequate radiographic workup. It would be wise to examine the patient after suitable therapy with antispasmodics.

Total Gastrospasm. Here the entire stomach is involved. A scirrhous carcinoma is closely simulated. The differential diagnosis again rests on a normal mucosal contour and some variation of the outline as different portions of the stomach become filled with barium. This is opposed to the permanent narrowing and deformity of malignancy which refuses to show any change as the barium passes through, maintaining its same narrowed contour.

The administration of antispasmodics in functional defects may aid in arriving at the diagnosis by diminishing any spastic manifestations.

Hour-glass Stomach (figs. 253–258). No discussion of gastric spasms would be complete without a word on hour-glass stomach.

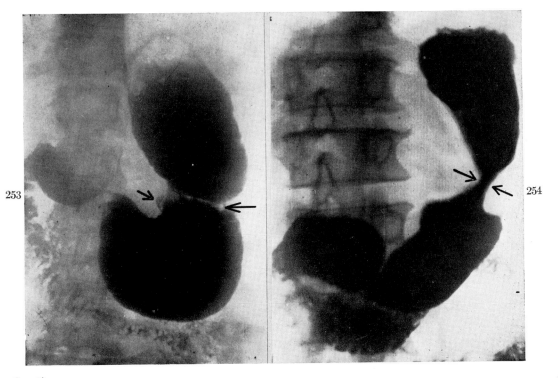

253   254

Question:

Both stomachs reveal deformities in the pars media (arrows). Which is malignant?

Answer:

253

A letter "B" type of deformity (constriction from *one* side); the middle of the letter produced by the spasm is characteristic of a benign ulcer.

254

A figure "8" type of deformity (constriction from *both* sides) suggests malignancy.

A spasm on the greater curvature of the stomach as in fig. 253 should be differentiated from (1) malignancy, (2) spasm secondary to ulcer. When both curvatures are involved and the stomach assumes a "figure eight" appearance, a malignant constriction should be considered (fig. 254). When, however, only the greater curvature is involved and the lesser curvature s relatively straight (i.e., a letter "B" appearance, with the spasm forming the mid-indenture of the "B"), a benign spasm opposite a peptic ulcer should be considered. Note that the middle of the "B" is deep enough almost to reach the lesser curvature.

Another cause of hour-glass stomach is the normal impression of the ribs (fig. 188), or perhaps spleen on the greater curvature

of the stomach in a thin individual. This is easily diagnosed by acquaintance with this defect and the knowledge that the defect may be corrected behind the fluoroscopic screen by the palpatory manipulations of the examiner.

Gastric syphilis is an important cause of hour-glass deformity of the stomach.[10] The constriction is central, producing a "figure eight" type of hour-glass. The constricted portion is usually smooth without evidence of an invading tumor (fig. 258).

The cascade type of stomach, as described previously, may also take on an hour-glass contour. Other causes of this deformity are spasm, adhesions, or pressure from extrinsic tumors.

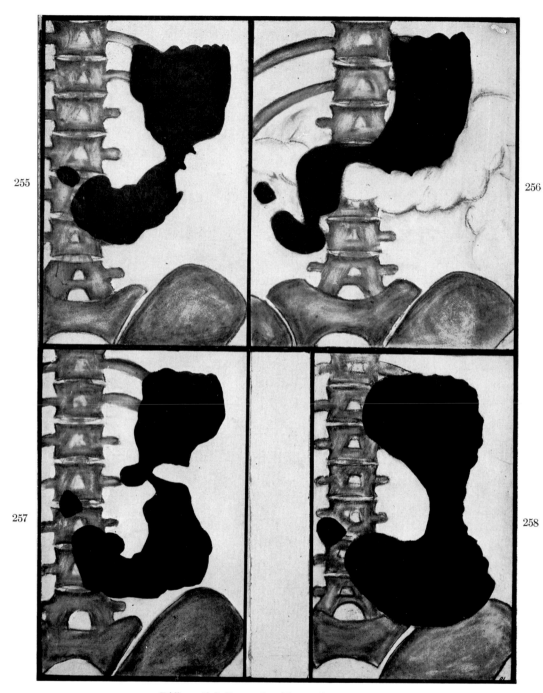

Differential diagnosis of hour-glass stomach.
(*See opposite page*)

INFLAMMATION (GASTRITIS)

In hypertrophic gastritis the rugae are said to be thickened, rigid and tortuous (fig. 259). It is often a matter of great difficulty to determine whether a given degree of mucosal thickening is physiologic or pathologic. It is often wise not to make a diagnosis after observing the relief pattern with the stomach relatively empty. As has been said, the stomach in an empty state permits more wrinkling of the mucosa, and thus the mucosal folds become more prominent. If, however, this tortuosity and thickening of the folds are present when the stomach is filled and the mucosa stretched, a diagnosis of gastritis receives more support. Diagnosis often depends on gastroscopic examination.

Gastritis often exists in conjunction with a gastric ulcer or neoplasm.

HERNIATION OF GASTRIC MUCOSA

This condition occurs in the presence of a hypertrophied and thickened pre-pyloric mucosa. Characteristically the thickened rugae produce a *central defect* in the antral region, leaving both the lesser and greater curvatures uninvolved (fig. 260). The hypertrophied and thickened rugae, being loosely attached to the submucosa, act similarly to a foreign body and are propelled through the pylorus by peristaltic waves. Within the bulb the prolapsed gastric mucosa becomes evident as a mottled defect (fig. 261). It should be emphasized, however, that the margins of the bulb remain smooth and intact. With the antral mucosa in the cap the antrum itself becomes narrowed. This entire sequence can easily be overlooked on the fluoroscopic screen. It is best demonstrated in the recumbent and right oblique positions.

Differential Diagnosis. The most common abnormality in the stomach which will tend to simulate this condition is a prolapsing antral polyp. This too presents a *central defect.* A polyp, however, which is small enough to pass through the pyloric sphincter will usually not produce an antral defect.[12]

GASTRIC ULCER (BENIGN)

The fluoroscopist in examining the stomach seeks for contour defects representing ulcers. Peristalsis is observed, and "skip" areas noted. *He examines the mucosa, and attempts to fill up and discover any craters with opaque media.* Mucosal studies are particularly valuable in discovering small shallow ulcers, or ulcers so situated that defects in gastric contours are difficult to demonstrate.

The barium mixture within the stomach should be manipulated as previously de-

Differential diagnosis of hour-glass stomach.

(See opposite page)

255
Carcinoma.
1. Figure "8" shaped. Constriction ragged and irregular.
2. Region of narrowing is aperistaltic,
3. No undue gas distention in region.
4. Not correctable during examination.

257
Benign ulcer.
1. "B" shaped construction.
2. Region of narrowing duriog active phase of ulceration usually aperistaltic. When activity ceases peristalsis returns.
3. No undue gas distetion.
4. Does not correct itself during examination.

256
One variety of cascade stomach.
1. Constriction smoouh.
2, Region of narrowing permits peristalsis.
3. Usually prominence of gas distention in region.
4. Often corrects itself during examioasion.

258
Gastric syphilis.
1. Constriction smooth (figure "8").
2. Region of narrowing aperistaltic.
3. No undue gas distention.
4. Does not correct itself during examination.

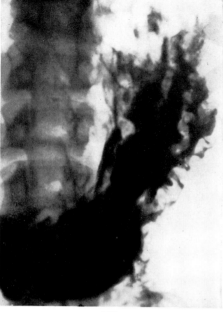

259

The various indentures and serrations seen on the greater curvature aspect and within the stomach are due to heaped up thickened mucosal folds. This is characteristic of hypertrophic gastritis.

Question:

Under what conditions may the normal stomach be made to appear in a similar manner?

Answer:

The stomach when insufficiently filled with barium permits more wrinkling of its mucosa. This increase in wrinkling renders the mucosal folds more prominent and may simulate the picture above.

Comment: To make a diagnosis of hypertrophic gastritis the stomach should be properly filled.

scribed, to demonstrate the rugal folds of the entire stomach. Attention should be given to even slight variations from the normal configuration and these should be evaluated. The direct visualization of an ulcer crater is usually possible if one is present (fig. 262). However, if there is a spastic incisura, shortening of the lesser curvature, or spasm of the gastric antrum without a crater being visible, its presence should still be suspected and a re-examination should be made after administration of anti-spasmodics, if neces-

sary, to confirm or rule it out.[11] Sharply localized tenderness is also a suspicious finding.

A chronic ulcer should be suspected when the folds appear star-like and radiate from a central crater.

Secondary Signs of Gastric Ulcer. A persistent spasm either of the entire antrum or a single incisural defect on the greater curvature is an important secondary manifestation of gastric ulcer. Thickening and tortuosity of gastric rugae, as with gastritis, may be present. Peristaltic waves are usually obliterated in their passage through a crater but reappear when the benign ulceration has healed. Any attempts to coordinate further signs with gastric ulcer depend upon the stage at which the ulcer is seen and its site.

Difficulties in Outlining the Crater. When, because better mucosal relief studies are desired, insufficient barium mixture is used, a crater may be missed. In this case, the barium may not enter every nook and crevice, even with the guidance of the palpating hand. Also, with inadequate filling of the stomach, the various gastric rugae and folds are not completely spread apart. A thick-walled crater with its margins more or less puckered and drawn together lying deep between such approximated rugae may not be discovered (figs. 267–272).

The crater may be shallow and thus not permit barium to be trapped within it.

Debris or blood clot may be found within the crater which will not allow barium mixture to enter. Adequate massaging will overcome this difficulty. For this reason it has also been recommended not to perform gastric radiographic studies until two weeks after a gastric hemorrhage has been stopped.

The crater may be high up in the fundus, perhaps in an inaccessible area, and unless opaque media can be massaged up into the crater, it may not become evident. It is thus important to stress the examination of the patient in both horizontal and erect positions. In this region the Schatzki

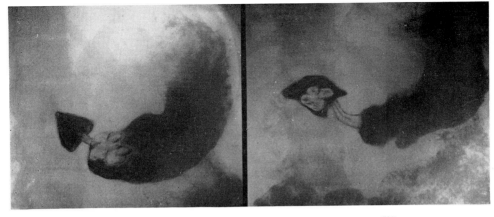

260   261

Question:

An area which fails to fill is seen in the antrum. What are the most probable causes?

Answer:

1. Carcinoma.
2. Thickened antral mucosa.
3. Polyp.

Fluoroscopic findings:

The defect in the antrum was seen to travel through the pylorus and into the cap.

Comment: Findings as above are characteristic of a prolapsing thickened antral mucosa. A *carcinoma* would not herniate through. A *polyp* large enough to be seen, as in figure 260, would be too large to pass through the pylorus.

maneuver is valuable, as described above (page 187).

A crater, although filled with opaque material, may remain undiscovered if the patient is not rotated with sufficient obliquity (figs. 195 and 196, also figs. 269–272). A crater may be present and seen when the patient is prone, but empty itself of barium when the patient is erect. Thus it may not be seen (fig. 245B). Proper massage is therefore essential.

Differential Diagnosis. Once a gastric ulcer is determined to be present, malignancy must be ruled out. Various guides have been set forth and are useful:

A lesser curvature ulcer is usually benign, a greater curvature ulcer is usually malignant.

A large ulcer with an irregular base may be malignant. This, however, is extremely variable, since ulcers of this description have been proved benign.

When ulcers are found both in the duo-

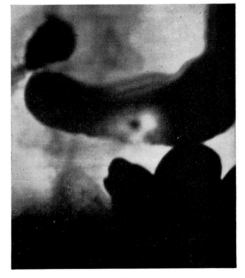

262

The examiner presses away the barium and finds a crater.

Question:

Is it a true or a false crater? (See figs. 211 and 212, p. 170.)

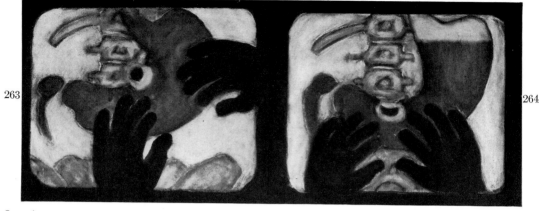

263   264

Question:

The palpating hands press overlying barium away and discover a *crater*. Which of these two demonstrate a malignant ulcer?

Answer:

263

The island of varium with a halo around it projects *out from* the gastric profile (*positive defect*). The halo is due to an edematous mucosal collar. This is a benign ulcer.

264

The island of barium is situated *within* the gastric profile (*negative defect*). This is a malignant gastric ulcer.

denum and in the stomach, it is likely that we are dealing with a benign process.

The response to healing is important. A benign ulcer should, with proper therapy, heal and disappear. A malignant ulcer may allow some granulation or perhaps neoplastic growth into the crater, which may tend to fill in and obliterate it, but opposed to a benign process, this will *never completely* heal.

The surrounding border of an ulcer may be demonstrated by applying sufficient pressure with the palpating hand to rid the area of the excess barium which obscures it. The *benign* crater is thus seen surrounded by a translucent zone produced by its edematous, inflamed margins (fig. 263). The *malignant* crater on the other hand is seen surrounded by a translucent zone produced by the indurated and heaped-up edges of the growth (fig. 264). Further, a *benign* ulcer projects from the gastric lumen as a positive defect (projecting from the gastric contour—fig. 263). A *malignant* ulcer is more apt to be present as a negative defect (within the gastric contours). Carman[11]

summarized these findings in his "meniscus sign."

In order for this sign to be useful in the diagnosis of malignancy, the fluoroscopist must first find the halo surrounding the crater, and next make certain that the crater is *within* the gastric contours. It cannot be determined that the crater is actually within the gastric contours until it is seen in *true profile*, since with slight rotation it is possible to throw a protruding benign ulcer and its surrounding translucent zone *into* the shadow of the gastric lumen (figs. 265, 266). Second, in order to be certain that true profile studies are made, the patient must be examined in the *erect position* since it is possible in the prone or supine position for the stomach wall so to distort itself, i.e., fold in upon itself, that an ulcerative process projecting out from the gastric contour may be folded within the gastric contour.

(*Note:* A posterior wall ulcer even when benign may mimic a malignant ulcer and produce Carman's "meniscus sign.")

The diagnosis of a malignant ulcer is amplified further if an irregularity of con-

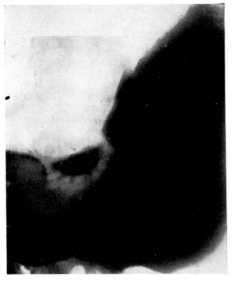

265

The island of barium with a halo around it is barium trapped in a crater. Is this a malignant or benign crater? (See fig. 266.)

tour as well as additional defects are noted *at some distance* from the crater itself.

When in the erect position the ulcer has a fluid level which is topped by air, a benign ulcer should be suspected.

DUODENAL ULCER (Figs. 275–280)

Deformed Duodenal Bulb as a Sign of Ulcer. Very often a duodenal ulcer will manifest itself by a deformed cap. A crater may or may not be visualized. It is perhaps a safe rule in the presence of a suitable clinical picture and in the absence of adhesions to diagnose a persistent abnormal configuration of the cap as a duodenal ulcer.[10]

The most frequent cause for an *apparent deformity* in a *normal bulb* is an incompletely filled bulb. Normalcy here is readily established by watching this bulb fill and empty. With filling and emptying, a *normal bulb* becomes larger, distends, assumes its normal smoothly triangular appearance, and the *deformity disappears*. But what about the scarred, contracted bulb of a duodenal ulcer, especially when associated with

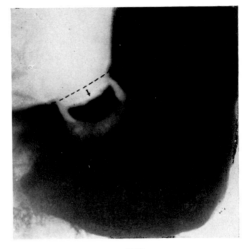

266

1. The crater is inside the gastric contour (dotted line is a continuation of the gastric profile and the crater is inside or beneath the dotted line).
2. To be certain that the crater was not inadvertently "tucked" beneath the gastric profile:
   A. The examination was performed in the erect position.
   B. The crater was examined in true profile.

Comment: The above findings are indicative of Carman's meniscus sign and at operation a malignant ulcer was found.

spasm? The more active the ulcer and the more contracted and scarred that it is, the less does this bulb dilate and expand with barium filling. The contraction, fibrotic scars and spasms do not permit this. The importance of this lies in the fact that the organically deformed bulb, as opposed to the normal bulb, *maintains its deformity* with filling and thus distinguishes it from the normal.

It should be stressed that by direct inspection on the fluoroscopic screen an appraisal can be made of the relative states of filling and emptying of a duodenal bulb. Although it is not recommended that fluoroscopy be omitted, yet, there are occasions when an examination has not been successful and the patient cannot be called back for reexamination. In such circumstances, it is

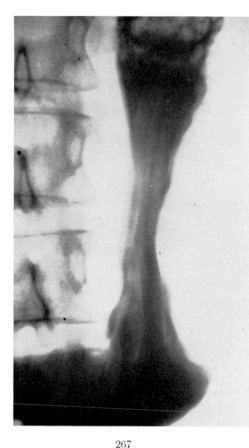

267   268

Question:

Figure 267 reveals a normal mucosal study of the vertical portion of the stomach. Does this entirely exclude ulcer within the region?

Answer:

Figure 2C8 is the same stomach and in the same position as figure 267. It is filled with barium and reveals an ulcer.

Comment: The stomach in figure 2C7, though revealing a normal mucosa, must not lead the examiner astray. Fluoroscopically, the examining hand must still try to push the barium into any hidden ulcer craters. Occasionally the ulcer crater may open and admit the barium only when the stomach is completely filled (as occurred here).

useful to observe on the *films* the barium in the apical and descending portion of the duodenum, which is *contiguous* and continuous with the barium in the bulb (figs. 273, 274).

Barium in varying amounts will enter into the *contiguous* descending duodenum as the bulb fills and empties. Further, barium in the descending duodenum by antiperistalsis will travel backwards and occasionally fill the duodenal bulb. Thus, varying degrees of filling of the *contiguous* descending duodenum point to varying degrees of filling of

the duodenal bulb which is *contiguous* and continuous with it and are hence diagnostically important: (1) If a deformity in the duodenal bulb remains *deformed in specifically the same fashion* during these various degrees of filling of the *contiguous* descending duodenum, that duodenal bulb probably is an *organically* deformed bulb, as for example, in duodenal ulcer. (2) If, with different degrees of filling, the duodenal bulb remains deformed and never becomes smooth and triangular but the deformity is *changeable and not constant*, this would suggest an

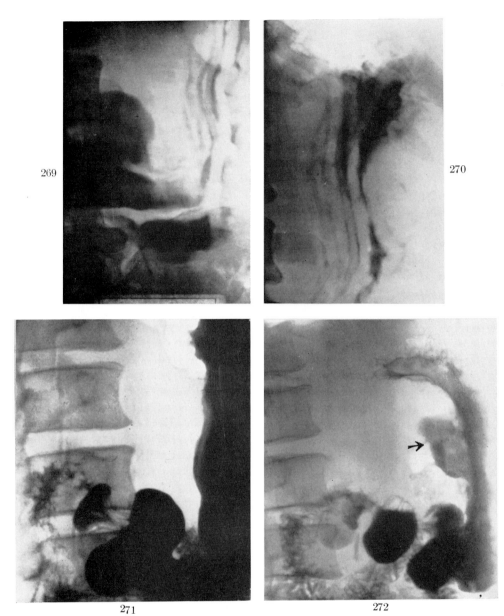

269   270

271   272

Question:

The gastric mucous membrane pattern in figures 269 and 270 is of the same stomach filled in figure 271. Figures 269, 270 and 271 appear normal. May an ulcer still be present?

Answer:

Figure 272 is the same stomach and in the lateral projection reveals a large gastric ulcer (arrow). In figures 269 and 270 the ulcer was not seen because the opaque media had not gained entry into the crater. In figure 271, the opaque media has entered into the crater, since the stomach is completely filled. The crater is not seen in figure 271 because it is situated on the posterior wall of the stomach; i.e., the barium in the stomach lies in front of the ulcer, thus hiding it. In figure 272, the patient is turned so that the posterior wall is brought into profile and the ulcer is seen.

Comment: Note how large an ulcer may be and yet be missed unless properly examined.

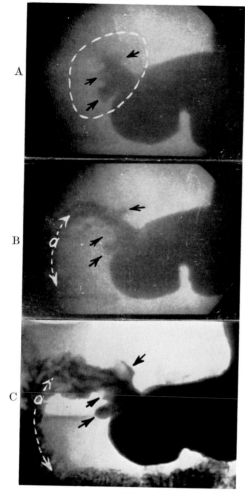

273

Question:

The duodenal bulb encircled in *A* appears deformed (arrows). Inadequate filling of the duodenal bulb permits the bulb to remain collapsed and improperly distended so that the bulb may *appear* deformed, when in truth it might be smooth, triangular and normal. How may one determine whether the deformity is due to inadequate filling or intrinsic pathology (as of ulcer)?

Answer:

If the duodenal bulb as it fills becomes larger and changes shape and contour, eventually achieving a smooth, triangular shape, it is normal. However, a scarred, contracted, deformed bulb will not permit itself to dilate with filling and thus achieve normal shape. Seeing the different degrees of filling by direct observation on the fluoroscopic screen and recording the findings on a spot film

irritable duodenal bulb such as is found with duodenitis. This latter type bulb would fill and empty quickly. (Cf. figs. 273, 274.) (3) If, with different degrees of filling, the duodenal bulb becomes dilated and smooth, this would be normal.

Crater as a Sign of Ulcer. The most definitive sign of a duodenal ulcer is the actual visualization of a crater.

A crater within the duodenum may not only deform the cap but also on occasion render this deformity characteristic.[12] Just as in the stomach a puckering of an old ulcer with radiating folds may be seen, also sometimes a central crater may exist with surrounding high thickened mucosal collar.

The examiner must be aware that when an *anterior or posterior* wall duodenal ulcer exists, the crater in the frontal projection (or right anterior oblique position) may be obscured by overlying barium and the bulb appear normal. With proper compression the ulcer niche may be seen "en face."

In the left anterior oblique position such an ulcer may manifest itself by projection from either the anterior or posterior walls (figs. 231, 232). This position, however, may be unsuccessful, for bulbs located high beneath the ribs (obese individuals)[17] are for the most part directed posteriorly and

is the method of choice. Observing the *contiguous* descending duodenum can also furnish an important clue (see text).

A reveals none of the opaque media has yet entered into the *contiguous* descending duodenum, i.e., the descending duodenum is not seen. In proceeding from *A* to *B* and next to *C*, the barium in the duodenal bulb becomes progressively more dense, but the bulb itself does not vary greatly in its size. Note, however, that in progressing from *A* to *B* to *C*, increasing amounts of barium are poured into the contiguous descending duodenum. This would indicate that the bulb as viewed in *A*, *B*, and *C* had different amounts of barium in it. This in turn would be evidence of *different degrees of filling of the bulb.* Note, however, that the *deformity* in the duodenal bulb remained *persistent* during these various degrees of filling. Thus, it can be assumed that the deformity was *not* produced by *inadequate* filling, but by an organic defect, i.e., ulcer.

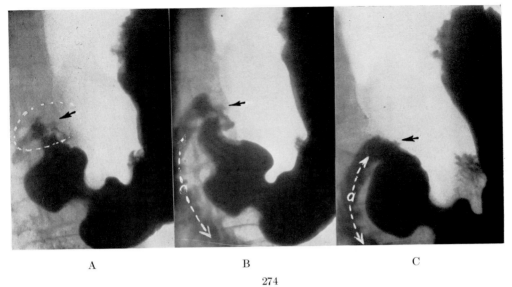

A   B   C

274

Question:

The duodenal bulb in *A* appears deformed (see legend, fig. 273). Is this deformity produced by inadequate filling of the bulb?

Answer:

As discussed in figure 273, if the duodenal bulb reveals the same persistent deformity as it empties and fills, this would indicate the deformity to be organic. Emptying and filling of the duodenal bulb can often be appraised by seeing the varying amounts of barium in the *contiguous* descending duodenum (a). *A* reveals the bulb before barium has spilled into the descending duodenum (a). *B* and *C* reveal the same bulb. The barium appears more densely packed, but the bulb itself is not larger. Note that the varying amounts of barium in the descending duodenum, together with the increased density in the bulb, demonstrate the relative filling and emptying of the bulb. Throughout *A*, *B*, and *C*, the deformity is persistent—despite the different degrees of filling. Thus, the defect can be considered organic (i.e., ulcer).

may be concealed by the *overlapping* barium filled antrum.

In regard to the duodenal compression, it is recommended as a routine that the bulb be compressed when the patient is erect as well as when he is recumbent. In the prone position, the use of a pneumatic compression paddle is advised.

Air Contrast Studies of the Duodenal Bulb
  (figs. 242–244)

Compression studies of the duodenal bulb, as noted above, cannot always be obtained because of the bulb's inaccessible position. Occasionally, too, marked abdominal muscle spasm may prevent effective compression. Even competent examiners may be unable to examine and compress the bulb properly.

In other cases, compression of the bulb may be dangerous, and, if done, must be performed with extreme care. Thus, in recent duodenal bleeding, the crater should be demonstrated by air contrast studies. In such cases, manipulation and compression of the bulb is to be avoided.

Thus, air-contrast visualization of the *crater* may be the only *certain* way to diagnose an *active* duodenal ulcer.[18] Having visualized the crater, its healing may be followed radiographically by periodic examination until it disappears.

It might be pointed out that air contrast studies are particularly useful in demonstrating those ulcers which are on the posterior wall. When the patient is supine, barium, with the aid of gravity, will remain in the crater, and air rising and entering the

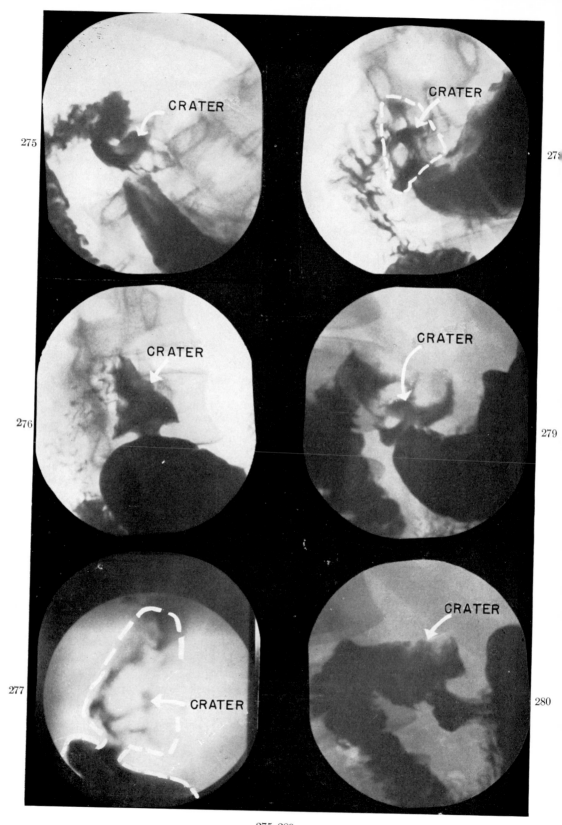

275–280

Different varieties of duodenal bulb deformities due to ulceration.

bulb (fig. 244) will permit contrast visualization of the ulcer. On the other hand, with the patient supine, barium in an anterior wall ulcer may "fall out" of the crater. In this event, a ring-like shadow, i.e., the opacified marginal ulcer wall, may be seen in air contrast.

Further Signs of Duodenal Ulcer

Other more or less characteristic deformities of the duodenum secondary to a duodenal ulcer are the existence of prestenotic diverticuli and the pylorus entering the duodenal cap in an off-center position. But descriptions of such deformities can more properly be left to radiographic texts.

Important secondary fluoroscopic signs of duodenal ulcer are hyperperistalsis, hypersecretion and, occasionally, antral spasm. Just as in the stomach, so in the duodenum: to coordinate any further signs would prove unsuccessful. Whereas hypertonus, hyperperistalsis and rapid emptying may be present at one time, the reverse may be present at another.

Duodenal Ulcers Not in the Bulb

Extrabulbar ulcers occur in about 5 per cent of cases. They occur more commonly in the descending portion of the duodenum between the apex of the duodenal bulb and the entrance of the ampulla of Vater.[12] The ulceration is usually single and large. The diagnosis is difficult and is commonly made by observing a marked irregular deformity which is persistent. The lumen within the region is narrowed and the duodenal bulb itself may often be irritable, although dilatation and stasis proximal to the stenotic area may also occur. The patient may reveal some sensitiveness over the ulcer area. The ulcer niche is often difficult to demonstrate.

A good technic for filling the second part of the duodenum is to occlude the third portion of the duodenum distal to the suspected abnormal areas. The examiner then waits for the second portion of the duodenum to fill as a result of a few successive gastric and bulbar peristaltic waves. The maneuver is carried out under fluoroscopic control and spot x-ray films are taken. This procedure is difficult in large, obese or muscular abdomens. The method may be attempted in the upright position with manual compression. It has been recommended that the procedure be performed in the prone or prone-oblique position.[21] Pads made from ordinary surgical gauze may be wound into oval balls and, under fluoroscopic control, placed between the patient and the table. Such a pad so positioned that when the weight of the patient rests on it, the third portion of the duodenum is occluded. This method requires a little patience and manipulation during fluoroscopy.

Ulcers of the genu are often well seen with the erect patient slowly rotated to an almost lateral position. Sometimes, with the patient prone, he must be rotated so that the left shoulder touches the screen, thus, practically lying in the right lateral decubitis position.

In all instances, spot filming the involved area is integral to the study.

Healing of Gastric and Duodenal Ulcers

In observing the healing of peptic ulcer, the size of the niche gradually recedes until eventually, in most cases, radiographically it may entirely disappear.

With chronic long standing gastric ulceration, some distortion secondary to fibrosis may result and a small projection from the gastric lumen be left behind. The healing of a duodenal ulcer cannot be studied with as great efficiency as the healing of a gastric ulcer, since the deformity in a scarified cap may prove persistent, this even in the presence of a healed crater. The last temporary deformity to disappear within the bulb is the spasm. When the ulcer heals with a cicatrized deformed cap, cure can be appraised by certainty, first that the deformity itself is constant and unchangeable, secondly, that the patient is symptom-free; both criteria necessitate a prolonged period of observation.

DUODENITIS

Duodenitis is a chronic inflammatory condition with little or no induration and an absence of chronic ulceration.[13] Konjetzny[11] believed that this condition is a pre-ulcerous condition. Its roentgen diagosis is not always possible.

It is characterized on the fluoroscopic screen as an irritable, unstable, writhing, fibrillating, rapidly emptying bulb. The *changing* irregularity of the cap is the prominent fluoroscopic feature (figs. 273–274). Although the cap even when filled is deformed, the deformity *changes* constantly. The deformity due to an ulcer is constant and without change (figs. 273–274). With duodenitis, a crater is never seen and the duodenal bulb is almost always tender on pressure.

DUODENAL STASIS

Duodenal stasis is characterized by a dilatation of the duodenum and a tendency of all portions to be filled at the same time. Compression of the duodenum by the mesenteric vessels is considered a prominent cause.[14] Other causes are congenital redundancy as well as mechanical sagging of portions of the duodenum.

Stasis is best demonstrated by examination in the erect position. Normally, the opaque meal remains in the bulb for only a few seconds and is then expelled quickly by peristaltic action. When the entire duodenum remains filled simultaneously this can be considered as fairly authentic evidence of obstruction and stasis. When a diagnosis of superior mesenteric artery occlusion is suspected, it is recommended that the patient be examined during an attack. There are periods when duodenal emptying may be temporarily satisfactory and a marked dilatation may not be discovered. In order to diagnose this condition, it is recom-

mended that the following criteria be met:[22]

1. There should be a constant dilatation of the duodenal sweep proximal to the midpart of the transverse portion corresponding to the point where contact with the superior mesenteric arteries should be.

2. There should be normal undilated duodenum demonstrated distal to this site.

3. There should be retention of barium beyond the normal time limit.

4. To-and-fro movements of barium should be seen within the duodenal loop.

Changes in duodenal peristalsis are commonly seen in duodenal stasis. The peristaltic waves are exaggerated and accompanied by antiperistalsis. Widman[15] noted that writhing and antiperistalsis is more intense when stasis is caused by duodenitis.

5. Other frequently associated findings are dilatation of the pylorus of the stomach, ptosis of the colon and small intestines, and ptosis of the right kidney.

Occasionally the disturbance may be functional. This is suggested (1) by failure to relieve distress by lying on the abdomen, thereby relieving tensions of the vessels on the duodenum or (2) when it is noted that symptoms appear only during emotional disturbances.

Puddling of the opaque meal may occur in various segments of the duodenum in asthenic individuals with atonic organs. Thus in these individuals the first portion of the duodenum may fail to empty after it is filled and the barium mixture may be seen here sometimes for quite a while afterwards. In other individuals of this habitus, stagnation occurs in the second and third portions when the patient is erect.

WIDENING OF THE DUODENAL LOOP

In individuals with a "steer-horn" type of stomach (hypersthenic obese people) the duodenal loop appears normally widened and thus in these individuals, appraisal is difficult when an apparent opening or widening of the loop is present. A common cause

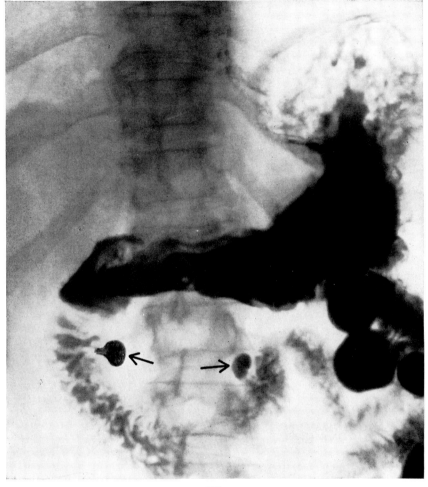

281

Grape-like shadows on duodenal sweep are indicative of duodenal diverticula. Note their presence *inside* the duodenal loop: this is characteristic.

for pathological widening of the duodenal loop is a tumor at the head of the pancreas. In arriving at a diagnosis of cancer of the head of the pancreas, in addition to seeing the widened duodenal loop the observer must seek for evidence of malignant invasion elsewhere in the vicinity, i.e., the antral region of the stomach and the descending portion of the duodenum. In large sized tumors of the pancreatic head the pylorus may also show signs of extrinsic pressure. The lumen of the duodenum may be encroached upon and become narrower and its contours, especially the descending loop, become irregular (fig. 282).

Acute pancreatitis may also cause widening of the duodenal loop. Roentgenological methods of diagnosis are of value in patients seen three or more days after onset of illness, when serum amylase values have returned to normal. The enlarged pancreas in this case may cause anterior displacement of the stomach and flattening of the medial duodenal mucosal folds. As the patient is rotated, fluoroscopically the distal portion of the stomach appears to move across the abdomen more rapidly than normally, due to its anterior displacement. (See law of the circle, p. 19ff.) Also, as a result of peri-pancreatic inflammation and edema there may

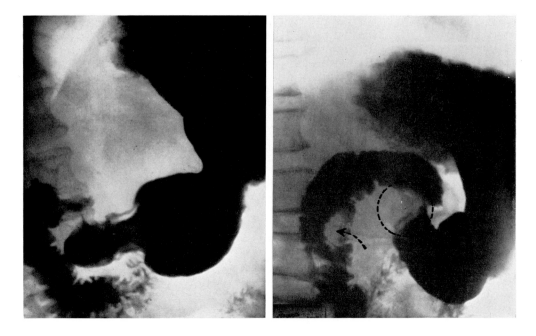

A   B

282

The descending duodenum in *A* (right anterior oblique position) is normal. The base of the duodenal bulb and antrum in *B* appears normal.

B (lateral projection) is the same patient as in *A* and reveals a defect at the base of the bulb and antrum as well as in the descending duodenum.

Comment: A pancreatic tumor was found at surgery, sitting in the duodenal sweep. It produced both deformities. If the examiner had been content with the study in *A*, the lesion would have been missed. It is urgent that all portions of the gastro-intestinal tract, when examined, be viewed in *all* directions. Even a tubelike structure as narrow as the descending duodenum does not show itself completely unless seen in *all* directions.

be some dilatation of the duodenum with local ileus.[25] Gastric emptying begins with little delay. However, subsequent abrupt stasis of barium in the descending duodenum may be striking on fluoroscopy.

On the other hand, narrowing due to spasm may be seen in the descending duodenum secondary to the pancreatic inflammation. However, it should be borne in mind that the narrowing may be due to compression—not spasm.[26]

In pancreatitis, the diagnosis must be confirmed by subsequent return to normal findings. This may take from a few weeks to a few months.[27]

DUODENAL DIVERTICULUM

Duodenal diverticulum is asymptomatic and is usually an incidental finding. It may be single or multiple, and arise from or occur in almost any portion of the duodenal sweep on its medial or pancreatic side (fig. 281). Retention of some of the opaque material in the sac is common. The length of time that barium is retained, however, is variable.

GASTRIC NEOPLASM

Certain findings during fluoroscopic examination should make the examiner suspicious of neoplastic disease. A negative defect (fig. 184) or failure of part of the

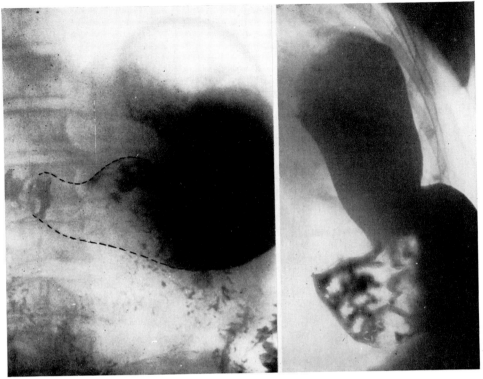

283   284

Question:

What are the important gastric mucosal configurations in the presence of carcinoma?

Answer:

Obliteration or disappearance of rugal pattern, as evidenced in the antrum.

An abnormal configuration which refuses to change when palpated.

stomach to fill should arouse suspicions of neoplastic disease (figs. 223–226). The defect is usually ragged and irregular, often presenting a typical "fingered" deformity. Other negative defects may also be seen in the region due to extension of the growth.

The mucosal examination with the thin barium mixture reveals varying patterns in malignant disease of the stomach. The folds tend to atrophy and disappear (fig. 283). Barium clinging to the various crevices in the growth may reveal a bizarre relief pattern of the tumor itself. However, for practical purposes, carcinoma should be suspected when the mucosal pattern is bizarre and rigid and refuses to distort itself by pressure with the palpating hand (fig. 284). Moreover, when this same defect does not

permit a normal peristaltic wave to pass through it, this can be taken as further evidence in arriving at such a diagnosis (fig. 285).

An ulcer crater with malignant characteristics has previously been described.

A smooth antral defect with free mobility may be a polyp (fig. 186). This on occasion may need differentiation from a foreign body. The greater mobility of the latter is to be sought for by applying pressure with the protected palpating hand.

Changes in peristalsis will occur with gastric carcinoma. Changes in peristalsis when present must be appraised critically. When the innervation is involved from any condition, changes in peristalsis may occur in areas not infiltrated with tumor.[23] Thus,

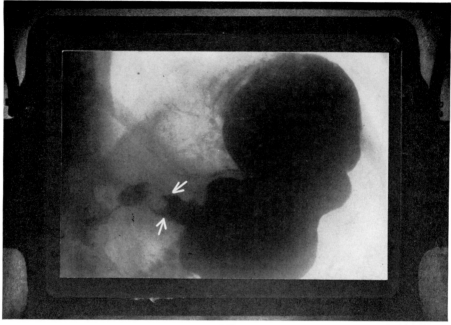

285

Question:

An area of narrowing is found within the antral region (between arrows). What may produce such a configuration?

Answer:

    1. Antral carcinoma.

    2. Antral spasm.

    3. Antral gastritis.

Question:

What were the fluoroscopic findings?

Answer:

    1. No peristalsis passed through the narrowed region.

    2. The narrow region did at no time dilate; i.e., *lack of changing contour*.

    3. When the mucosal pattern was examined it was found disrupted and with an abnormal pattern. This abnormal pattern (fig. 285) was persistent and could not be changed by the palpating hand.

Comment: In order to make certain that these findings were persistent, the patient was re-examined ten days later, with the same results. At laparotomy an antral carcinoma was found.

peristalsis may be diminished at the lesion and in areas where a lesion may not even be present. Occasionally a passive wave may occur in the region of a lesion as a result of transmitted peristalsis either around or through the infiltrated area.

NEOPLASTIC DISEASE OF THE FUNDUS

Neoplastic disease within the fundus frequently involves the cardia, the lower end of the esophagus and the adjacent portion of the pars media of the stomach. Because of its location, the principal clues to its existence may be detected at the *lower end of the esophagus* or when barium first *enters* the stomach (figs. 286, 288). Since the recognition of the normal is an essential prerequisite to the diagnosis of the abnormal, and since carcinoma of the fundus is so frequently associated with carcinoma of the lower esophagus, it would be valuable to review briefly the normal pasage of barium through the esophagus and entry into the stomach.

It should be stressed that familiarity with this entry is important, a familiarity gained by fluoroscopic study of many known normals and such variations as hypertonic, atonic, cascade stomach, etc. (see pp. 157 and 196).

Examination of the Normal

At this point, pages 113–117 should be reviewed. In summary, the space occupied by the esophagus is first examined for fluid levels or mass formations. Normally the space behind the heart and in front of the spine, occupied by the esophagus, presents no significant opacities, no fluid levels, no soft tissue densities. After viewing this space and finding it normal, the fluoroscopic screen is lowered and the normal gas-distended fundus is examined. (See fig. 27, p. 27.) Note should be made of any encroachment on to the stomach air bubble which cannot be explained. The distance between the superior margin of the gastric fundus and the lung above should be appraised. The normal thickness should be between 5–15 mm.[24] Any encroachments, if present, should again be checked when the region is examined with opaque media as described below.

Examination of the Abnormal

At this point, pages 117ff should be reviewed.

Before Contrast Media. After examining the esophagus, the screen is next carried downwards and signs within the fundus are sought. The stomach air bubble is carefully scrutinized. The distance between the superior margin of the fundus and the base of the lung above should be appraised (see fig. 227, p. 175). Irregularities in the fundus should also be noted. At this point the patient should be instructed not to belch during the balance of the examination. The

examiner must be aware that the distance between the fundus and the lung above must be appraised when the fundus is *distended* with air and the patient is in the *erect* position. The normal thickness of 5–15 mm. may be increased, due to incomplete distention of a normal fundus (figs. 227–230). Also, the incompletely distended fundus may present some irregularities in its roof, simulating a tumor. In truth, this may be nothing more than infoldings of normal mucosa. Usually the air swallowed during the normal ingestion of the barium mixture is enough to adequately distend the fundus and clear the dilemma. At times the examiner may have to introduce larger amounts of air. This is described below.

A soft tissue mass with irregular or lobulated outline projecting into the lumen is characteristic of tumor (fig. 286*B*, also fig. 287*B*, p. 215).

The question frequently arises as to whether a suspicious shadow is or is not located in the stomach fundus. A lesion, in order to be determined as *within* the gastric lumen, must be seen as *intraluminal* in *all* degrees of obliquity. A good procedure is to position the patient so that the profile of the suspected shadow is best seen against the air contrast offered by the stomach air bubble. The patient is next turned through an angle of 90 degrees. The angle of rotation should be in two directions, i.e., right and left. The purpose of rotating in both directions is the possible removal of overlapping shadows (spine, liver, spleen, etc.). Spot films are taken to confirm all findings. If, in these degrees of rotation, the suspected shadow is *still* found to be within the lumen, it is probably intragastric in position. Further maneuvers are described presently under "Useful Aids in Examining the Fundus."

With Contrast Media (compare figs. 286 A and 286 B). A mouthful of the barium suspension having been swallowed, its course down the esophagus and entry into the stomach air bubble is studied. Its down-

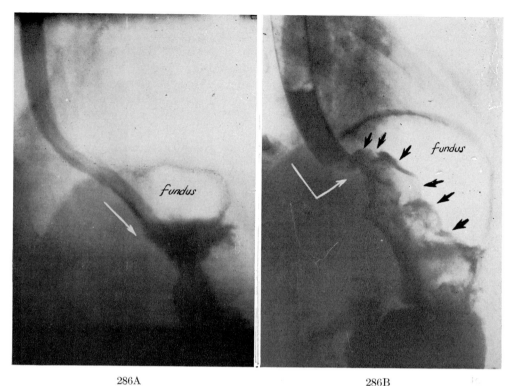

286A   286B

Normal entry of barium into the stomach fundus shown in figure 286A.

Question:

What signs in figure 286B indicate the presence of a fundal carcinoma? (Cf. fig. 286A.)

Answer:

a. Soft tissue mass with irregular contours (black arrows) projecting into the stomach fundus.

b. Fluoroscopically, one can see the abnormal irregular course (arrows) followed by the contrast material as it trickles down over the tumor.

c. Retention of barium in the esophagus (note fluid level within esophagus, which is absent in fig. 286A).

d. Irregularity at the lower end of the esophagus.

e. Entry of the esophagus into the stomach at right angles (bent arrow) as compared with normal (straight arrow in fig. 286A).

ward descent into the pars media is observed. This procedure is repeated with several mouthfuls. It should be borne in mind that barium coming into a normal stomach enters in a single stream (figs. 207, 208), but if there is a projecting tumor, its entry may be split (fig. 209). To see the barium column split as it enters the cardia, an amount of barium large enough to travel through all channels and portions of the suspected tumor must be given. When such precautions are not taken, the examination may pass as normal (figs. 291–296). A small sip may travel to *one* side or through the region of the tumor and enter as a *single* stream. This is especially apt to happen when a patient has a lesion at the cardia, causing dysphagia, since he has learned that he cannot handle large amounts of ingested material comfortably. The normal inclination of such a patient is to sip small amounts. This (or any) patient must be told

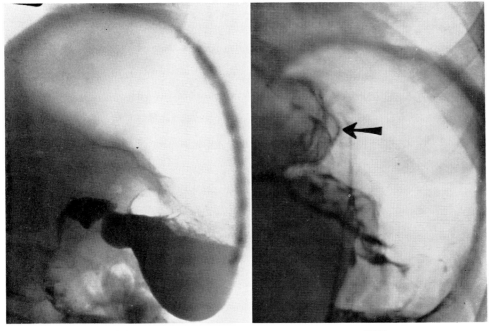

287A   287B

Fig. 287A is the same fundus shown in fig. 287B. In fig. 287B (an *enlarged* spot film of fig. 287A) a mass is seen projecting into the fundus (arrow), but not in fig. 287A.

Question: Why was the mass found in fig. 287B but not seen (missed) in fig. 287A?

Answer:

In fig. 287A the patient was not fluoroscoped and was routinely given a Seidlitz powder. The fundus distended, the patient was placed in a standing position, and the picture was snapped.

The degree of fundal distention in fig. 287A is too great, i.e., a mass which without fundal distention occupies ⅒ of the fundus would, if the fundus were distended 10 times, occupy ¹⁄₁₀₀ of that fundus. This would be harder to find.

The patient was not fluoroscoped. The tumor might thus have been photographed "en face," i.e., not in profile. The tumor "en face," if it were not large enough or not covered with barium, might not have offered sufficient contrast to be seen—i.e., it would be "blotted out" by the large distended air pocket of the fundus.

The tumor, being small and made smaller by the comparatively overdistended fundus (explained above), would have offered more contrast if properly coated with barium. The technician made no real attempt to coat the tumor properly with barium.

Answer:

In fig. 287B the examining physician took the film with fluoroscopic spot film control.

The degree of fundal distention is not too great. In this patient the normal amount of air swallowed while drinking the barium mixture was sufficient to distend the fundus (16 oz.). Note that the *enlarged* spot film may falsely imply that the distention is as great as in fig. 287A.

The patient was rotated until an *"apparent mass"* was seen projecting into the fundus. This was spot filmed. The mass, having been found in profile, could now be followed fluoroscopically on further rotation, and at no time could it be rotated out of the fundus. Its position *within* the fundus was thereby proved.

The patient took 16 oz. barium and was then placed in a supine Trendelenberg position to coat the fundus. Barium may not adhere to a smooth fundus, but enough is apt to adhere to a "roughened" tumor surface to make that tumor visible.

to drink large amounts—enough to demonstrate the defect—and to drink rapidly.

Other modes of abnormal entry into the

cardia in the presence of a tumor may also be seen. Thus, barium may be observed rebounding off a projecting neoplasm. Also

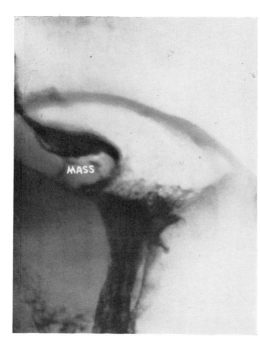

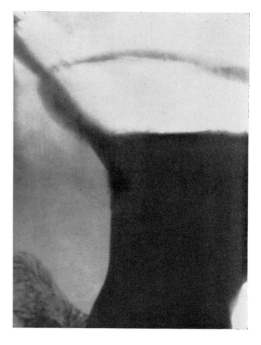

288A   288B

The stomach is being examined. The first few mouthfuls of barium are observed entering the stomach. The opaque material is seen coursing over a tumor mass.

Question:

This is the same stomach as in figure 288A. Why does the entry now appear normal?

Answer:

This demonstrates the "penalty" of observing too late. The stomach is now filled and the flooded area blots out the tumor. If the examiner had missed observing the first few mouthfuls of barium traveling over the tumor, he would now no longer see it.

Comment: In any gastro-intestinal study, the actual entry of barium into the stomach must be observed with the first few ingested mouthfuls.

barium may be seen traveling *around* a projected neoplasm (figs. **297–299**). This traveling around a projecting neoplasm should be distinguished from the entry of barium into a cascade stomach (carefully cf. figs. **289, 290**).

The barium, in its entry into the stomach, may also be regurgitated back up the esophagus in the presence of a tumor.

All findings should be confirmed with spot films.

The importance of seeing the *initial entry* of the opaque media through the cardia and into the fundus bears repetition. If visualization here is delayed, the upper pole of the stomach may quickly become partially filled and significant fundal irregularities may become inundated by the barium and hidden (figs. **288A,B;** cf. figs. **289, 290**). This is especially serious since palpation and thin layer compression studies are not possible in the highly placed gastric fundus.

During the time that the fundus is examined, the examiner keeps an eye on the lower end of the esophagus. As already noted, abnormal retention or deformities here are *important clues* in the diagnosis of fundal carcinoma (fig. **286B**). Having ex-

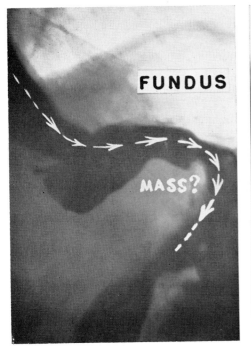

289

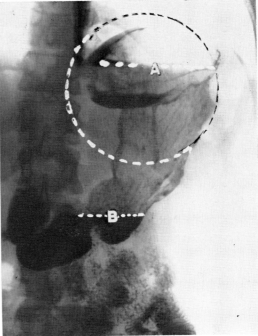

290

Question:

(Area viewed is portion encircled in figure 290.)
The patient is in the erect right anterio oblique position. Barium is seen entering the stomach, then winding its way over an apparent mass to descend into the stomach. How may this occur without a lesion being present (as opposed to the situation in figure 288A)?

Answer:

In a cascade or "cup-and-spill" type stomach, as the barium pours from the "upper cup" into the lower portion of the stomach it may sometimes appear as if it were traveling over a mass. The examiner will recognize this appearance by being familiar with the "cup-and-spill" effect. Moreover, separate fluid levels in the fundus and at the lower portion of the stomach would also inform the examiner as to this cascade effect.

amined the fundus, the examiner next raises the screen and makes final direct observation of the opaque media in its passage through the esophagus. In summary, important signs to look for which may betray the presence of an underlying tumor are:

1. Esophageal dilatation. Fundal carcinoma not infrequently involves the lower esophagus, causing partial obstruction. The widened lumen is produced secondary to the involvement.

2. Esophageal retention. The underlying partial obstruction producing the increased caliber of the lumen may also be responsible for a temporary holdup of some of the

opaque media after the major portion of the barium suspension has passed into the stomach. In more severe degrees of obstruction, reflux of the retained barium upwards into the esophagus and reverse peristalsis may be seen. The vallecula sign may also be positive.

3. Deformity and narrowing of the esophageal contours. As a result of the involvement of the lower end of the esophagus, its contours may be deformed or narrowed.

4. Intraluminal masses in the gastric fundus. An intraluminal mass within the fundus may occasionally be seen as a filling defect in the barium-filled fundus. This is

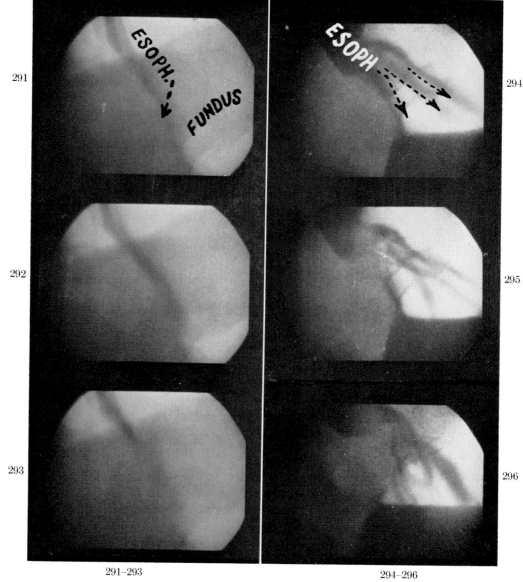

291–293   294–296

Question:

Is the entry of barium into the fundus normal?

Answer:

Yes. Barium enters into the gastric fundus in a single stream directed downwards, and thus appears normal.

Question:

The *same* gastric fundus as in figures 291–293. Is the entry of barium into the fundus normal?

Answer:

No. The barium entry is now split into many streams. This is characteristic of a neoplastic lesion at the site of entry.

Comment: In figures 291–293, the patient had been instructed to take a *sip* of the opaque media. The patient followed instructions and swallowed an amount *not sufficient* to fill *all* of the channels—which, when filled out properly as in figures 294–296, yielded the diagnosis.

During every esophageal study, the examiner must make certain that he has seen the esophagus when *enough* of the opaque media has been swallowed to *completely* fill out the region in question. For this, sipping is insufficient; the patient *must* be instructed to *drink rapidly* and take *large mouthfuls* at a time.

best demonstrated by placing the patient with a barium-filled stomach in the supine Trendelenburg position. As shown in figures 169–171, the defect in the barium-filled fundus must be appraised critically. Some minor deformities may occasionally occur to confuse the examiner. When difficulty arises, air contrast studies of the fundus should be performed to confirm the diagnosis.

Useful Aids in Examining the Fundus

1. Because of the ready availability of air within the fundal region of the stomach and since a large percentage of the neoplastic diseases within the stomach is of the polypoid type, air contrast studies are particularly suited to this region (figs. 227–230).

Many technics have been devised to perform air contrast studies of the fundus more efficiently. Thus, Seidlitz powder and various carbonated drinks have been given. If a patient is asked to swallow air, the request may confuse him and he may not be aware of his ability to do so. A recommended method is to ask the patient to drink through a glass tube while the examiner himself holds the glass containing the barium suspension. Without the patient being aware of the maneuver, the glass is slightly lowered away from the tube, and, instead of barium suspension, he draws in and swallows air. This "fooling the patient" is often successful in distending the gastric fundus with air.

A precautionary measure in securing good air contrast studies of the fundal portion of the stomach is to advise the patient to try not to belch throughout the examination. The fundus should be coated with barium. The patient is given 8 oz. of a thick barium mixture, then placed in the supine position (fig. 199C). In this way, the fundal wall, and any lesions on it, are coated. Air next administered must not overdistend the fundus (fig. 287).

2. Diaphragmatic movements may sometimes aid in the diagnosis of fundal neo-

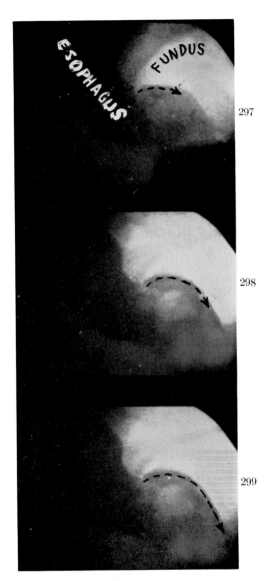

297

298

299

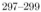

297–299

Barium is seen entering the stomach (dotted line), and winding its way over a mass. Since normal entry should carry the barium more or less in a straight path downwards, the course of the barium traveling over a mass is abnormal. In this case, it is produced by a tumor. This is a similar situation to that seen in figure 288, but no blotting out took place.

Question:

When may such an entry be simulated in the normal?

Answer:

See figures 289 and 290.

plastic disease.[19] Thus, with inspiration and expiration, the shape of the normal fundus changes. A shadow within the fundus may constantly retain its own peculiar shape even when the rest of the fundus alters appearance. This constancy in appearance may indicate fundal neoplastic disease. Assessing the significance of this lack of change of course demands a thorough understanding of the effect of inspiration and expiration on the *normal* stomach and the examiner should bear these changes in mind when studying the stomach suspected of an infiltrative or neoplastic lesion.

3. Any density encroaching upon the stomach air bubble must be appraised. An important question is whether the shadow is intra- or extraluminal. This, as described above, is determined by continued rotation of the patient until either the lesion is rotated out of the fundal lumen or the examiner is convinced that rotation alone will not cause the shadow to rotate clear of the stomach air bubble. When, in certain cases, it is difficult to decide whether a lesion projects into the air bubble, coating the suspected shadow with opaque media and viewing it in air contrast may resolve the question. *If the seat of the suspected shadow is within the lumen, barium can be made to settle on it,* outlining its margins with a pencil-like line. If it is located *outside* the gastric wall, opaque media within the stomach cannot possibly coat it.

To perform this test, the patient is positioned so that the suspected lesion presents its most *irregular* margin in profile. *Careful note is made of this position.* The patient, with his stomach half filled with contrast material, is next placed in the supine Trendelenberg position. The opaque media thus fills the fundus. After this, the patient is again arranged in the upright position, thereby permitting the barium suspension to descend into the stomach, leaving a thin coating to outline the fundus. The patient is now placed in the degree of obliquity previously noted as best demonstrating its most irregular margin in profile. These *irregularities*, if *intraluminal*, are now coated and outlined by the opaque media. If *extraluminal*, they will not be coated nor outlined by the opaque media, and in such case the deformity is produced as a result of indenture from the outside.

4. When a fundal tumor extends downwards into the pars media, its presence must first be detected *before* the involved region is completely covered over with opaque media. In order to revisualize this downward extension, after its inundation, the patient should be examined in the erect position. The examiner must now wait until the gastric fluid level sinks low enough to permit the lesion to appear above it (fig. 97). At this time, a thin coating of barium remains, outlining the lesion.

5. Tumors localized to the fundus and not extending downwards often betray their presence by producing a thickening of the space between the stomach air bubble and the base of the lung (see fig. 27, p. 27 and figs. 227–230).

6. In rare instances, it is possible to palpate the cardiac end of the stomach. The patient is asked to breathe in deeply. With inspiration the diaphragm descends and pushes the cardiac region of the stomach downwards beneath the costal arch. This maneuver can be performed with the patient in the erect as well as horizontal positions.

7. The examination should be performed with both thick and thin barium mixture. The splitting of the stream by a tumor projecting into the path of the opaque media is best seen with thinner mixtures (figs. 207–209, p. 169).

8. In the process of film taking, no definite routine is followed. Films are taken in those positions which fluoroscopically elicited the most information.

Summary

Carcinoma at the fundus of the stomach is most difficult to diagnose. Suspected cases must be examined with painstaking care.

One of the chief difficulties is the decision as to whether some of the irregularities in the fundal mucosa are due to early tumor or some anatomic variation. Suspected cases where a decision cannot be reached immediately must, therefore, be re-examined at 2 to 3 week intervals.

Esophagoscopy and gastroscopy are important aids. Early, small carcinomas of the fundus can be extremely difficult to detect radiologically. It should be remembered that if the cardia is involved, the lesion may be seen with the esophagoscope.

PYLORIC OBSTRUCTION

In the presence of pyloric obstruction the stomach is large. It is distributed transversely across the abdomen with the antral region far to the right of the spine and the duodenal cap directed backwards and to the left. This first portion of the duodenum is often well hidden behind the antrum and most often can be seen only in a true lateral position. Obstruction due to a stenosing duodenal ulcer usually gives rise to such an appearance. Peristalsis in this type of stom-

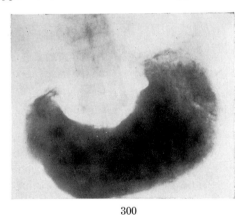

300

Question:

What may produce the multiple dark and light shadows within this stomach cast?

Answer:

These multiple defects may be produced by either polyps or food residue. The free mobility of these defects, as found by palpation behind the fluoroscopic screen, pointed to food residue.

ach may at first be active, but soon the gastric musculature tires and the dilated stomach lies quiet and grossly distended. Negative defects with wide mobility in such stomachs are frequent and due to food residue (fig. 300).

Extremely large stomachs are usually caused by benign obstructive processes, since a patient with a carcinoma obstructing the gastric outlet does not live long enough for the stomach to attain so large a size. This rule is not infallible.

In cases of complete obstructive lesions, it is often impossible to state whether the lesion is in the pre-pyloric, pyloric or post-pyloric regions.

EXTRINSIC PRESSURE ON THE STOMACH

Extrinsic pressure exerted on the stomach will cause a displacement and spreading of the mucosal folds in exactly the same manner as the examiner can produce with the palpating hand (fig. 301). In other words, the stomach will be distorted in a characteristic fashion depending upon the pressure exerted upon it. With sufficient pressure the gastric mucosal folds may even disappear. On fluoroscopic examination the examiner will note that the stomach may be in an abnormal position, and that distortion of the mucosal pattern presents a characteristic extrinsic indenture, the stomach draping itself, or being stretched over, the applied pressure.

A diagnosis, however, is not always simple, and other clues must be sought for, e.g., lack of crater formation within the gastric lumen. Normal rugal folds when seen are highly important in arriving at an accurate diagnosis.

PERIGASTRIC ADHESIONS

Perigastric adhesions occur most frequently along the lesser curvature of the antrum and lower body of the stomach. The most frequent adhesions are gallbladder,

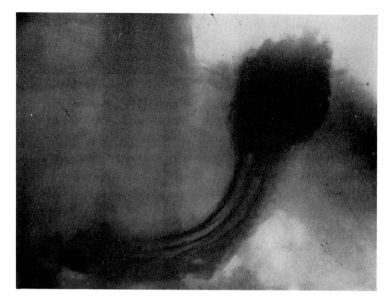

301

Question:

Is the hollowed out smooth contour of the lesser curvature due to *intrinsic stomach pathology* or is it produced by pressure from an *extrinsic mass?*

Fluoroscopic examination:

1. Stretched-out appearance of the normal rugal pattern as if it were being indented by a mass outside the stomach.
2. No defects in the mucosal pattern or gastric contours.
3. No ulcer craters.
4. Peristalsis was seen passing through the region.
5. The entire stomach was flexible, pliable, and mobile.
6. The stomach generally appeared as though it were draped over a mass situated in the region of the lesser curvature.

Answer:

Laparotomy revealed an *extrinsic* mass pressing and indenting the lesser gastric curvature.

pancreas, liver or diaphragm. The adhesions may produce deformity, irregularity, fixation and elevation of the stomach wall. This deformity and iregularity of the stomach may be difficult to distinguish from the carcinoma.

It is significant that with adhesions as opposed to carcinoma, the stomach wall is soft, pliable and peristalsis passes through the deformed region. A "trapped-air" sign has been described as diagnostically valuable when adhesions are present which elevate and fix the antrum. When the stomach wall is soft and pliable and the patient is placed in the erect position, adhesions may pull on the lesser curvature wall and produce a tenting and trapping of air beneath. Peristaltic constrictions aid in the formation of this tenting. Since a soft stomach wall is essential for this tenting to take place, it is not expected when an antral irregularity is produced by a stomach wall stiffened by carcinoma.

SUMMARY: PROCEDURE

Since fluoroscopy of the stomach is considered the most complicated of all fluoroscopic procedures, it would be wise for the examiner to prepare for himself an outline of his expected findings. A suggested form for such an outline is indicated directly below.

1. Were gastric and duodenal contours adequately studied? Were there any undue dilatations, projections, positive or negative filling defects? Are fundus and cardia normal?

2. Was there any abnormal change in the position of the stomach?

3. Was peristalsis present on both curvatures?

Recommended Fluoroscopic Sheet to be Filled Out

Stomach: Hypertonic   Orthotonic   or Hypotonic

Position:

Peristalsis:

Defects or other irregularities:

Mobility:

Pliability or Flexibility:

Duodenal cap: Well visualized   Not well visualized

       Small or large:

       Filled completely or incompletely:

       Misshapen

       Defects

Duodenum: 2nd, 3rd and 4th portions visualized

       Normal or abnormal

Examination of the Small Bowel

General Principles

INTRODUCTION

THE SMALL BOWEL is the longest portion of the digestive tract. It is the most physiologically active. In the main it is readily accessible. Yet, progress in the radiographic diagnosis of small bowel lesions has not been as satisfactory as that in other portions of the gastrointestinal tract. Several factors may be held responsible.

1. Its very length is a disadvantage. Thorough examination is tedious and time consuming and the dividends are often small. The incidence of organic disease in this portion of the bowel is lower than in any other part of the gastrointestinal tract.

2. In order to accommodate the twenty-odd feet of small bowel within the abdomen, considerable coiling and overlapping of the various loops take place, making accurate visualization of individual loops difficult.

3. Preparatory to examination, fasting alone or in combination with cleansing enemas from below is insufficient to cleanse the small bowel. The retained secretions and small bowel contents cannot be adequately eliminated. These contents may mix with the opaque media and even in a normal individual may produce bizarre patterns simulating disease (figs. 302–304).

4. In truth the line of division between the normal and the abnormal may be so narrow and a definite diagnosis so difficult that *unless the positive findings of any disease process can be duplicated in at least two different examinations, no diagnosis of a small bowel lesion should be assumed as certain.*

The fluoroscopic examination is helpful in counteracting some of the disadvantages.

1. The loops of bowel, although overlapping, are situated chiefly in the center of the abdomen, without any viscera overlying the main portion, and are thus readily available to palpation. One segment can be separated from another, fluoroscopically studied, and spot filmed.

2. Portions of the small bowel when trapped and compressed within the pelvis are unattainable for adequate examination.

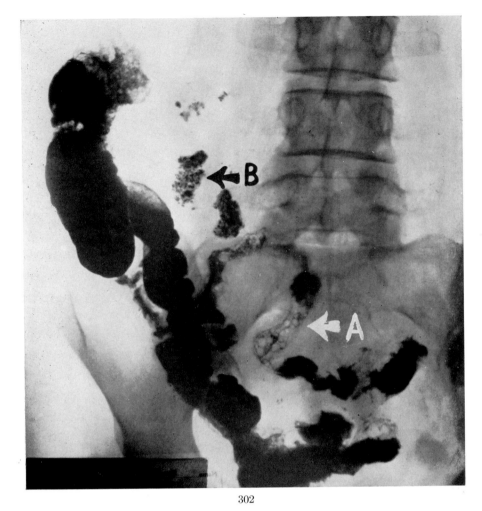

302

Question: What produces the bizarre mucosal patterns at *A* and *B*?

Answer: A demonstrates a mixture of air, fluid and barium. The mucous membrane is not properly coated and, therefore, not really outlined. *B* demonstrates barium gathered in floccules. The barium in this form is incapable of homogeneously layering out on the mucosa to outline its true pattern. These changes must not be confused with abnormalcies of the mucosa.

They may be shifted or dislodged upwards out of the true pelvis and into the abdomen, however, by simple maneuvers such as placing the patient in the Trendelenberg position. These loops, now more accessible, lend themselves to more accurate examination.

Loops of bowel failing to shift with this maneuver may often be palpated via the rectum or vagina during the fluoroscopic examination. Other methods useful in reaching these loops are described below (page 258).

3. The radiographic film appearance of the small bowel may on numerous occasions be confusing. It may be difficult to arrive at a decision as to whether a disease process is present. Fluoroscopic examination may prove extremely helpful. A good rule to follow is to develop and study the film immediately while the patient is still on the x-ray table. If a suspicious loop of intestine is found on the film, the patient is immediately refluoroscoped. The involved loop found behind the fluoroscopic screen is now

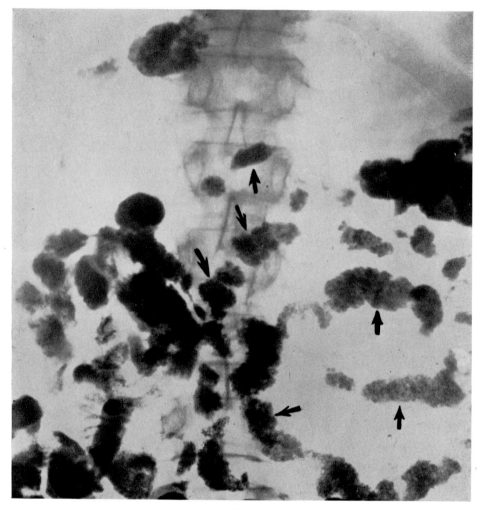

303

Segmentation (Cf. figs. 313-315, page 231).

Question: The feathery upper and lower margins of the opacified jejunum are absent. Does this indicate that the Kerkring folds are absent or flattened?

Answer: No. The barium has become lumpy and in the form of *lumps* is not capable of entering into the crevices between the folds to form a mold outlining the Kerkring folds.

subject to various observations not otherwise possible (fig. 332). Thus, finding the involved segment tender or rigid is an important factor. By means of graded compression, the mucosal pattern may be more adequately studied. *It should be stressed that confirmation of the fluoroscopic findings by conventional or spot filming should be the rule.*

4. As in other portions of the intestinal tract, study of the peristaltic wave is important. A loop suspected of being infiltrated with neoplastic disease may be examined behind the fluoroscopic screen. The direct visualization of a peristaltic wave arriving at the segment, and *failing* to pass through, is indeed indicative of abnormalcy.

5. The stomach tube as well as the long

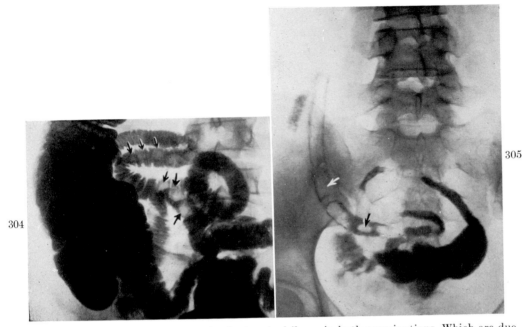

Circular negative defects are seen in the terminal ileum in both examinations. Which are due to structural changes in the small bowel?

304

Fluoroscopically, the ileum in this case was found nontender, and the defects could be shifted about freely. Characteristically this type of defect is produced when the ileum is filled in a retrograde fashion during the course of a barium enema. Such defects are caused by fecal material being washed back from the colon. The exaggeration of the transverse folds in the ileum is also a result of retrograde filling.

305

These defects were seen fluoroscopically to be part of a tender mass. They were constant in position and did not move about freely. These are the polypoid changes found in regional ileitis.

intestinal tube may be used to study the small bowel. Their passage and management may be performed more efficiently with the aid of the fluoroscope, as described in the second section of this chapter and in Chapter VIII.

It should be stated here that there is some small amount of duplication between the present chapter and the chapter on Intestinal Obstruction, since repetition of information at logical points of discussion seemed likely to be a more helpful measure to the user of this volume than excessive cross references. An attempt has been made, however, to keep such repetition to a minimum.

ANATOMY

The small intestine is in the main a freely movable, coiled, tube-like structure occupying most of the abdomen. It extends from the pyloric sphincter of the stomach to the ileo-cecal valve located within the cecum.

The small intestine is the longest part of the gastrointestinal tract, being some 20-odd feet in length. It consists of two portions; the *first*, called the *duodenum*, has previously been discussed. The *second*, a longer coiled portion attached to the posterior abdominal wall by a convoluted or fan-shaped mesentery, is called the *mesenteric portion*. This portion of the small bowel is the part we shall discuss here.

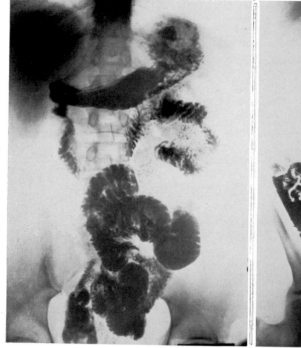

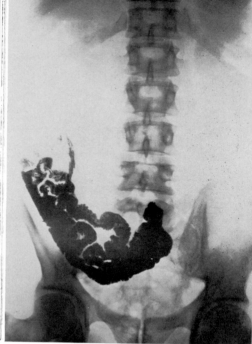

306

Gastric emptying and small bowel filling. Note total amount of barium in stomach and loops of small intestine; compare this with the amount of barium seen in figure 307.

307

Same patient as in figure 238.

Question:

Patient has neither vomited any of the barium seen in figure 306 nor passed any by rectum, yet the quantity of barium now appears diminished. How does this come about?

Answer:

Dehydration of the barium mixture in the ileum makes it appear more concentrated and lessened in amount. This is a normal finding.

This mesenteric portion of the small bowel is again divided into an upper two-fifths called *jejunum*, and a lower three-fifths, the *ileum*. No sharp line of division exists between these two portions, and one passes imperceptibly into the other.

Jejunum Contrasted with Ileum. The loops of the mesenteric portion are freely movable and not fixed in position. Its various loops may shift and slide about on each other so that no *true* constancy of position can be attained. Finding constancy of position of an individual loop, except perhaps in the terminal ileum, is extremely suggestive of abnormalcy (figs. 311, 312). Yet, *as*

groups, various portions of the small intestine are more or less confined to their own sections in the abdomen.

A rough and ready rule as to the distribution of the small bowel loops would place the *jejunum* in the left upper quadrant and central portions of the abdomen; the *ileum*, in the pelvis and right lower quadrants of the abdomen; the *transitional* small bowel, *i.e.*, that portion wherein the small bowel gradually changes from jejunum to ileum, would be expected to occupy the right upper quadrant immediately beneath the liver (fig. 320, p. 234).

As seen on the fluoroscopic screen then, a

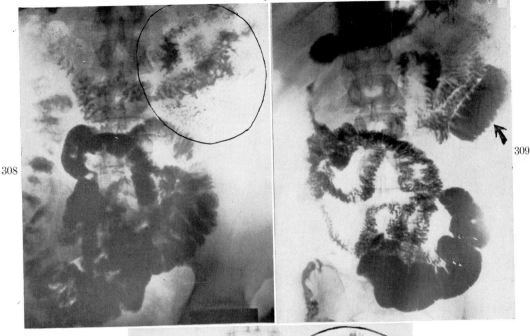

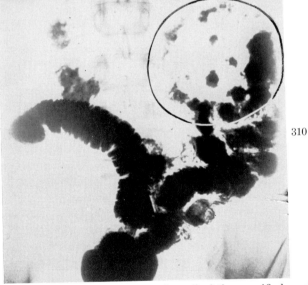

Some normal variations that may occur at the tail of the opacified small bowel.

308

Segmentation at the tail (encircled loops) due to incomplete filling, i.e., irregular emptying of the last gastric residues.

309

A dilated segment (arrow) may be a trailing segment and produced by partial obstruction. To confirm the presence of a "trailing segment" it must *retain* its dilated appearance at interval studies. Also, localized holdup of the opaque media must take place *at this segment*, and the holdup should be seen as a damming back of the barium during repeat studies. Since none of these were present, the segment here arrowed is considered normal.

310

Clumping of barium at the tail (encircled loops).

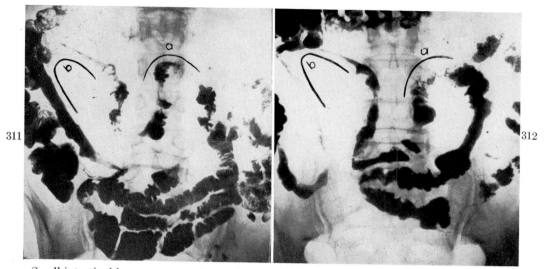

Small intestinal loops are normally freely moveable and do not maintain the *same position* on interval examinations. A *fixed* configuration or position in the abdomen should suggest abnormalcy. *In comparing any interval studies, a certain attitude of mind is necessary. The examiner should concentrate on detecting loops which are fixed and do not change their configuration or positions.*

311

First interval study: Loops *a* and *b* palpated fluoroscopically are rigid, masslike and tender.

312

Second interval study (one hour later): Loops *a* and *b* retain the *same position and configuration.*

Comment: Fixation of loops may be produced by adhesions, extrinsic tumor or cyst, or, as in this case, regional ileitis.

segment of bowel occupying the left upper quadrant would be expected to be jejunum (fig. 313). As compared to a loop of bowel in the right lower quadrant or pelvis, the jejunum would be wider, varying from 2 to 3 centimeters in diameter. Its margins would be typically feathery or herring-bone in appearance. This feathery or cross-hatched appearance is determined by the character of the mucosa lining the lumen. The basic pattern of the mucous membrane within the jejunal portion of the small bowel is formed by the valvulae conniventes or Kerkring folds. These are large transverse circular *folds of mucous membrane* which project into the lumen, i.e., perpendicular to the direction in which the lumen runs. They are really folds, i.e., reduplication of mucous membrane, the two layers of the fold being bound together by submucous tissue.

A loop of bowel occupying the pelvis or

right lower quadrant would be expected to be ileum (fig. 315). As compared to the diameter of the loops of bowel higher up, the ileum is narrower, varying from 1.5 to 2.0 centimeters in diameter. Its margins are relatively smooth and the inner walls or mucosal pattern less vertical. Especially in its terminal portion, the mucosal folds are practically linear or disposed in a fashion parallel to the lumen.

The folds within the ileum require further discussion. Although anatomically, as discussed above, they are basically transverse, as seen radiographically they are subject to change. At one time they may appear cross-hatched and vertical and at another time linear and parallel to the lumen. The cross-hatched type of mucosal fold is especially seen after a barium enema when the ileum is filled in a retrograde fashion (fig. 304). Perhaps this transverse arrangement of folds is nature's method of erecting

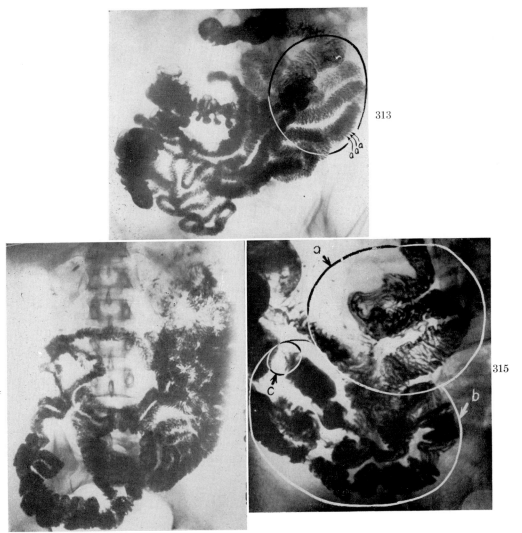

Continuity.

313

Continuous small bowel pattern revealing the feathery (*a,a,a*) jejunal margin. This feathering represents barium *between* the folds. This examination was performed one hour after the barium left the pylorus.

Question:

Is the transit time normal?

Answer:

Yes. The barium is seen entering the cecum. The normal time for this is 1½–2 hours.

314

Normal continuous small bowel. Compare with figure 322, page 239 and figures 325–327, page 242.

315

Transitional small bowel (*a*). Ileum (*b*). Normal or physiologic narrowing, produced by either segmentation or peristalsis (*c*).

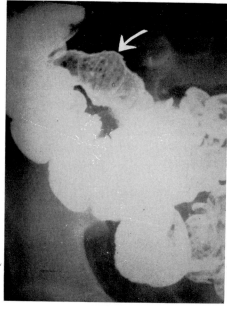

316

Small polka dots in the terminal ileum are a
normal variant in children and are produced by
local lymphoid polypoid thickenings.

a barricade in order to help obstruct the
retrograde flow from the cecum.

The terminal ileum in children presents a
pattern different from the adult. In a child
the terminal ileum presents a cobble-stone
appearance, produced by regional aggrega-
tions of lymphoid tissue called "Peyer's
patches" (fig. 316). This is a normal variant
and does not indicate the presence of disease.

Portions of the small bowel within the
right upper quadrant and central portions
of the abdomen would possess characteristics transitional from the jejunum and ileum
(figs. 317–320).

*Mechanism Producing Mucous Mem-
brane Pattern.* The normal mucosal pattern
is relatively fixed within the jejunum;
within the ileum it may be variable. The
mechanism controlling the pattern in jejunum and ileum is similar to that within
the stomach. It is primarily dependent on
the muscularis mucosa, which contracts and

relaxes, thereby changing the small bowel
pattern as an independent mechanism. Some
changes in the small bowel pattern may occur, however, secondary to contraction and
relaxation of the longitudinal or circular
muscles in the wall of the small intestine.
As in the stomach, a more linear distribution of the folds appears when the circular
muscle contracts, i.e., as sticks tied in a
bundle. When the longitudinal muscle contracts, the length of the involved segment
shortens, and just as the folds in an accordion, the mucosa becomes cross-hatched
or vertical.

Terminal Ileum and Cecum. The lateral
margin of the terminal ileum and the medial wall of the cecum may be fused for
varying distances. However, if the mucosal
pattern is normal or there is no history of
adhesions, this must be considered a normal
variant.

The termination of the small bowel at
the ileo-cecal valve deserves special mention. Commonly, the freely movable terminal ileum ascends in a more or less vertical
fashion and ends as it inserts into the *medial*
aspect of the cecum. It should, however, be
emphasized that the terminal ileum may
also end by inserting into either the *posterior* or *lateral* walls of the cecum.

MOVEMENTS OF THE
SMALL INTESTINE

Introduction—Gradient Movement. As
the barium enters the small bowel, a great
deal of activity, restlessness and churning
movements seem to take place in those coils
of jejunum which first receive the opaque
media. As the barium is transported and
distributed into the coils lower down, the
activity appears to lessen, albeit still present. The closer the head of the barium
column comes to the ileo-cecal valve, the
less movement is seen. Finally, at the terminal ileum, a degree of inactivity is
reached strongly akin to that in the colon.
Indeed, it requires patience, persistence, and

painstaking examination to see peristaltic waves within the terminal ileum. If movement within the terminal ileum is seen at all, it will be of two varieties; (a) The non-propulsive type, where contraction or pendulum movement takes a few seconds to develop, meanwhile traveling at a very slow pace in one direction or another and finally fading out. The rate of travel is so slow that such movement within the terminal ileal segment must be carefully sought. (b) Propulsive waves, which are deep, rapid peristaltic waves causing rush movements that carry the ileal contents into the cecum.

This gradient type of movement within the small bowel is not unexpected. The restless activity and relatively faster transport of contents taking place within the jejunum is in keeping with the rapid emptying of the stomach. It would appear as though the contents were speedily removed from the higher jejunal coils to keep them empty and in readiness for further gastric emptying. In the lower coils of ileum, however, this same immediate necessity for rapid transport does not exist. This slowing down of the lower small bowel is more in key with the slow colonic movement, and not only acts as a further check to too rapid passage of ileal contents into the cecum but permits more time for absorption (figs. 306, 307). In order to slow the passage through the ileum still further, anti-peristaltic waves may occur within the terminal ileum for a variable distance above the ileo-cecal valve.

Gross Movements. On the fluoroscopic screen, general inspection of the small bowel reveals two types of movements. First, a slow, deliberate, up and down, rhythmic, mass-like movement, resulting from the upward and downward movements of the diaphragm during respiration. Secondly, especially in the upper jejunum, a restless, milling about movement; this, as has been explained by Barclay, is due to the action of the muscularis mucosa, which not only breaks down the food more finely but also aids in transport of the bowel contents.[1]

Peristaltic Waves. These are chiefly responsible for the forwarding actions of the intestinal contents. They are seen as ring-like constrictions, starting high up in the duodenum or the upper loops of jejunum, traveling at a relatively rapid rate through several loops of bowel, pushing bowel contents on in front. They are called peristaltic rushes. Alvarez[2] described these waves as sometimes originating in a swallowing movement and at other times starting in the duodenum at about the time that a peristaltic wave within the stomach reaches the pylorus.

Reverse peristaltic waves may normally be seen in the first and last portions of the small bowel, i.e., duodenum and terminal ileum. When seen in other portions of the small bowel, the examiner must seek explanation. Any irritative focus, either functional or organic may be responsible for such reversal of the peristaltic waves. Belching, nausea, vomiting may produce such reversal. It may be seen proximal to a small bowel obstruction.

Scavenging waves, i.e., surges up and down the bowel, and peristaltic waves in the more distal intestinal loops, are associated with peristaltic rushes.[2]

Segmentation. This is a process wherein localized constrictions occur with some regularity throughout the small bowel. The constriction is at right angles to the long axis of the bowel and squeezes the barium to either side, so that the contents are divided into segments. After an interval, a similar constriction occurs in the portion of the bowel into which the barium has been squeezed. The net effect is to return the bolus of barium to its original situation. These segmentation movements are more numerous higher up within the small bowel. They are more easily seen, however, in the lower ileum, where the superimposed peristaltic waves are less frequent and thereby cause less confusion.

Another type of segmentation may be called *progressive segmentation*.[3] A ring-like contraction occurs and divides an opaque bolus into two segments. One of these segments is squeezed or pushed over a fair length of bowel. As a general rule,

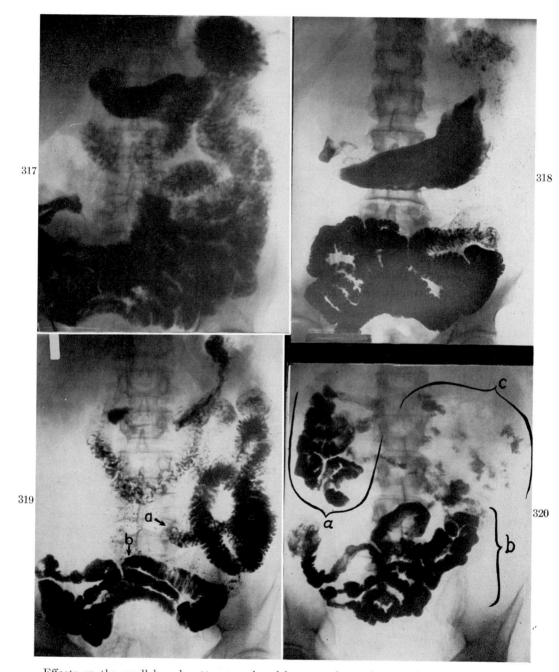

Effects on the small bowel pattern produced by normal gastric emptying and variations in jejunal-ileal transit time. Figures 317–320 show the same patient followed at half-hour intervals for 2 hours. (*See legend, facing page.*)

this segment is again divided by a constricting ring and continues to make progress in the initial direction. Hence the term progressive segmentation. In the main, it produces a forward progress of the opaque meal. Occasionally, and especially in the duodenum, it may move in a retrograde direction.

Frequently the examiner may note a mass of barium which travels rapidly through several loops of intestine. At its onset, it may appear as a progressive segmentation, but once started the intact mass travels much farther.

Pendulum Movements. Another type of movement seen behind the fluoroscopic screen is pendulum movement. These appear as back and forth or side-to-side swaying movements of individual loops of bowel, and are not seen as readily as other movements described so far. They are probably due to intermittent contractions in different parts of the loop of bowel, resulting in to-and-fro movements of the intestinal contents.

Contractions Involving Only Portions of the Small Bowel. Golden[4] described indentations of the ileum, from one-fourth to one-third the diameter of the bowel, which persist for a short period of time. He further quotes Puestow,[5] who described similar contractions, ascribing them to rhythmic segmented movements. Localized ring-like contractions can occur in a column of barium. The ring may be complete or incomplete.[4]

Tonus Waves. Changes in calibre may be noted in a barium mass outlining a well filled intestinal loop. Associated with this there is no actual movement of barium or any other type of contraction. It may be a manifestation of the bowel accommodating to movements elsewhere, or may indicate a change of bowel tone.

BASIC OBSERVATIONS FOR THE X-RAY EXAMINATION

In order to obtain all of the information that an examination can offer, the examiner must first be acquainted with exactly *what* information that type of examination can provide. Without previous knowledge of *what* to look for, some information may be obtained, yet much will be missed. With a systematic planned approach, the examiner should look for certain information he has determined will make that examination complete.

In examining the small bowel, these are the essentials upon which the whole examination rests. The examiner should actually ask himself these questions:

Is the small bowel pattern continuous or

317

One-half hour interval. Gastric emptying is continuous. Small bowel pattern is continuous.

318

One hour interval. The stomach is aperistaltic and has stopped emptying. A short distance downward the barium is lodged in the small intestine. Interruption of gastric emptying here can be produced by the "gastro-ileal" reflex.

319

One hour and a half interval. Resumption of gastric emptying. The head of the *faster* moving jejunal contents (*a*) catching up to the tail of the *slower* moving ileal contents (*b*).

(*Note:* Transitional small bowel between ileum and jejunum not yet filled at this time. Compare with figure 320.)

320

Two hour interval. Stomach has emptied. Barium has moved forward. Barium from the jejunum (fig. 319) has moved forward and entered into the transitional small bowel (*a*) located in the right upper quadrant. The next forward progress of the barium will join up with the slower moving ileal loops (*b*). The last gastric residues (*c*), now in the jejunal loops, appear flocculated.

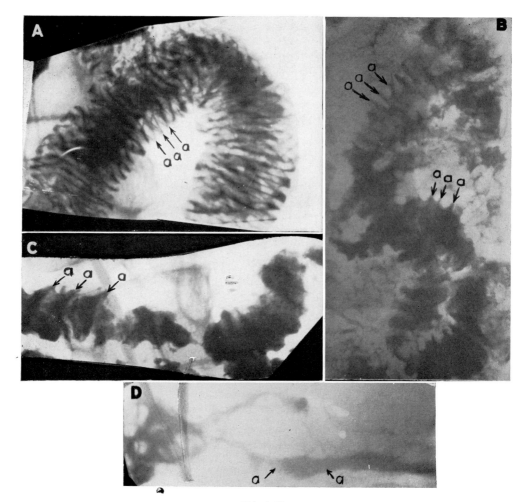

321 A–D

A. Normal small bowel, *a,a,a* are crevices between folds and are normally spaced.

C. Further inflammatory changes reveal narrowing of the lumen, the folds spaced farther apart.

B. Inflammatory thickening of folds. Crevices between folds reveal increased spacing. The transverse folds themselves are coarser and not as fine as in A.

D. Further inflammatory changes reveal destruction of the folds with fibrotic narrowing of the lumen.

segmented? Is the mucous membrane pattern normal? Is the motility or time consumed as the opaque media travels from the stomach to the cecum normal? How long does it take for the last residues of barium mixture to leave the small bowel? Is the bowel lumen narrowed or dilated? Are the loops of small bowel in their normal position or are they displaced? Are the loops of bowel fixed in position? Are they tender? The examiner must be prepared to make specific observations that will answer these questions.

The following description offers a basic

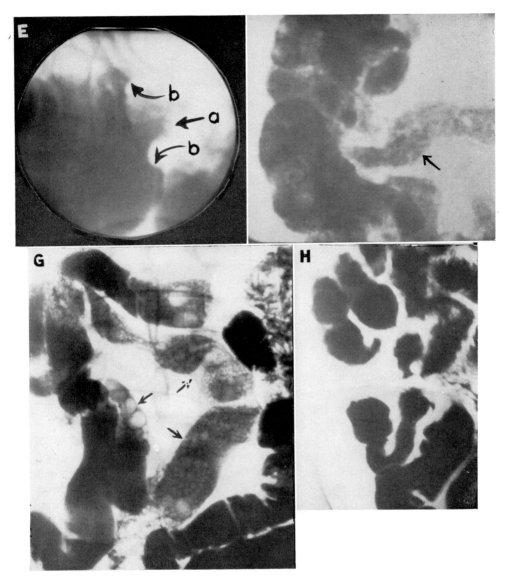

321 E–H

E. Segment *a* starts abruptly at *b-b,* is short in length with no mucous membrane pattern present. This is a carcinoma of the small bowel.

G. Artefacts in small bowel produced by mixture of barium, air and secretions. This must not be confused with mucosal destruction.

F. Mottled irregular densities present in ileum (arrow) produced by flocculated barium. This is a normal finding and not to be confused with mucosal destruction of regional ileitis.

H. Segmentation in ileum produced by lump formation of the dehydrated barium. Normal.

understanding of these phenomena and some of their variations. It should be borne in mind that such fluoroscopic observations must always be confirmed by either con-ventional or spot film examination. With this warning we can take up (1) segmentation—its various causes and forms, (2) scattering of barium, (3) mucosal patterns,

(4) motility (transit time), (5) dilatation, (6) narrowing of the small bowel, and (7) displacement, fixation or tenderness of bowel loops.

SEGMENTATION

The barium mixture normally winds its way through the various loops and coils of the small intestine as an elongated, rope-like, continuous column. For descriptive purposes, this column may be looked upon as having a head, body, and tail. The most distal and (leading the rest of the column) is the *head*. The middle is the *body*, and the proximal end is the *tail*. With the progressive addition of opaque mixture into the small bowel, the body becomes progressively longer (figs. 313–315).

An important characteristic in the appearance of this opacified column is its *continuity*. At least two factors are important in its formation.

First, the *steady*, free-flowing increments of barium mixture from the stomach into the small bowel help render the appearance *continuous* by filling and packing the intestinal loops.

Secondly, as already mentioned, a gradient difference in speed of transport exists within the small bowel. It is more rapid in the higher jejunal loops and becomes progressively slower in the lower ileal loops. The net effect of these unequal speeds is that while the head of the barium column situated farther on in the intestine is slowing down, the newer increments of barium at the tail of the column normally can catch up. The tail, thus, is linked with the body and the column appears *continuous* (figs. 317–320).

Segmentation may be defined as a discontinuity or interruption of the continuity of the barium column which has just been described. Although it *may be present* in normal individuals, it is *so frequently* associated with the abnormal that thorough acquaintance and ready recognition with this phenomenon is *extremely important*.

The discovery of an interrupted or broken column *must make* the observer cautious. This *may be* an important clue to an underlying disease process. The causes of segmentation, then, and its various forms, will be discussed in some detail.

NORMAL SEGMENTATION

Loss of Fluidity as a Cause of Segmentation. Interruptions or breaks in the column may be produced by the opaque mixture losing its fluidity and the barium being converted into lumps. Normally, this is apt to happen when the opaque mixture reaches the last loops of ileum. In this location, the fluid may become absorbed and the dehydrated barium may appear as a dense, elongated, tightly packed column, or divided into *segments* (fig. 322).

Clumping of the Barium as a Cause of Segmentation. Mucus: In *children*, it is normal to find the typical small bowel pattern to be discontinuous or segmented (fig. 303). This may be produced by the comparatively poor muscular development, and resultant maladjustment of transport speeds of small intestinal contents.[6, 7, 8] More recently it has been shown that in infants the *mucus content*, when combined with the barium mixture, forms clumps, thereby destroying the continuity of the column (fig. 303). Flocculation and clumping of the opaque media in newborn infants may even be present prior to the first feeding. Normally, infants appear to have a relative excess of mucus within the small intestine as compared with the adult.[9, 10, 11]

In healthy adults, a discontinuity of the opaque column may also occur from clumping or flocculation of the barium solution owing to its mixture with upper intestinal mucus. This often takes place at the head of the barium column and may remain there as the meal progresses through the small bowel. The snowflake appearance at the tail of the barium column may be the result of flocculated or clumped barium from the same cause[12] (figs. 308–310).

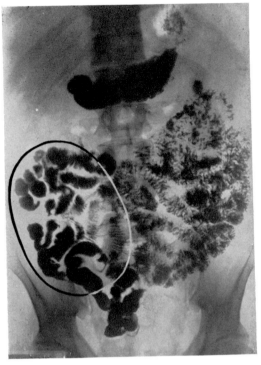

322

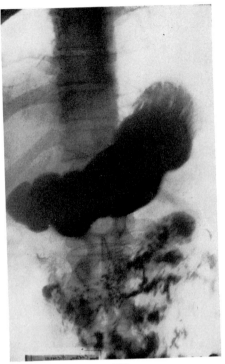

323

The terminal ileal loops (encircled) appear segmented.

Question:

How is such an appearance produced normally?

Answer:

The barium mixture reaching the ileum forms dehydrated lumps. The segmentation is due to a lumpy distribution of barium in the ileum. Normal.

Fats: Pendergast et al.[13] found that adding fatty material to the barium meal in normal individuals resulted in a segmented pattern. In the examination of infants, fatty food residue may well be present in the intestine from previous feedings. In infants, the period of starvation before examination is 8 hours or less. Bruslag[8] in 1935 pointed out that almost half of his series of children had a gastric residue after 8 hours.

In this regard, it is important to be sure that the segmentation or disruptions of the small bowel pattern sought for when testing the patient for allergic manifestations are not instead due to clumping of the barium

Question:

Segmentation of barium is seen in the small bowel loops immediately beneath the stomach. What may produce this change?

Answer:

Irregular gastric emptying of the first small portions of barium may produce a discontinuous or segmented pattern. Normal.

mixture because of the type of food used as an allergen. If it contains fats, clumping would result.

Segmentation because of Poor Filling of the Small Bowel. As the stomach begins to empty, that is, as the first few small amounts of barium pass through the pylorus and start forward progress through the small bowel, the initial quantities of opaque material may be so sparse that the result will be only partial filling of the intestinal loops. This poor filling will hinder the packing effect and thereby render a segmented pattern (fig. 323). If an inadequate amount of barium is given in the first place, this same poor filling of the small intestine and segmentation will result. A similar effect is obtained if adequate amounts of barium mixture are given but its exit from the stomach is held up by either irregular or poor gastric emptying, or a spastic pylorus. The stomach may be full yet the supply of barium into the intestines may be inadequate. The net effect would be the same as though small amounts of barium had originally been used and a segmented or discontinuous pattern would result.

Finally, although no interference with gastric emptying be present during the passage of the bulk of the opaque material out of the stomach, *inadequate emptying* of the *last* gastric residues of barium may produce a segmented type of pattern *at the tail of the barium column* (figs. 308–310).

Reflex Segmentation. The gastro-ileal reflex, wherein distention of the ileum causes reflex closure of the pylorus with consequent holdup of gastric emptying, produces irregular gastric emptying and thus discontinuity of the small bowel pattern (figs. 317–320). Perhaps this reflex is a mechanism whereby the ileal loops are permitted time to deal with their contents while the stomach holds up its evacuation. It has been shown that not only *distention* but *irritation* of almost any portion of ileum or jejunum can delay gastric emptying and thus become a potent cause of the segmentation pattern. This could explain at least one of the mechanisms responsible for a segmented pattern in association with partial obstruction from small bowel tumor or some irritant factor producing inflammatory disease.

Reflex segmentation of the small bowel pattern is also present in the group of diseases to be discussed under disordered motor function (page 272). Here, as elsewhere, no clear etiology for the pattern has been determined, but considerable importance must be given to disturbances in the autonomic nervous system.

Segmentation because of Mode of Transport in the Small Bowel. Distribution of the barium mixture into narrowed and wide segments has also been considered as segmentation.

During the normal packing and transport of the opaque material, one portion of the intestine may momentarily become overdistended with resultant widening of the involved loop and flattening of the mucosa. The peristaltic waves, or the normal rhythmic segmentations responsible for this overdistention, may render the appearance of the adjacent loop of bowel narrow and spastic. The distal portion of this overfilled region may be fortuitously narrowed either because of normal bowel emptying or because of a normal turn in the loops of bowel. Thus, an area resembling segmentation, as evidenced by the alternate presence of narrow and wider segments, may appear, but as an expression of normal small bowel activity.

SEGMENTATION AS A MANIFESTATION OF THE ABNORMAL

Segmentation as a manifestation of the abnormal may result from either functional or structural lesions. The fluoroscopic and radiographic appearances of the segmented or discontinuous small bowel when produced by an abnormalcy may be indistinguishable from the normal variant patterns described above.

Segmentation Resulting from Interruption of the Smooth Continuous Flow of Opaque Material.

1. Partial Obstruction. As described above, irregular emptying of the stomach may result in an irregular distribution of opaque material within the small bowel. In similar fashion, a lesion producing partial obstruction within the duodenum or early jejunum may produce an effect similar to an obstructive mechanism at the pylorus. And, as already described, this partially obstructive lesion prevents the *regular* passage of barium. Because of the resultant poor filling the intestinal loops distal to the lesion are not properly packed and a segmented pattern results (figs. 337, 338).

2. As has been pointed out, the *stretched walls* of overdistended small intestinal loops as well as *irritative phenomena* within the

small bowel can reflexly close the pylorus, producing an irregular supply of barium mixture into the small intestine. This can occur with inflammatory foci of the small bowel as well as distended small intestinal loops proximal to an obstructed lesion. In each case, irregular entry of the barium into the small bowel results in a segmented pattern.

Segmentation occurs prominently in the presence of intestinal adhesions. The explanation may be either partial obstruction or irritation.

3. Malnutrition. Malnutrition is also capable of producing a break in the continuity of the barium column.[14] Roentgenologic continuity of the small bowel depends upon the stronger or speedier intestinal movements *above* rushing the new barium contents to catch up with the barium increment in the lower loops where movement is slower (figs. 318, 319). With malnutrition, peristalsis in the upper loops becomes diminished and therefore insufficient to produce the packing effect necessary to keep the column continuous.

4. *Clumping of Opaque Media as a Cause of Segmentation.* As indicated above, freshly secreted mucus from any part of the gastrointestinal tract may cause flocculation or clumping of the opaque media.[11] The observation of large clumps of barium in the small intestine in the presence of sprue, etc. (for a more complete listing see Disordered Motor Function, page 272) may be due, then, to excessive secretion of mucus within the intestinal tract. Since the ileum normally secretes more mucus than jejunum and also, as pointed out above, dehydration of the barium mixture resulting in lump formation is more apt to occur in the ileum, interpretation of segmentation as abnormal within this region requires considerable circumspection and caution.

Similarly, as already noted, clumping may be caused by the mere presence of abnormal amounts of fat, producing a segmented appearance of the opaque media in the small bowel (fig. 303).

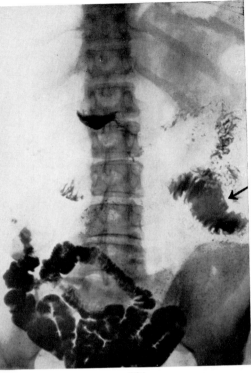

324

Question:

What may arrowed segment represent?

Answer:

1. Normal segmentation at tail of small bowel.
2. Irregular emptying of last gastric residues.
3. Trailing segment? This would be difficult to prove, for to be characteristic of a "trailing segment," a hold-up at this point would have to be evident on the other films during hourly study, and barium tends to be held up at this point for 10 hours or more.

5. *Disordered Motor Function* (figs. 325–327 and page 272ff). Disordered motor function is a name given to the radiographic pattern exhibited by a number of different diseases. These are listed and described elsewhere. At this point it should be pointed out that the exact etiology of the segmentation taking place as part of this phenomenon is unknown. Some authors have attributed the cause to spasm, either neurogenic or muscular. Certainly the autonomic nervous system plays an important part in the behavior pattern of the small bowel. Disturbances in nervous control may produce a pro-

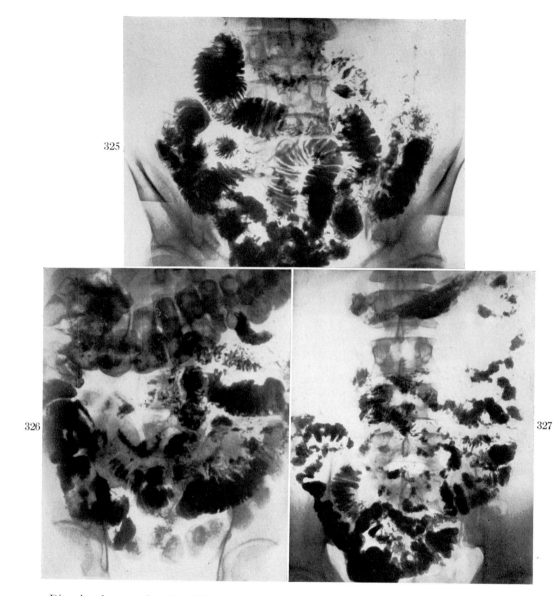

Disordered motor function. Note the breaking up of the continuity of the small bowel into segments. The border between normal and abnormal is not clear and distinct. Any of these may be found in a normal individual and yet be the only radiographic finding pointing to some abnormalcy in certain functional or organic small bowel disorders. (Cf. fig. 313, p. 231.)

found effect on the opacified small bowel, including the formation of a segmented pattern. But though the nervous system plays a significant role, yet the abnormal quality and quantity of secretions and the presence of excess fat in the intestine are also important etiologic factors.[11]

Summary. It deserves emphasis that a segmented pattern should place the examiner on his guard. It may be an important clue that pathology is present. It must not be disregarded. But to be accepted as an abnormalcy, it must be duplicated on repeat examinations.

SCATTERING (FIG. 320)

Scattering is a normal phenomenon found within the small bowel. It is a descriptive term given to the small residues of barium seen at the tail of the barium column as it travels through the small intestine.

After the greater portion of the opacified column has passed, small boluses of the barium suspension remain behind, probably within the crevices of the Kerkring folds. The appearance of these small residues at the tail of the column has been likened to "snow flakes." Marshak has pointed out that in the sprue pattern, instead of the small barium deposits, larger amorphous deposits resembling larger snow flakes may be left behind (described *as a coarse or amorphous type of scattering*).[15] He has also described a more linear type of scattering in the same illness. In sprue, these findings are usually associated with pronounced segmentation, dilatation, and increased secretions within the small bowel.

MUCOSAL PATTERNS

Abnormal Mucosal Patterns (fig. 321). It should be borne in mind that the small bowel is seen on the fluoroscopic screen as a barium cast of the intestinal lumen. The feathery peaks which are the upper and lower margins of the opacified intestinal lumen are formed by the barium within the crevices *between* the folds.

In the presence of inflammatory disease, the folds become thick. The examiner should expect the feathery peaks, i.e., the region *between* the folds, to become *spaced farther apart* (figs. 328–331; compare fig. 313). With further inflammatory changes the thickened mucosa continues to encroach on the lumen and the cast-like shadow of the intestinal lumen narrows, the feathery appearance becoming flatter and eventually lost (figs. 328–331).

The inflammatory changes may go on to ulceration. Ulcers in this portion of the intestinal tract are not different from ulcers elsewhere, e.g., in the stomach. Filled with opaque media they form projections outward from the bowel wall. When multiple, these projections form long, irregular intestinal segments. Early ulceration is generally associated with narrowing of the lumen because of the inflammatory edema of the bowel and overlying spasm. *Later ulceration* is also associated with narrowing of the lumen, but chiefly because of fibrotic replacement of the bowel wall. The lumen may become sufficiently narrowed to appear as an elongated string (Kantor's string sign) (fig. 332).

In the later stages, the mucosa within the involved segment is largely shed and the retained mucosa goes on to become thickened and polypoid (fig. 305).

Neoplastic disease also causes alterations in the mucous membrane pattern. As elsewhere in the intestinal tract, the most common change produced by a malignant tumor is complete destruction of the involved mucosa (figs. 333, 334).

Destruction produced by inflammatory diseases must be distinguished from that produced by malignancy. Mucosal changes arising from inflammatory disease occupy longer segments, and the change from normal to abnormal is gradual. Malignant neoplastic changes occur more abruptly and in shorter segments (compare figs. 333, 334).

Pitfalls in the Interpretation of Mucous Membrane Pattern.

1. The barium mixture in any portion of the small intestine may form irregular floccules or clumps, and in this lump-like manner cannot properly outline the bowel wall (figs. 303, 322).

2. Special attention has already been given to the terminal ileal loops. Here not only can mucous secretions cause clumping but because of water absorption the barium normally becomes thick and pasty. The barium can become tightly packed into irregular clumps (fig. 322). It should be emphasized that especially in the ileum, proper outline of the lumen requires that the fluidity of the barium mixture be retained.

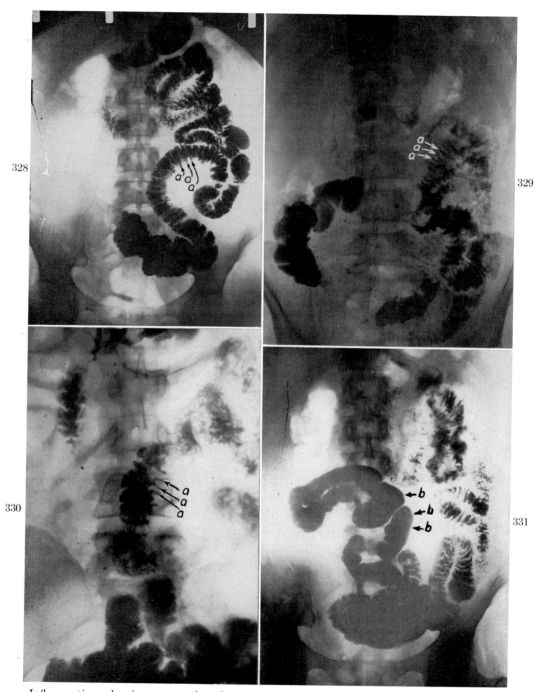

Inflammation, showing progressive changes in the Kerkring folds. The feathery appearance is produced by barium in the crevices between these folds. Inflammatory thickening of the folds will spread the crevices *a,a,a* (feathers) further apart. Progressive inflammation (evidenced by progressive widening of the folds) is shown in figures 328–331. (*See legend, facing page.*)

To help overcome these difficulties, preparation of the barium mixture with isotonic saline may be useful. Another maneuver when study of the last loops of ileum is desired is to fill them via retrograde barium enema. A leak through the ileo-cecal valve and opacification of the terminal ileal loops is thus secured. Fecal material or air bubbles carried from the colon back into the ileum may produce a false impression of polypoid or other mucosal changes (figs. 304, 305).

MOTILITY (TRANSIT TIME)

Introduction. Transit time as applied to the radiographic examination of the small bowel refers to the time consumed by the opaque media as it traverses the small bowel, i.e., from the duodenum to the cecum. It is assumed that the barium suspension recommended here (page 254) is administered.

It should be emphasized that this time interval does not start at the moment the barium is ingested. An abnormal hold-up within the stomach may prolong the time necessary for the opaque media to reach the cecum. In such an instance, a *prolonged transit time* would find its etiology in the *stomach* and *not* in the small bowel. Small bowel motility may be unduly prolonged by a full colon. This is a physiological type of obstruction and is best seen when fecal impaction occurs.[33] Conversely, small bowel motility may be increased by good colon evacuation. Small bowel transit time starts as the examiner sees the first boluses of opaque media pass into the duodenum. It terminates when the head of the barium column reaches the cecum.

Small bowel transit time is normally ap-proximately one and a half to two hours. Up to five hours is within normal limits. A time interval shorter than one hour can be considered as an accelerated transit time. A time interval delayed beyond six hours may be considered a prolonged transit time.

In observing the passage of the opaque media through the small bowel, it is important that the examiner determine the time at which *all* of the barium has left the small bowel, i.e., when all of the small bowel loops are clear of opaque media. This time interval should be approximately nine hours after the initial entry of the opaque media into the duodenum.

Study and observation of this transit time is not theoretic but has practical value. A thorough understanding should yield important clues as to the existence of disease processes.

Delayed or Prolonged Transit Time. In the main, delayed transit time may be either organic or functional in origin.

Finding a delayed or prolonged transit time, the examiner should immediately think of a hold-up, either organic or functional. Almost reflexly must the eye set out looking for either narrowed or dilated loops. It is these dilated or narrowed segments which, if present, may be the clue to the cause of the hold-up (figs. 332, 335).

Dilated loops should be followed to their distal terminations and may lead to the site of a lesion. Often the narrowed segment of bowel responsible for the hold-up or partial obstruction may be found at this point. A narrowed segment may often be found by careful inspection without first finding dilated loops (fig. 333).

Important *organic causes* responsible for

328

Some spreading of folds as indicated by separation of *a,a,a.*

330

Further inflammation of mucosa, blunting of folds and further separation of *a,a,a.*

329

Further inflammatory change, further spreading of folds.

331

Further progress in the inflammatory process shows shedding of the mucosa and smoothening of the bowel wall (b,b,b).

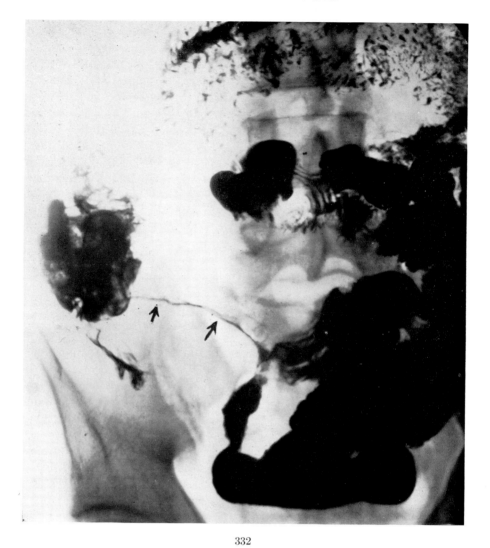

332

Question:

The findings on the film suggested regional ileitis (arrows). Fluoroscopically what confirmatory signs could be obtained?

Answer:

Under direct fluoroscopic observation:

1. Palpation revealed the narrowed ileum (arrows) as part of a tender mass.

2. No manipulation or pressure could fill the *narrowed segment*, confirming "Kantor's string sign" (arrows).

3. Spot films with pressure confirmed the destroyed mucosal lining.

4. Even with manipulation, the terminal ileum remained relatively constant in position and *well separated from the rest of the bowel*. The thickened mesentery acts to produce this latter change.

Note: (a) These findings must be duplicated on repeat examination to be confirmatory. *Temporary spasm* would reveal the segment filled on re-examination. (b) The cecum should be checked for possible involvement.

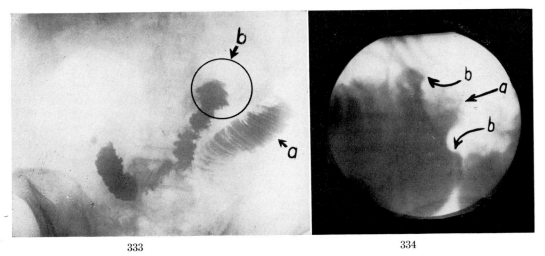

333   334

Question:

Will the Kerkring folds (*a*) become obliterated when the jejunum is distended?

Answer:

Within the jejunum, no amount of distention can obliterate these folds (*a*).

Comment: In the presence of intestinal obstruction, the widened loops should be followed to the point where the bowel is no longer distended (*b*). The cause for the obstruction may be located at this point. (See fig. 334.)

Spot films taken at *termination of distended* bowel (*b*, fig. 333) reveal a carcinoma by its undermined edges (*b*) and constricted segment (*a*).

this partial obstruction are adhesions or bands, chronic sclerosing or fibrotic inflammatory small bowel, disease, and tumors either benign or malignant. Delayed small intestinal motility has been described in patients with metastatic malignancy in the abdomen.[12] Scleroderma is another important cause producing a prolongation in transit time, but here partial obstruction is not the precipitating factor (fig. 335).

The second important subdivision causing prolonged transit time are diseases which are *functional in origin*. These are varied. They may be emotional,[16] psychogenic or reflex in etiology. A prolonged transit time is found in reflex or paralytic ileus (page 321), hormonal deficiency states such as hypothyroidism, severe hunger, and the advanced stages of all of the various diseases capable of producing the small bowel pattern associated with disordered motor function (page 372) such as sprue, etc.

Acceleration of the Transit Time. Acceleration of the transit time within the small bowel has been found in the *early* stages of inflammatory lesions. Hypermotility of the small bowel has been described in *early* cases of carcinoma of the cecum and ileum.[17] In the main, during the *earlier* stages of other disease processes such as sprue, or even in severe hunger, the transit time seems to be accelerated. In the *later* stages of these same diseases it is slowed or prolonged. It is possible that the acceleration of the transit time in early inflammatory conditions may be produced by increased irritability of the bowel wall.

Other factors responsible for acceleration in the transit time may be psychogenic or emotional. A hormonal etiology is also described and is present in hyperthyroidism.

It should be pointed out that in some cases of gastroenterostomy, when the stomach empties through a large stoma the con-

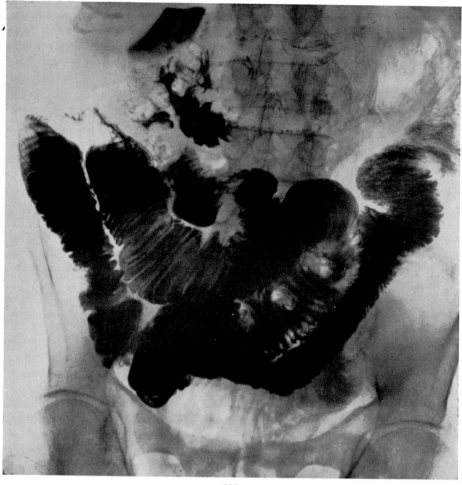

335

Question:

Eleven hours after the barium first passed through the pyloric sphincter, it was located in the segments above demonstrated. Is this normal?

Answer:

No. The cecum is generally reached within 2 hours and the small bowel is empty in 10 hours. Neither requirement appears fulfilled in this case.

Comment: The bowel wall is dilated. This is a case of scleroderma, possessing the small bowel characteristics of this disease, i.e., a dilated bowel wall and hypomotility.

tents may pass rather rapidly into the small bowel and produce a hypermotility.

DILATATION OF THE SMALL BOWEL

Introduction. The jejunum ordinarily should not measure more than 2.5 cm. in diameter and the ileum not more than 2.0 cm. If dilatation beyond these limits were to indicate the presence of a disease process within the dilated segments, then any portion of *over-filled normal bowel* could be interpreted as being abnormal. This is not the case. Widening of the lumen in itself does not necessarily indicate the presence of pathology. The increased caliber must be more or less constant, not transitory in appearance, to indicate a lesion. This same constancy should apply to the mucosal folds, which, in the presence of small bowel dilatation, are generally more widely separated and thicker than normally seen. In acquiring a mental image of this change, no amount of descriptive material can really be as instructive as actually viewing multiple films demonstrating these changes (figs. 333–335).

An indication of the diagnostic value of recognizing increased caliber of the intestinal lumen is that the *first* clue that many organic diseases of the small bowel yields is dilatation of the segments of bowel proximal to a lesion. Often, if this clue were absent, the very presence of the lesion would be entirely overlooked.

Having recognized that abnormal dilatation of the small bowel either in portions or in its entirety is present, the examiner must proceed to search for the cause.

The causes for abnormal dilatation of the small bowel may be divided into three groups:

1. Dilatation proximal to an obstructive lesion (fig. 333).

2. Dilatation at the site of a disease process within the bowel wall.

3. Dilatation as a result of functional or nervous derangement.

1. Dilatation Proximal to an Obstructive Lesion. This subject is discussed in the chapter on Intestinal Obstruction, but deserves brief repetition here.

Dilatation proximal to an obstructive lesion is evidenced radiographically by a widening of the lumen of the bowel. As already described, when the lesion is in the jejunum, the Kerkring folds are more widely spaced and, being stretched, may appear thicker. The examiner should then direct his eye *distally*. By following the expanded loops downward the narrowed or stenotic segment responsible for the proximal dilatation may be found (figs. 333, 334). Because of the holdup and consequent irregular passage of the opaque media through this narrowed segment, the column of the barium suspension *beyond* the lesion may appear broken into segments and disorganized.

Other possible etiological causes for such a segmented pattern in the presence of an obstructive lesion are discussed under segmentation.

When dilatation is associated with intestinal obstruction, numerous air and fluid levels within the distended loops may also be present (fig. 399, p. 324).

Fluoroscopically, the dilated loops of bowel proximal to the lesion reveal increased activity and hyperperistalsis. Reverse peristalsis may also be present.

The more common organic causes for obstruction of the small bowel are adhesions, inflammatory diseases, tumors (either benign or malignant) and sclerosing enteritis, to be discussed in the final section of this chapter. Volvulus and intussusception are important causes of acute obstruction.

2. Dilatation at the Site of the Disease Process within the Small Bowel Wall. Various diseases of the small intestine make themselves evident by dilatation of the *affected* loops.

Sarcoma within the small bowel not infrequently produces dilatation of the involved region.

Although scleroderma is more apt to involve the esophagus, it may appear within the small intestine and produce dilatation *at the site of involvement* (fig. 335). Amyloidosis has been described as capable of producing dilatation of the affected bowel wall. Replacement of muscle tissue by scleroderma or amyloid deposits results in dilatation of the affected segment. In amyloidosis, amyloid deposits have also been found present within the intramural nerve ganglia.[18]

Distention of the small intestinal lumen may also be produced by organic disease of the mesentery. Response of the small intestinal segments to the adrenalin within the intestinal wall may explain this phenomenon.[19, 20] Denervation of the intestine must first take place and this may be accomplished by infiltrative disease of the mesentery; e.g., carcinomatous infiltration, sclerosing mesenteritis and regional enteritis with secondary fibrosis of the mesentery.[21]

3. Dilatation Associated with Functional Dilatation of the Small Bowel. Dilatation and narrowing of the small intestine are closely related to the muscular tonus of the small bowel wall, which is controlled by the sympathetic and parasympathetic nervous systems. Normally a balance between these two is present. Stimulation of the *parasympathetic* fibers produces increased tonus with resultant *narrowing of the lumen of the bowel, increased peristalsis and hypermotility*. Stimulation of the *sympathetic* has the opposite effect; it produces a *dilatation of the lumen of the bowel* with *decreased peristalsis and hypomotility*.

This balance of the sympathetic and parasympathetic may be destroyed, without direct stimulation of nerve fibers. For example, the sympathetic nervous system will predominate if the parasympathetic nervous system is inhibited through a *lack* or relative *failure in the production of acetyl cholines*. Administration of excessive amounts of intravenous fluid is associated with hypoproteinemia and lessened amounts of acetyl choline. Paralytic ileus after operation is not infrequently produced by this mechanism. A low blood potassium may also produce dilatation of the small bowel by the same mechanism. Ross Golden, quoting Arae,[22] indicated that the effect of peritonitis on the intestine may be a result of overstimulation of the sympathetic nervous system.

Stimulation of the sympathetic nervous system with widening of the bowel wall may be present in psychoneurotics. It may also be hormonal in origin, being present in hypothyroid states.

Finally, as previously mentioned, dilatation of the bowel wall has been found in sprue and in a host of diseases which are capable of producing the radiographic pattern seen in those illnesses exhibiting a disordered motor function. (See page 272.)

NARROWING OF THE SMALL BOWEL

Introduction. Narrowing of the lumen of the small bowel, as is emphasized in various parts of this book, may be an important sign indicating the presence of disease. It is important, however, not to judge *every small intestinal segment that is narrowed as pathologic*. A portion of bowel which may be momentarily underfilled or perhaps a segment recently emptied may appear narrowed yet be entirely normal (fig. 336). A normal fold or bend in the bowel wall may cause the opacified lumen of the bowel to appear narrowed.

Narrowing of the small bowel just as dilatation can be either organic or functional in origin, the latter being closely associated with parasympathetic involvement.

Organic Narrowing of the Small Bowel. Narrowing to be considered as organic in origin must, first of all, be present whenever the segment is filled with opaque media. This finding must be confirmed by repetition on two separate examinations. Overlying spasm exaggerating the degree of narrowing must be borne in mind. Certain indicative or confirmatory findings should be looked for. (a) The bowel may maintain its same relative *configuration* on duplicate examinations (figs. 311, 312). (b) Organic narrowing is often associated with some dilatation of the proximal loops. Within these dilated loops, increased peristalsis and reverse peristalsis may be present. (c) Destruction or other significant changes within the mucous membrane of the narrowed segment will confirm the presence of a lesion. (d) Tenderness or mass formation in the narrowed region will also be confirmatory.

Causes of Organic Narrowing of the Small Bowel (figs. 311, 312, 332). Organic narrowing of the small bowel may be produced by sclerosing enteritis, carcinoma, and even infarction.

The bowel may also appear narrowed as a result of extrinsic pressure, such as adhesions, tumors, etc.

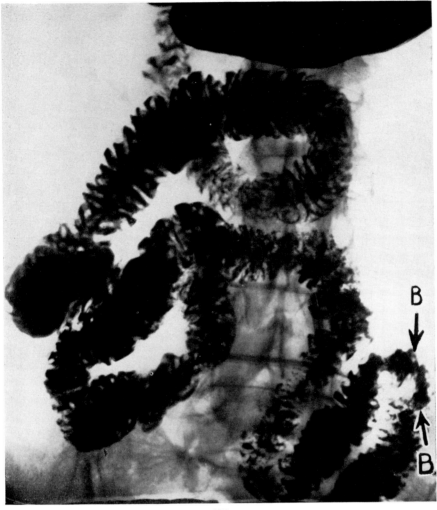

336

Question:

Segment *B-B* appeared on film examination. Is it normal?

Answer:

1. The segment was located behind the fluoroscopic screen, palpated and observed. It was seen to fill normally, and was determined as normal.

2. The narrowing is thus produced by either temporary poor filling, or physiologic contraction of the bowel wall, or a bend in the bowel.

Comment: If the segment was the site of a constricting lesion, the proximal loops would be more dilated. Further hourly study would reveal retention of the barium loops proximal to this segment.

Functional Narrowing of the Small Bowel. Stimulation of the parasympathetic nervous system produces narrowing of the small bowel lumen and increased peristalsis. Psychosomatic and emotional states may stimulate the parasympathetic nervous system and thereby narrow the intestinal lumen. Friedman[16] has demonstrated the effect of emotion on the gastrointestinal tract. The breaking up of the opacified barium

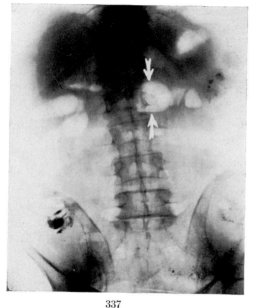

337

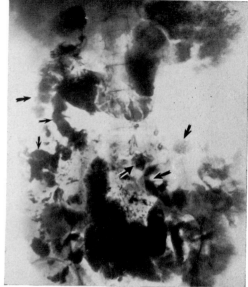

338

Question:

Patient was ambulatory, with a history of intermittent vomiting. Can the air-containing loops in upper abdomen be explained?

Answer:

(All of the air except that between the arrows *might* be in the colon or stomach and thus be normal). The air bubble between the arrows appears ball-like, alone, and localized. In view of the history, this was accepted as a possible sign of air-distended small bowel loop, deserving of further study. (See fig. 338.)

Same patient as in figure 337.

Question:

The small bowel pattern (arrows) is not continuous (see figs. 313, 314, page 231). How may this segmentation pattern (arrows) be produced?

Answer:

Irregular passage of the opaque media through a carcinomatous constricted area may result in irregular filling and segmentation beyond the lesion. See section on segmentation for further reasons.

Comment: Although a carcinoma was found high up in the jejunum, it is not seen on this film, but the breaking up of the small bowel pattern is produced by its presence.

column with resultant segmentation as well as acceleration of the transit time are important features.

It is important for the examiner to bear in mind that often a localized region of narrowing may be present and yet difficult to discover. It may be considerably overlapped with adjacent loops of bowel. Methods for overcoming this difficulty are discussed in the next section and in Chapter VIII.

DISPLACEMENT, FIXATION, TENDERNESS OF SMALL BOWEL LOOPS

Gross displacements of small bowel loops are judged by *persistently* finding areas in

the abdomen free of any intestinal loops, which areas normally are occupied by the small bowel. The examiner must have a certain attitude of mind when looking at the various intervals of study of the small intestine. *At least once* during the examination, he must see *every* section of the abdomen which normally should be occupied by small intestinal loops to be occupied by these loops. When an area is discovered which should show such loops, but does not on *any* of the interval studies, the discovery is important (figs. 343–350, pages 262–266), and generally indicates a mass pushing the loops to the side. Generally, no amount of manipulation can move intestinal segments into these "empty" areas. Further appraisal of displacement is made by seeking the loops adjacent to this entry area narrowed and positioned so as to appear to be displaced or pushed by the pathology causing the displacement.

Fixation is appraised by palpation and determining the segment as immovable. It is possible for a loop to appear fixed when in truth the examiners hand may never really have reached or palpated the loop of bowel under question. This is apt to occur when the patient holds his abdomen rigid and

although behind the fluoroscopic screen the two dimensional view appears as though the hand both overlies and touches the bowel when actually the rigid musculature acts as a wall preventing the hand from palpating the structure beneath. Similarly, loops of intestine which are deeply placed in the pelvis and inaccessible cannot be reached by the examining hand.

Tenderness. The various intestinal loops are not tender to palpation. Discovering a painful or tender region should put the examiner on his guard for a possible underlying lesion.

Methods of Examination

INTRODUCTION

The main roentgenologic methods for the examination of the small bowel are:

A. Routine ingested barium meal (motor meal).

B. Duodenal intubation and small bowel enema.

C. Use of the Miller-Abbott tube (see Chapter VIII, page 326ff).

A basic rule in examining the gastrointestinal tract is to to certain that *all* portions of the part examined are clearly visualized. This means that, ideally, in the examination of the 20-odd feet of small intestine, not even a tiny segment should miss careful scrutiny and observation. This aim can often be carried to a successful conclusion in examination of the esophagus, stomach and colon, since these organs are opacified and may be seen in their entire length within a matter of minutes. Such is not the case with the routine type of small bowel examination. Its greater length makes the usual type of gastrointestinal fluoroscopy too lengthy. If *continuous observations* were made of the *progressive* filling of the entire small bowel during *routine* examination, the time would vary from one to six hours, and the amount of radiation received by the examiner and the patient would be dangerous. Thus in the *routine type of ex-*

amination of the small intestine, the ideal of observing the progressive filling of the various loops, and seeing every portion and tiny segment, can not really be attained. For this the small bowel enema, to be described below, may be used.

Another difficulty is the arrangement of the small bowel. When the relative smallness of the space within the abdominal cavity is contrasted with the length of small intestine contained therein, the degree of twisting, curling, approximation and overlapping of the various loops must indeed be great. For this reason it could almost be called the "no man's land" of diagnostic radiology.

The examination should be planned and follow a routine aimed at being complete, while still allowing a certain amount of flexibility. The examiner should be ready to alter the plan and attack the problem with an alternative method if need be. Rarely do two consecutive patients present the same problem. A clinical picture strongly suggestive of a small bowel tumor might necessitate a small bowel enema if the routine small bowel examination were indecisive, whereas a patient suspected of having sprue or some functional disease could be adequately studied by oral administration of barium. Indeed, a patient suspected of having a functional illness is better examined by giving oral barium since it is more physiologic than the enema. For example, motility, either rapid or slow can better be appraised. Segmentation of the barium column, when present, can be clearly demonstrated by the routine ingested meal but not by small bowel enema.

Finally, various types of intubation may be utilized. The long intestinal tube (Miller-Abbott) has its special uses, both diagnostic and therapeutic. A patient distended as a result of an obstructive small bowel lesion can undergo deflation by means of this tube. He could next be studied by instilling opaque media through the tube and a diagnosis made as to the cause of the obstruction.

The routine barium meal and duodenal intubation are described in the following section. The technic for the long intestinal tube, because of its importance in intestinal obstruction, is given in considerable detail in Chapter VIII.

ROUTINE INGESTED BARIUM MEAL (THE MOTOR MEAL)

This is the commonest roentgenologic method of gastrointestinal study. Normally the same mixture is employed as used in examining the stomach and duodenum. The amount of barium suspension used varies with different examiners, from as little as 2, 3 or 4 ounces to as high as 16 to 20 ounces. Here it is recommended that 16 ounces of mixture be used (equal parts, by volume, of water and barium).

Before starting the actual examination, the examiner should secure a brief but detailed review of the patient's history and other pertinent data as the basis on which the roentgenologic procedure is planned.

Survey Examination of Abdomen and Chest

Before the opaque media is given, the abdomen is examined fluoroscopically. Where possible, a film should also be taken at this time. This may often, especially if the film is taken in the erect position, immediately indicate the diagnosis, e.g., intestinal obstruction. In the presence of obstruction, oral administration of opaque media might be contraindicated. (See Chapter VIII, page 336.)

Fluoroscopic examination of the chest can also help in excluding pathology within the thorax as etiologic factor. The diaphragmatic excursions should be watched for abnormalcy below. Thus, an inflammatory lesion on one side of the abdomen may cause a reflex diminution in the excursion of the diaphragmatic cusp on the involved side.

The esophagus, stomach and duodenum are next fluoroscopically examined with opaque media. The technic is as detailed in this chapter on Stomach. It is of advantage at this point, while the stomach is still in a relatively *empty* state (only 1 to 2 ounces being used up to this time), that the *duodenal jejunal flexure and the adjacent jejunal loops be seen, examined, and spot filmed* (fig. 342). It is important that this be done with only a *few ounces* of barium solution in the stomach and *before* sufficient barium is taken to fill the stomach. The stomach in a filled state hangs down and covers the duodenal-jejunal flexure and adjacent loops of small bowel, often making it impossible to properly examine the region.

This part of the examination being completed, the patient is next asked to drink the balance of the mixture and its further progress through the intestinal loops is observed.

During the first hour it is recommended that observations be made at 15-minute intervals. The timing should start as the first quantities of opaque media pass through the pyloric sphincter. At these first four examinations, search is made for any existing pathology and observations are made of the rate of gastric emptying and the concomitant speed with which the head of the barium column is filling the small bowel. The various bowel loops are separated with the protected hand and examined individually. Mobility and flexibility of the segments are determined, abnormal displacements noted, and the mucosal pattern where possible is viewed with graded compression. Any undue narrowings or widenings should also be noted. Roentgenograms, with the patient in the supine position, should be taken immediately after each of these 15-minute interval fluoroscopic examinations.

After these first four examinations, further fluoroscopic observations are performed periodically, the time interval between each periodic examination being determined by observations made in the previous examinations (i.e., by appraising the rate of gastric emptying and the speed of small bowel filling). This appraisal and time interval determination will be discussed at greater length below. For the present it is important merely to stress that the time elapsing between these intervals should not be too prolonged, lest loops of bowel not yet reached by the barium at one period be passed by the barium at the next period and thus miss examination. Generally, these periodic examinations are performed every 45 minutes.

Each of the periodic examinations should consist of fluoroscopy and filming, the roentgenogram being developed and examined immediately. An apparent abnormality appearing on the film and not detected in previous fluoroscopy should immediately be checked by again fluoroscoping the patient, followed by new spot films.

The examination should proceed in this manner until the cecum is reached. Where possible, further fluoroscopy and filming should continue until the small bowel is completely emptied. Emptying is delayed if barium is still present at 10 hours after its initial entry into the small bowel.

Golden[34] permits food when the opaque column has reached the cecum, continuing the examination until the small bowel is emptied. He concludes the study by examining 24 hours after the barium administration.

EXAMINATION OF THE TERMINAL ILEUM

The methods to be described below for accelerating the speed of the barium mixture through the small bowel are especially indicated when the terminal ileum is to be examined. The examiner using only conventional methods, without employing special aids, is often confronted with extreme difficulty in visualizing the terminal ileum. The rate of the forward progress of the barium solution through the ileal loops is extremely slow. Just before entering the terminal ileum, it approaches the almost standstill rate of the colon. Perhaps in the visualization of the terminal ileum, even more important than accelerating methods is patience and perseverance on the part of the examiner.

In practically all instances where the terminal ileum is especially to be studied, retrograde filling by colonic barium enema should be performed in addition to this routine type of study.

Several films with compression study of the terminal ileal loop must always be secured for satisfactory study of the mucosa.[34]

SPECIAL FACTORS IN SMALL BOWEL EXAMINATION

Various factors in this routine small bowel examination require further elaboration for a more thorough understanding.

1. The above method for routine small bowel examination is devised to subject the small intestine to a careful examination. It may, however, be too time-consuming when examining large groups of patients. *Screening practices* may be employed to determine which patients need more exhaustive studies. One such screening method is herein recommended. Fluoroscopy is limited to the time of giving the barium by mouth and its observation through the first loops of jejunum, *being mindful to keep the stomach relatively empty until the duodenal jejunal flexure has been seen and filmed* (fig. 342). At the completion of fluoroscopy, filming is again performed. Next, further films are se-

cured at specified intervals. Intervals of 1 hour, 2 hours, 3 hours, 4 hours and 5 hours have been found to provide much information regarding the small bowel status.

2. A *time table* describing the progress of the barium mixture follows: Within limits, the examiner should expect that the normal stomach may be almost empty at the 3-hour film, and the head of the barium column should be at the ileum. He may further expect filling of the right colon at the 5-hour examination, and that barium remaining in the small bowel will be confined to the terminal ileum. More or less all of the administered barium should be in the lower half of the abdomen and to the right of the midline at the 5 hour film.

(This time table is a generalization and is subject to exceptions. However, when profound disturbances are found in this timing, abnormalities should be carefully sought.)

3. *Speeding up the small bowel study.* In certain instances it may be desirable to speed up the examination. For example, as described above, the examiner desirous of seeing the terminal ileum may be unduly delayed by the slow progress of the barium meal. During this waiting period, administering 8 ounces of ice water, or perhaps an additional small amount of barium mixture may produce the desired effect. Pansdorf[23] advised giving four separate doses of 1 ounce barium mixtures at approximately 15-minute intervals. Weber and Kirklin[24] advocate 8 ounces of a mixture consisting of equal parts (by volume) of barium and water prepared with a mechanical mixer. The patient is instructed to take the entire 8 ounces at the outset. He is examined immediately thereafter and again at intervals of 15 and 30 minutes after the initial drink. The next 30 to 45 minutes the patient is instructed to rest. It is believed that lying on the right side during the intervals helps the stomach to empty more rapidly. With the stomach then almost empty, additional barium mixture as above and in the same amount (8 ounces) is given. In some cases,

a palatable meal of the patient's own liking is given. Films are again taken periodically. These maneuvers are intended to speed up gastric emptying and cause an increase in peristaltic activity within the ileum. This increased peristaltic activity is important in helping avoid delay in filling the terminal ileum.

Certain other maneuvers may be used to speed up the examination. Weintraub and Williams[25] suggested the use of a barium meal made with cold normal saline. This resulted in more rapid passage of the barium solution from the stomach and through the small bowel. Cold isotonic saline has been shown to hasten the motility and gastric evacuation. Thus, the patient may be given such a drink immediately after the ingested barium, and one-half hour later another glass of the same isotonic saline can be given. For patients on salt-free diets, ice cold water without salt may be given. This is not as efficient, but will increase the small bowel motility.[35] When these procedures are successful, the ileo-cecal region can be reached in from one-half to one hour. Additional diluent has the disadvantage, however, of making contrast and detail less distinct. In addition, speeding up motility lessens the opportunity to detect motor dysfunction.

4. *Approximation of small bowel loops and quantity of opaque solution used.* Some examiners prefer to give small amounts of barium solution. With small amounts, e.g., 4 ounces, one or two segments are opacified at a time. With fewer loops opacified it is easier to separate and examine each individual segment than when large amounts of opaque material have been administered and many more loops opacified. With the bowel lying free in the abdomen, and *many* loops of bowel opacified by these larger quantities of barium solution, the various coils overlap to such a degree as to make examination difficult.

There are, however, disadvantages in the use of smaller amounts of barium. Thus, smaller amounts of opaque material may not adequately *pack* the intestinal loops, which are then difficult to investigate. A loop inadequately filled is not properly outlined, and may give false impressions (e.g., segmentation). It should be remembered that the barium forms a mold of the lumen, and that only when every portion of the lumen is lined with the modeling material can a true rendition of its inner surface be secured.

To overcome these difficulties, larger amounts of barium suspension are given. With resultant better filling of the small bowel loops, it becomes important for the examiner to use certain maneuvers to separate the overlapping, well packed segments. This may be accomplished under direct fluoroscopic visualization by careful manipulation and palpation. By manually applying various degrees of compression, the barium within the lumen may be thinned and the mucosal pattern seen.

5. *Examining the total length of small bowel.* It is important in examining the small bowel to attempt to see every segment or portion in the *entire length* of the small intestine. The motor meal in the routine type of small bowel examination does not allow efficient observations of progressive filling and examination of all segments of the small bowel. Yet, since a well planned and efficient routine examination of the small bowel must have this for its aim, an informed approach is particularly important and special maneuvers must be resorted to as necessary.

Barium solution having been taken by mouth, the examination then proceeds as successive loops of bowel are progressively filled. This opaque column, as a plaster mould outlining the interior of the small intestine, demonstrates lesions which may be present. With forward progress at the head, emptying of the loops at the tail must take place. Loops emptied and no longer opacified can no longer be visualized either fluoroscopically or radiographically—

a fact that, although quite obvious, should be dwelled on for a moment. Even if some opaque residue remains in some of these loops, the filling by these last residues would be partial and inadequate to outline the lumen properly. Certainly, fluoroscoping or filming a loop of bowel wherein only a part of its interior is opacified is not of any great use for diagnostic purposes. The problem is, therefore, at what intervals should the patient be fluoroscoped and radiographs taken during the routine type of examination, so that the examiner may be reasonably certain that the column has *not* passed on and left certain segments unexamined.

The answer lies in estimating how rapidly the opacified column is making progress through the small bowel. The examiner achieves this by observing the speed of gastric emptying and at the same time gages the rapidity of small bowel filling taking place at the head of the column. During the first hour, after the drinking of the barium suspension, then, frequent observation of gastric emptying and small bowel filling is made. The recommended method of examining at 15-minute intervals during the first hour may seem arbitrary, perhaps even haphazard, but with experience it can be quite efficient.

6. *Skipped Segments.* Another difficulty which may present itself is that during any of these interval examinations certain segments of bowel within the *body* of the opacified column may be temporarily empty (as discussed under Segmentation). If the examiner is to see the small bowel in its entirety, he must be aware that these skipped segments exist, and during fluoroscopic examination try to fill them. If such a segment cannot be filled, and a lesion is still suspected, repeat examination is indicated. A small bowel enema may be performed if the segment persistently fails to fill.

7. *Skipped Areas.* Areas may be found in the abdomen where small intestinal loops should normally be found but at no time during the conventional interval studies are

they seen as occupied with small intestine. Persistence on the part of the examiner may elicit the cause for these skipped areas. It may be necessary for him to wait until the loops immediately proximal or leading into this skipped area are opacified. When this occurs, he stations himself beside the fluoroscopic table while the patient is behind the fluoroscopic screen and every few minutes looks to see if barium is entering into this area. This is time-consuming, but often the diagnosis may rest upon the findings so obtained. The examiner's patience may be rewarded by eventually seeing a loop of bowel go through the questionable region, and presenting all of the characteristics of regional enteritis, and thus determining that the mass displacing the small intestinal coils is produced by the thickened mesentery and nodes associated with this disease (figs. 343–350). On the other hand, he may instead be rewarded by finding a circling loop of intestine not typical of regional enteritis. This circling loop may act as the guide which leads the palpating hand to discover the edge of a mass which previously the examiner could not be sure of. The clinical conclusion that a mass is present may rest entirely on the finding of this definite edge.

8. *Dilatation or narrowing of segments* (fig. 336). Loops of bowel *momentarily* possessing an unusual form will appear pathologic and pose the same problem as in true dilatation or narrowing previously discussed. The solution of this difficulty is the same as already advised in such cases: Fluoroscope prior to each film exposure, and, with the patient remaining on the table, process and read the radiograph immediately. Should a discrepancy arise between the fluoroscopic and film findings, refluoroscope immediately in conjunction with confirmatory conventional or spot films. It is important that the question arising on the film be cleared immediately.

9. *Unattainable loops.* Loops of small bowel situated deep within the pelvis, as noted earlier, cannot be studied properly because they are not accessible to palpation. In such regions, overlapping and failure adequately to visualize individual loops is common. An attempt can be made to raise these loops out of the pelvis by administering two large glasses of water about 2 hours before the examination. Consequent distention of the urinary bladder may lift loops of bowel out of the pelvis. The rectum and sigmoid colon can be distended by a water enema, which will displace some of the small bowel loops up into the abdomen and may thus position them more suitably for examination. A simpler method is to place the patient in a rather deep Trendelenberg position. It is important to bear in mind that a 10 to 15 degree tilt is not sufficient to cause the small bowel loops to slip from the pelvis into the abdomen.

10. *Examination of the terminal ileum and ileo-cecal region.* We have already seen that the terminal ileum presents an important problem in examination because the forward progress of the barium mixture approaching this terminus is extremely slow. (See maneuvers to speed up examination, page 256.) Proper examination demands proper filling. Routine examination of the terminal ileum should be supplemented by barium enema studies and retrograde filling of this loop of intestine. When the barium enema method is used, the terminal ileum should be examined both before and *after* the patient evacuates the barium mixture. Occasionally, the ileum may fail to fill *prior* to evacuation, but becomes filled afterwards. The opaque media entering the terminal ileum by means of this retrograde enema is not dehydrated, and, in a more fluid state than oral barium from above, permits more accurate examination.

The insertion of the terminal ileum into the cecum must be established. It is well to remember that the ileo-cecal sphincter may be located on either the medial, posterior, or lateral walls of the cecum. The defect produced by the sphincter may simulate a tumor. Its identification under such conditions is important. Finding the ileo-cecal sphincter fluoroscopically is not difficult. It entails only proper dark adaptation, proper patient positioning and correct *graded* compression over the cecum at the expected site of ileal entry. In practically every case with the cecum filled and the proper degree of pressure applied, the ileo-cecal sphincter can be brought into view (figs. 339–341).

When seen, the two lips of the sphincter help distinguish that this is a normal structure, not a tumor. It is also important that the ileum be seen entering into the *center* of the apparent defect. *This entry must be equidistant from the superior and inferior margins of the sphincter* (fig. 341). Establishing this mode of entry is important in distinguishing the ileo-cecal valve and differentiating it from tumor or other masses capable of producing a similar defect within the cecum (figs. 339–341).

The ileo-cecal region should be studied after the oral administration of contrast material as well as after retrograde filling of the colon. The ileo-cecal valve can fluoroscopically be appraised most efficiently after evacuating the barium enema. Enlargement of the ileo-cecal valve is best seen at this time. In a question of such enlargement, certain secondary signs are of some value and should be sought.[36] These would include dilatation of the terminal ileum and its failure to empty when the colon and cecum themselves empty well.

Intussusception may occur with an enlarged valve. This is best seen on the evacuation study. The enlargement of the valve should be considered significant only in the presence of associated symptoms and localizing signs and in the absence of any other cause for the abdominal distress.[37]

DUODENAL INTUBATION AND SMALL BOWEL ENEMA

Small bowel barium enema consists of passing a short intestinal tube through the stomach into the duodenum and next opacifying the entire small intestine through it.

INDICATIONS AND CONTRAINDICATIONS

The first question regarding duodenal intubation and small bowel enema is *when* to use it. The procedure is not pleasant, though not painful. The examiner would like to avoid it when simpler forms of examination will suffice. It is an alternative diagnostic procedure which can be used after careful routine barium meal study of the small intestine has been indecisive, and where distinct lesions such as tumors, inflammations, kinks, adhesions, bands and diverticula are still suspected.

Functional conditions such as sprue and other illnesses characterized by a disordered motor function do not lend themselves to examination by this method. Transit time and segmentation, important changes looked for to diagnose these functional ailments, cannot be properly demonstrated when the small bowel is studied by intubation and enema. For example, true transit time is controlled by intestinal peristalsis or motor power. The forward progress of the opaque media when given by intubation and enema is not controlled by physiologic activity but by the simple addition of more solution and hydrostatic pressure, i.e., the barium solution above the patient.

Since intubation is not physiologic it also causes vomiting if the barium is given too rapidly. Inasmuch as patients with peptic ulcerations or duodenitis may be adversely affected by mechanical trauma, especially when the duodenal lesion is in an active stage, it would be wise not to subject them to intestinal intubation. It is likewise not recommended in cases of acute obstructive or paralytic ileus (see Chapter VIII).

Its chief value is that it permits visualization of the *progressive* filling of each individual loop of small intestine, which can be observed under fluoroscopic vision. The length of any lesion, its relationship to nearby structures, and the presence or ab-

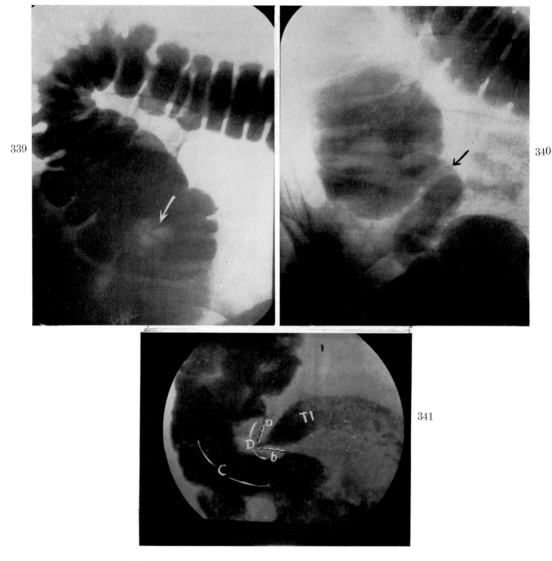

339

340

341

339

A defect (arrow) is present within the cecum. This may be due to tumor or ileo-cecal valve. How may a decision be reached? See figures 340, 341.

340

The terminal ileum is filled (arrow) by retrograde fashion through barium enema. See figure 341.

341

Behind the fluoroscopic screen, the defect in the cecum is located and an attempt is made to demonstrate the terminal ileum entering into the defect. Under direct fluoroscopic observation the region is compressed. *If at no time can the terminal ileum be seen to enter into the defect, the defect is probably produced by a tumor. When the defect is produced by the ileo-cecal valve, as here demonstrated, the terminal ileum will be seen entering into it* and the point of entry is equidistant from the superior and inferior margins of the defect (*a* equals *b*). (*TI*, terminal ileum; *C*, cecum, *D*, defect.)

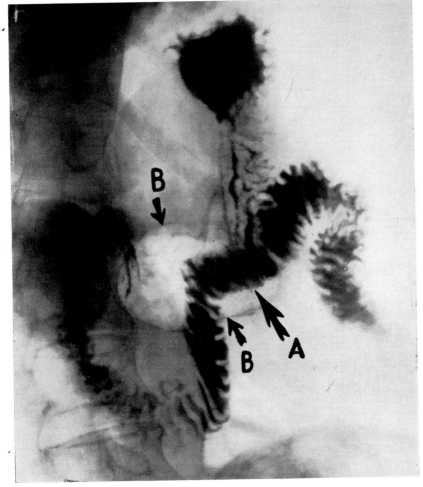

342

The stomach in a relatively empty state permits adequate visualization of the duodenal jejunal flexure. *B,B* indicates the outline of *empty* stomach overlying *but not blotting out* the
shadow of the underlying duodenal jejunal flexure, *A*.

sence of rigidity can be judged more easily
than with other methods. For example, in
an inflammatory enteritis, barium when
given by mouth may be sped through the
region of maximal narrowing preventing the
visualization of the actual *extent* of the
lesion. When *continuous* and *progressive*
filling of *successive* segments can be directly
observed, the filling of the involved segment *cannot* be missed. It may be seen in
its entire extent and immediately spot
filmed.

A small bowel enema may be used to ad-

vantage in the examination of the terminal
ileal coils. During the routine ingested
method, the barium solution may become
dehydrated and lumpy as the lower ileal
coils are reached (fig. 322). The barium in
this form only coheres and cannot efficiently
adhere to and outline the intestinal walls. A
truer impression of the lumen may be obtained by a mixture in a more liquid state.
A small bowel enema fills rapidly enough
that the barium mixture arrives in the
terminal ileal coils in such a liquid state.

If necessary, the ileo-cecal valve, cecum

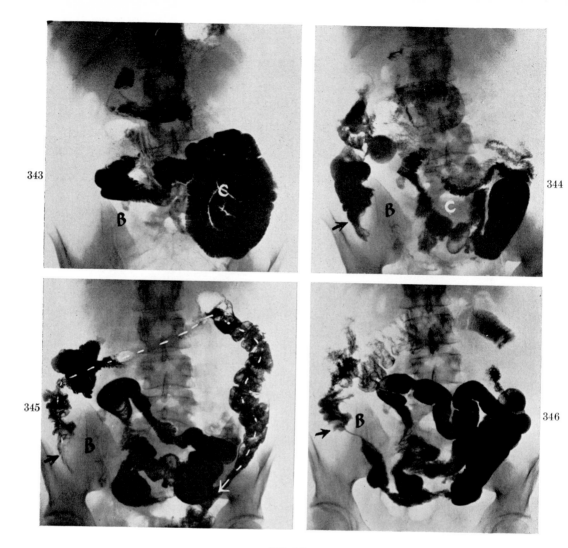

343–346

Question:

Regional enteritis is suspected. A barium meal has been given and a small bowel study performed. In figure 344 the cecum (arrow) is reached. In figure 345 the barium has reached well within the descending colon (dotted line). Often in small bowel studies, when barium reaches well within the colon the examination is concluded. However, is this examination complete?

Answer:

No. It is important that *all* spaces where small intestinal loops should normally be found be seen filled with these loops at least *once* during the study. Area "C" is seen free of small bowel loops in fig. 344 but filled with them in fig. 343; thus it can be passed as normal. Area B remains unoccupied with small bowel loops throughout the examination (figs. 343–346). Thus it is advisable that the small bowel examination be continued until all spaces where small bowel loops are expected to be found are actually seen so occupied or an explanation for their absence is made.

Question:

In figure 344, regions "B" and "C" appear to be relatively free of small bowel loops. What are some of the causes for this?

Answer:

(1) A normal small bowel study where the loops within "B" and "C" just "do not happen"

262

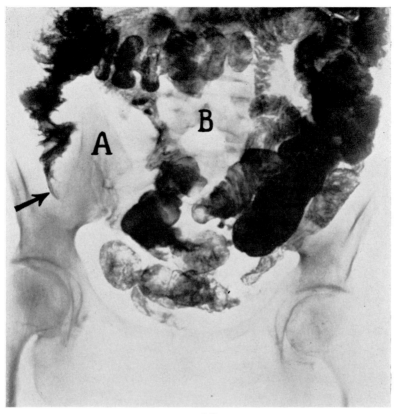

347

Question:

Regional enteritis is suspected. Are there any clues in figure 347 which might lead the examiner to suspect the lesion?

Answer:

Yes. Figure 347 reveals the cecum narrowed (arrow) and two spaces (A and B) not filled with small intestinal loops (see figs. 343–346). This examination was continued in figs. 348-349.

and ascending colon may also be examined quite efficiently by small bowel enema. This is especially important when examination of the right side of the large bowel by barium enema is either unsatisfactory or impossible (e.g., in spasm of the cecum or ascending colon or in anal insufficiency where the patient cannot retain the opaque mixture when given by rectum).

The procedure is also valuable in that it

to be opacified at the moment. Region "C" in figure 344 is such an area, since it is filled in figure 343.

(2) A tumor mass pushing the small intestinal coils to either side. Here the space would not fill, no matter how persistent the examiner.

(3) Thickened mesentery and nodes and involved loops of small intestine behaving as a tumor mass, usually found with regional enteritis.

Comment: This examination was at first terminated after figure 345. It is possible that if the examiner had pursued the examination until the small bowel had emptied itself, a loop might have been caught within space "B"—not shown before—and filled, and thus the cause for the space in region "B" would have been found. In this case, the patient was brought back and the small bowel restudied with the aim of determining the cause for space "B". Greater persistence on the part of the examiner revealed the cause of the space in region "B" when he elicited the *narrowing* (beneath B, fig. 346) of the terminal ileum as typical of regional enteritis.

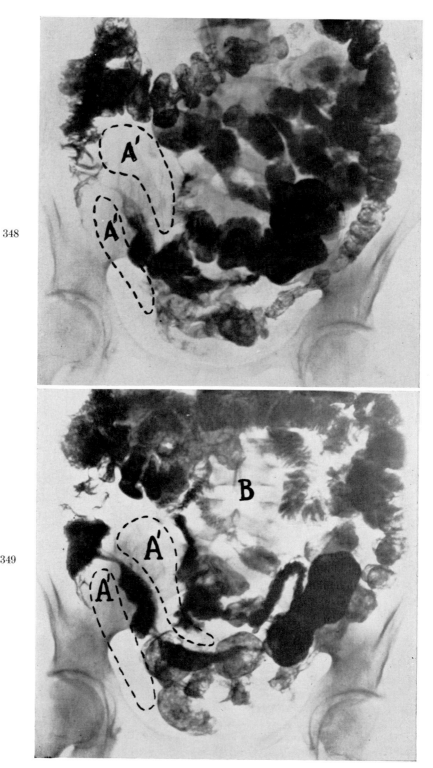

See legend, facing page.

not only shortens the time of examination but it reduces the number of times the patient must be fluoroscoped.

METHODS OF INTESTINAL INTUBATION

The method consists in the passage of an ordinary stomach tube into the duodenum and the subsequent administration of barium.

It is important that the stomach be empty. The examination can profitably start in the morning after approximately 8 hours of fasting. When it is intended likewise to study the right side of the colon, cleansing of the large bowel as described under colonic barium enema (see Chapter VII) should be performed.

The mixture used should be relatively dilute, being thinner than the type used for other gastrointestinal examinations. For the usual gastrointestinal series a mixture consisting of equal parts of water and barium is recommended. To this mixture can now be added two glasses of lukewarm water. This corresponds to 6 parts of barium to 18 parts of water by volume. From 800 to 1200 cc. of barium suspension is necessary to fill the bowel. In children, considerably less is used, and where marked reflux into the stomach is present, more than this amount is necessary. The mixture should be passed while warm. The respiratory passages may become irritated when the indwelling tube is made cold by injecting cool solution.

An ordinary duodenal tube (Einhorn type) is passed by the usual method. This part of the procedure may be facilitated by passing the tube with the patient on the fluoroscopic table.

The tube having been passed into the descending portion of the duodenum the barium suspension is next injected through its lumen into the small bowel (page 332). As the barium runs in, its rate of flow is controlled by the attendant who holds the container of barium over the patient's head. The hydrostatic pressure responsible for the speed of flow varies with the height of the can. It is recommended that this be elevated to approximately 10 inches. At this level a smooth slow continuous flow may be expected. The same precautions in controlling the height of barium solution during colonic barium enema should be observed here. Another precaution is to maintain the inflow. Interrupted injection will cause the forward progress of the opaque media to stop, and to start its forward movement anew the examiner must wait as though the barium first had to refill the entire portion of the small bowel already containing opaque media. The flow should be slow, continuous and as far as practical under constant fluoroscopic vision. *Accurate records of the radiation received by the examiner and patient should be kept to avoid exposure to dangerous amounts.*

1. Passage of the duodenal tube through the stomach into the duodenum may be

---

348–349 (Same patient as in fig. 347.)

During fluoroscopy the cecum was found tender to palpation, indicating an abnormalcy. Spaces which do not fill at least once during the examination should not be overlooked, and the examination should not be concluded so long as they are *unexplained*. Continue the examination to permit barium to enter these spaces, if possible. Give more barium if necessary. In figures 348 and 349, persistence of this type of study by the examiner elicited the cause for spaces A′ and B. Space B filled with normal loops (fig. 348) and proved to be a space which just did not happen to opacify in figure 347. Space A remained as a space, but became divided into two longitudinal compartments (A′A′) by a persistently narrowed terminal ileum. Fluoroscopically, the narrow terminal ileum was tender and typically involved with regional enteritis.

Note how the visualized terminal ileum stands alone, well separated from the other intestinal loops by spaces A′A′. Since an intestinal coil involved with the regional enteritis generally stands alone, well separated from the other intestinal coils, it has been referred to as a "proud" loop of intestine. It stands alone because the thickened mesentery and nodes associated with regional enteritis push the other loops aside.

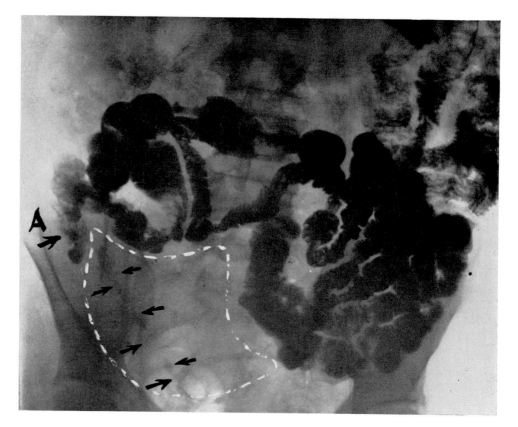

350

In this small bowel study, when the cecum (arrow A) was reached, a large space (dotted line) was found unoccupied by small intestinal loops (see figs. 343–346 and 347–349). Carefully looking into the space, the examiner could see the "proud" terminal ileum (arrows) (see also fig. 349) taking the entire space for itself. This was confirmed as regional ileitis by palpating while fluoroscoping and finding the loop tender and rigid, and by subsequent spot films revealing persistent narrowing and destroyed mucosa of the involved loop.

facilitated when performed on the fluoroscopic table. The technic is much the same as described in Stage I for the long intestinal tube (page **329**).

2. The examiner should carefully observe the head of the barium column as in its forward progress it canalizes and distends the lumen of the bowel. Any apparent narrowing, undue dilatation, or area of mucosal change, swelling or destruction should be noted. For clearer and more accurate visualization a *small port of observation* should be used, and the lead-protected hand be active in separating overlapping loops. Throughout the procedure, liberal use should be

made of spot films in order to confirm and record the fluoroscopic findings, especially in regions where pathology is suspected or discovered.

The duodenal jejunal flexure and the regional upper loops of small bowel should be examined and spot filmed as quickly as possible, since, as cautioned above, the stomach should be relatively empty. If any delay occurs in examining and spot filming this region, and if reflux from the small intestine back into the stomach takes place, the stomach will fill and the overfilled gastric shadow will hang down as an overlying curtain and make efficient examination of the duodenal-jejunal region difficult or impossible (fig. 336).

3. In those cases where filling of the right side of the large bowel is important, the barium after passing through the ileum is permitted to progress through the ileo-cecal valve. The cecum and the right side of the colon can thus be filled and studied.

4. In most normal cases it is easy to observe the flow of barium directly to the cecum. In other cases the flow is retarded because of the reflux of barium into the stomach, and in such instances forward progress of the opaque media may be so slow that the time necessary to fluoroscopically visualize complete small bowel filling can be dangerous and cause overexposure to both examiner and patient. The flow of barium in the average normal case is approximately 15 minutes. In rare cases, however, it can take up to 90 minutes. This is especially apt to happen where marked reflux of barium into the stomach causes delay. The average time consumed by examination when pathology is encountered is somewhat greater than the average time for normal examinations.

5. Reflux into the stomach cannot usually be remedied as might be expected, by lowering the level of the barium solution. In addition, lowering the barium solution may stop progress of the barium column. It has been thought that reflux was related to increased pressure within the duodenum. However, since it can also occur in a patient where the duodenal pressure is low, i.e., where the duodenum is incompletely filled, this theory is untenable.

Other maneuvers which the examiner may attempt in order to overcome this reflux include passing the duodenal tube further down into the jejunum, positioning the patient so he lies with his right side down (helping to carry the opaque media quickly away from the stomach) or suspending the barium in isotonic saline.

Slowing the rate of flow into the duodenum has been of some help. A syringe may be used to inject the opaque media, with the same syringe later employed to inject small quantities of air for air contrast studies.

It should be frankly stated, however, that in cases where reflux is an important complicating factor, the efficacy of none of these methods can really be counted on.

6. Performing the small bowel examination with the duodenal tube is a simple procedure and is practical not only for hospital but also for office procedure. Although accompanied by the usual annoyance and difficulties, it is successful in the great majority of instances. It should not be performed in any case in which routine examination of the gastrointestinal tract is contraindicated. Thus it would not be used in cases with marked mechanical or paralytic ileus. In these instances the long intestinal tube (Chapter VIII) should be employed. Where the emergency is such that time is of the essence and the life of the patient is at stake (suspected gangrene of the bowel, mesenteric thrombosis or strangulated external hernia), the problem itself should be handled without any intestinal intubation. This will be discussed in greater detail below.

Diseases of the Small Bowel

In large part, diseases of the small bowel should be suspected when symptoms point to the abdominal portion of the gastrointestinal tract and suitable examination has excluded stomach, duodenum or colon. The indications for small bowel study may be summarized as:

1. Diarrhea which cannot be explained by colonic study.

2. Intestinal bleeding when the colon, esophagus, stomach and duodenum have been excluded.

3. Pain in the abdomen located within the distribution of the small bowel when other causes have been excluded. This is especially indicated if the pains are cramplike and suggestive of either complete or partial intestinal obstruction.

4. When diseases capable of producing disordered motor function are suspected. These will be enumerated below.

INCOMPLETE OR PARTIAL INTESTINAL OBSTRUCTION[26]

Many of the pathological entities existing in the small bowel are capable of producing incomplete obstruction. Such diversified lesions as adhesions, sclerosing enteritis, tumors—either benign or malignant, and various types of extrinsic pressure, may make their presence known through this symptom complex. Intestinal obstruction is important enough and commonly enough encountered that an entire chapter has been devoted to the various forms of the condition, its causes, diagnosis and roentgenologic management (see Chapter VIII). There are, however, some special points regarding *partial* obstruction which should be made here.

1. Although dilatation of proximal small bowel loops generally increases as the degree of partial obstruction progresses, in certain obstructive processes there may be little or no dilatation of these segments proximal to the block. For example, narrowing of the intestinal lumen in the early stages of *inflammatory enteritis* is produced by a combination of spasm and mucous membrane swelling. This is generally not associated with dilatation of the proximal loops.

Dilatation is also frequently absent in *adhesions*. An explanation offered for this latter lack of dilatation in that some degree of hypertrophy occurs within the muscle of the proximal loops of bowel which adequately compensates for the constriction produced by the adhesions. When compen-

sation is lost, the *proximal* intestinal loops dilate.

2. Dilatation proximal to a constricting lesion is first localized to the segments immediately above the lesion. With continuing holdup the dilatation gradually extends craniad. *The dilatation may remain localized to a few proximal segments for prolonged periods of time.*

3. Peristalsis.[26] Fluoroscopically, increase in peristaltic activity is observed in those segments proximal to an obstructive lesion. Reverse peristalsis may also be present. This should not be confused with a to-and-fro appearance of the small bowel segments proximal to an obstructing lesion produced by the inability of a peristaltic wave to pass much of the opaque media through the narrowed segment so that the residue flows back into the proximal segment. The degree of peristaltic activity may vary. If the bowel becomes tired and atonic, peristalsis may not be as evident.

4. Mass formation or tenderness. The suspected lesion may be palpated under direct fluoroscopic visualization. The presence of a mass or localized tenderness may be elicited.

5. Trailing segments. Some separation or segmentation of the barium column is a normal finding at the tail of the barium column (figs. 309, 324). This is generally confined to poorly filled segments and, during interval studies, is inconstant in appearance and location. When, however, a segment which is *well filled* appears separated from the rest of the column, and during the periodic or hourly studies it *reappears as well filled* and the forward progress of the barium meal appears retarded at this point, it may be called a trailing segment. Trailing segments can be an important clue in lesser degrees of *partial obstruction.*

This fact emphasizes the importance of continuous observation of the filling of the small bowel and next its complete emptying. A diagnosis of partial obstruction may often be made after observing at several intervals a retardation of the forward passage of the barium at the same location (figs. 309, 324).

6. Gas accumulation. Any localized *persistently* gas filled loop or loops within the small bowel may be significant. This should make the examiner suspicious of an obstructive type of lesion, and may indicate stasis[27] (fig. 337, page 252).

In partial obstruction the mixture of barium, gas and fluid gives a characteristic mottled appearance. Under fluoroscopic palpation with the patient in the supine position, a succussion splash within the involved coils may on occasion be demonstrated.[28]

7. Segmentation. Segmentation associated with partial obstruction has been described above (see page 238 and fig. 338, p. 252).

REGIONAL ILEITIS

Fluoroscopic and radiographic findings are shown in figures 311, 312, 329–332.

Early cases of regional enteritis are not easily recognized. The thickening of the mucosa, tenderness of the various involved loops, and the demonstration of rigidity may be difficult to demonstrate and are nonspecific in character. It is more frequently diagnosed as the involved segments become narrowed as the result of either spasm or fibrotic stenosis. The radiographic signs become characteristic as the lumen narrows.

When barium enters into a normal loop of small bowel, the contours of the opacified loop should be smooth. If, as may happen in the terminal ileum, the barium has become inspicated or clumpy, the contour may occasionally appear irregular, but when this irregularity occurs in a *normal* loop of small intestine, the irregularity *changes* with different degrees of filling. The irregularity is not *constant*. However, an irregularity which persistently remains the same with different degrees of filling would be indicative of organic defects within the wall of a small bowel. The barium forming a cast model of the lumen would demonstrate the irregularity resulting from the defects in the wall (figs. 351–354).

To see the diseased loops of intestine in this illness, no great degree of manipulation or uncovering of overlapping loops of bowel is generally necessary. The narrowed loops of bowel are well separated from the adjacent small bowel loops by the thickened mesentery (figs. 332, 348–349). This thickened mesentery and the loops *well separated* form a characteristic tender mass (figs. 343–350). The rigid loops will be seen to be constant in position; i.e., with periodic studies their position will appear unchanged (figs. 311, 312, on p. 230).

Compression studies of the mucous membrane reveal mucosal changes consisting of either ulcerations or polypoid formations (fig. 321). Sinus tracts and adhesions of loops of bowel are common. Proximal to these cicatrized narrowed segments will occur some dilatation of the intestinal loops.

The examiner finding a localized small bowel lesion must not be content until the stomach, the entire small bowel and the colon have been examined. He must be aware that skip areas are frequent and multiple involvement, although not the rule, may be present. Local spasms of the cecum may be present, similar to those seen in tuberculosis or colitis.

TUBERCULOSIS

Peritoneal Involvement. Tuberculous peritonitis indicates its presence by irregular narrowings and partial obstructions of the small bowel. These are caused by extensive adhesions. The radiographic change is that of a breaking up of the continuous small bowel column by the adhesive processes.

Fluoroscopically and radiographically the findings are suggestive of the segmentation pattern seen with disordered motor function. In tuberculous peritonitis, since *fixed adhesions* are responsible for the broken pattern, intestinal loops which are

dilated or segmented *retain their same configuration each time they are filled.* A similar segmented appearance produced by
functional derangements, i.e., in the absence
of fixed adhesions, is incapable of repro-
ducing itself with the same exactness. (See
the section on adhesions, page 308.)

Luminal Involvement. Tuberculous disease of the small bowel produces mucosal
edema with thickening of the Kerkring
folds and narrowing of the bowel lumen.
Later, ulceration appears. In appearance
the condition may resemble regional ileitis.
As a rule, the cecum and ileum are involved
together. The regional plastic exudate produces a matting together of the regional
loops.

Fluoroscopically, the segments are not
overly tender but are often difficult to separate. Increased peristaltic activity is an
early finding, probably resulting from a
localized segmental irritability, barium
passing through quickly and not well retained. This is often accompanied by
atonicity of other segments, with concomitant weak peristalsis.

TUMORS OF THE SMALL BOWEL

(FIGS. 333, 334, PAGE 247)

When tumor is suspected the ideal would
be study of the small bowel by continuous
fluoroscopy, to be followed by filming. This
is presently not practical, although in the

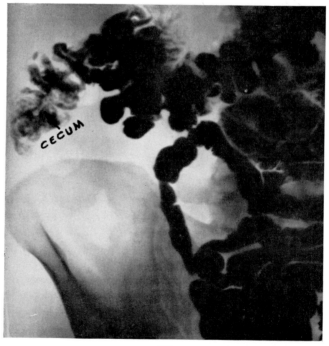

351

This patient had intermittent unexplained pain in the right
lower quadrant of the abdomen. In this first examination, the
cecum is reached, and a space unoccupied by intestinal loops
is shown present on the medial aspect of and below the cecum.

The persistent examiner then fills the terminal ileum (figs.
352–354), which is questionably tender to palpation. Still no
definite mass is palpable.

Question:

What further signs may the examiner seek to confirm the
terminal ileum as abnormal? (See fig. 352-354)

near future fluoroscopic image intensification will improve the method.

The type of examination recommended at this time is that described under routine small bowel study. This should be supplemented by retrograde filling of the ileal loops with barium enema. However, when a *definite* lesion is suspected and *routine study does not uncover the source of the patient's symptoms*, intubation type of examination must be performed.

Radiographic Signs. Radiographically, the important clues sought for are the signs of partial small bowel obstruction previously noted (see page 268).

The diagnosis of small bowel tumors is

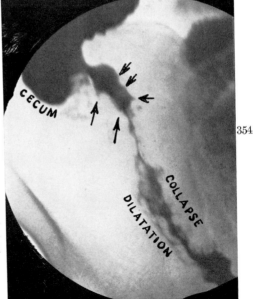

Answer:

Figures 352–354 reveal the results of further examination, in which the previous space is now filled. The terminal ileum is seen in different stages of distention with barium. Note how the dilatation is greatest in figure 352, somewhat less in figure 353, and relatively narrow and collapsed in figure 354. Despite these different degrees of filling, the contour *continues to remain the same* (compare arrow for arrow in figures 352–354). On the contrary, a *normal* soft bowel loop would *change contour* during different degrees of filling. Hence, abnormality is determined in this case, and clinical findings subsequently confirmed regional enteritis.

extremely difficult. In some cases even the most careful and painstaking technics may not uncover the lesion.

To search for the tumor when dilated loops of bowel are present, is to follow the dilated segments to their termination (figs. 333, 334). The lesion should be found at this point. The lesion, when found, most commonly presents as an annular constriction (figs. 333, 334). It should be examined by graded compression and spot filmed. Irregularity of outline and destruction of mucosa are indications that it is intramural. The involved segment is generally short and rigid; a sharp transition from the normal to the abnormal is characteristic.

Spot filming during fluoroscopy and the use of graded pressure is essential in the demonstration of these changes. It should be borne in mind that a definitive diagnosis, benign or malignant, lymphosarcoma or carcinoma, can rarely be arrived at, fluoroscopically or radiographically. The important diagnostic point is that the lesion be discovered.

DISORDERED MOTOR FUNCTION

(Figs. 325–327, page 242)

The term disordered motor function as applied to the small bowel[3, 9, 11, 29] designates a number of diseases characterized by either hypomotility or hypermotility, segmentation of the barium column, clumping and flocculation of the barium, occasionally dilated or contracted loops of bowel and thickening or flattening of the mucosal folds.

The various conditions observed as capable of producing this phenomenon may be classified as follows*:

I. Disturbances of Nutrition
 A. Pancreatic insufficiency
 B. Tropical sprue
 C. Idiopathic steatorrhea

---

* From a table compiled by J. Friedman.[16] Reproduced by courtesy of the author and the American Journal of Roentgenology, Radium Therapy and Nuclear Medicine.

 D. Celiac disease
 E. Hypoproteinemia
 F. Hypopotassemia
 G. Vitamin deficiency
 H. Intestinal parasites (hookworm)
II. Secondary to Organic Disease in Intestine or Mesentery
 A. Chronic peptic ulcer
 B. Ulcerative colitis, regional enteritis, tuberculous enteritis
 C. Intra-abdominal abscesses
 D. Tumors in intestine or mesentery
 E. Sclerosing mesenteritis and lipodystrophy of mesentery
 F. Mesenteric adenitis
III. Dysfunction Associated with Generalized Metabolic Disease
 A. Hyperthyroidism
 B. Lead poisoning
 C. Porphyria
IV. Dysfunction Associated with Neurologic Disease
 A. Diabetic neuropathy
 B. Pernicious anemia
 C. Tabes dorsalis
 D. Vagotomy and sympathectomy
V. Administration of Foodstuffs with Barium
 A. Fats especially fatty acid
 B. Hypertonic saline and sodium bicarbonate
 C. Carbohydrate
VI. Retention of Fluid and Mucus in the Intestine
VII. Autonomic Blocking Drugs
VIII. Allergy
IX. Emotional Disturbances

Etiology. The term disordered motor function has been suggested because it is believed that the changes present in this syndrome, i.e., segmentation of the barium column, dilatation of the loops, etc., result to a considerable degree from deranged motor function of the autonomic nervous system. The radiographic appearances are not primarily owing to structural changes in the small intestine, but to variations in the physiology. The presence of excess fat in the intestine plays an important part in the production of this pattern.

Clumping of the barium with resultant breaking up of the opacified small bowel column is a frequent finding in normal children up to the age of 14 and has little diagnostic significance[32] (fig. 303, p. 226). Below the age of 5, a segmentation pattern resulting from clumping of the barium suspension occurs in the majority of normal children. As mentioned earlier, normal mucus content in the infant bowel may be the causative factor.

Technic of Examination. The small bowel is studied as previously described by routine barium meal. Since the condition has been ascribed to physiologic variations, it is unwise to add any ingredients to the ordinary barium-water mixture. It is particularly important when disordered motor function is suspected that prior to examination all fat content be eliminated from the small intestine. At least fifteen hours should elapse between the last meal where fats were permitted and the examination itself. Where possible, this fat-free period may profitably be extended to twenty-four hours. When reporting for examination the patient should have nothing by mouth, i.e., no food, no drink, no smoking, no chewing gum. Because of the profound effect that the emotions have on the small intestinal pattern, it is important that the patient be kept in a calm relaxed state.

It is particularly important that adequate amounts of contrast media be given. Small or limited amounts of barium mixture may add confusion because this in itself is capable of producing an apparent segmented pattern (see section on Segmentation, page 239). The recommended meal is, again, 16 ounces of opaque media containing 8 ounces of barium by volume to which enough water has been added to make a total of 16 ounces of mixture.

No advantage has been gained by this observer's use of micro-pulverized powder.

During the course of the examination, large amounts of opaque media may become pooled in several segments of small intestine. Since this will interfere with proper visualization of the balance of the small bowel, an additional 4 to 6 ounces of mixture may be given.

Radiographic and Fluoroscopic Findings.

1. Segmentation. In a typically well developed case exhibiting disordered motor function the predominant finding is a breaking-up of the barium column into various segments.

2. Motility. Behind the fluoroscopic screen, in early cases, the small intestinal segments display hypermotility. The opaque media, gathered together into clumps or floccules, appear to be moving rapidly but aimlessly about. A to-and-fro irregular type of peristalsis is present. In more fully developed cases, the hypermotility changes to a hypomotility; forward progress of the opaque media slows, the barium at times seeming to lie more quietly in the large atonic loops.[30]

3. Tone. *In early cases* hypertonicity with resultant spasm and narrowing of the bowel lumen is present. This would result in the diffuse, irregularly spastic type of segmentation associated with hypertonicity. At this time, hypermotility is also present. The barium mixture may reach the cecum in less than half an hour. *In more advanced cases*, hypotonicity may be seen, and the small bowel loops now become dilated. Hypomotility is also seen at this time. At 6 hours, gastric retention may be present, with the head of the barium column not yet arrived at the cecum.

These changes, especially in sprue, are best seen in the mid and distal jejunum.

4. Disturbances of the mucosal pattern. Thickening of the mucosal folds, as evidenced by a widening of the spaces between the Kerkring folds, as well as lowering of their height is an important finding. However, a large part of the mucosal fold flattening previously described is probably due to clumping of the barium mixture, with resultant inability of the opaque media to *outline* the *true* mucosal pattern. In advanced cases, obliteration of these folds has been described.

5. Scattering. Normal scattering is feathery, resembling snow flakes. In the presence

of disordered motor function, however, *clumps* of barium may be left scattered at the tail of the barium column. This finding is generally associated with pronounced segmentation and increased secretions.

6. Hypersecretion and gas associated with the mucosal thickening and edema.

Gaseous distention is frequent, and occasionally gas and fluid levels are present. With hypersecretion, the barium suspension may appear granular, with areas of coarser flocculation dispersed through the segments. These changes may be due to diminished power of the mucosa to absorb both gas and fluid secretions.

Assessment of Radiographic Findings.

1. It is possible that the altered pattern of the small intestine may not be pathologic, but only a functional variation that is within normal limits. It should be emphasized that in order to establish a diagnosis the *constancy* of the findings *must be confirmed by repeat examinations.*

2. It has been shown that large amounts of mucus, as well as the presence of fats in sufficient amounts, are capable of producing the phenomenon exhibited in disordered motor function.

In sprue, fat absorption is interfered with, resulting in increased fat in the small bowel. This may explain the radiographic changes in that disease. Similarly, other disorders may interfere with fat absorption, i.e., enlarged mesenteric glands, acute or chronic inflammatory tuberculosis, lymphoblastoma, or malignant neoplastic disease— these by obstructing the lymphatics.

3. Sprue. The disordered motor pattern is well demonstrated in the sprue syndrome. Dilatation of the small bowel is an important finding, and is more marked in advanced cases.

4. Allergy.[31] With food allergy, the radiographic appearances within the small bowel depend upon whether the allergen is given at the same time that the opaque meal is given. When the allergen is *absent*, the small intestine which is allergic may show either (1) a normal appearance, (2) rapid transit with hypertonicity of the ileum, or (3) hypertonicity with delayed transit.[28]

The roentgen findings may be interpreted as allergic in origin only if they occur or are accentuated when the suspected food is added. In this event, marked alteration in the motility of the gastrointestinal tract occurs, associated with narrowing and segmentation of the small bowel.[31]

Examination of the Colon

Fundamentals

ANATOMY

THE LARGE INTESTINE is a tube-like structure approximately sixty inches long and of variable width. It is widest at its origin, in the cecum, measuring from two to three inches. As it courses distally it diminishes in caliber so that by the time it reaches the descending colon it is approximately two-thirds of its original width. Within the rectum it balloons out again to a diameter of two to three inches.

For convenience in description, the bowel is subdivided into various portions, i.e., cecum, ascending colon, hepatic flexure, transverse colon, splenic flexure, descending colon, sigmoid colon, and finally the rectum (fig. 355).

The Cecum. The cecum is the widest part of the colon except for the rectum. It is usually completely surrounded with mesentery, and thus freely mobile. Situated in the right lower quadrant, its shape varies from round and pouch-like to conical.[1] Its exact height tends to vary with the body build of the individual. In the hypersthenic it may be high, whereas in the hyposthenic, it may be low and deep down within the true pelvis. In addition to these norma variations, when the proximal part of the ascending colon is unusually free, the cecum

may point to the left and its tip may come to lie on the left side of the spine. The mobility of the cecum is on occasion so great that in one examination it is possible for it to lie in the middle of the abdomen and at another time in the right iliac fossa.[2]

Ascending Colon. The ascending colon starts at the level of the ileo-cecal valve, and passes upward to just beneath the liver, ending at the hepatic flexure. This portion of the bowel is usually covered by mesentery on three sides only, i.e., anteriorly, medially, and laterally. Posteriorly, it is related to the posterior abdominal wall. In spite of this the ascending colon usually maintains a moderate degree of mobility as determined with the palpating hand, behind the fluoroscopic screen.

Hepatic Flexure. The hepatic flexure is formed by the right-sided forward and medial bend of the large bowel. It has no firm attachment above and thus is quite variable in position. When the bowel is distended with barium it usually lies just beneath the liver. In the erect position, however, and also when the bowel is no longer distended with opaque material, it is usually found just a little above the iliac crest. This is its usual position on the film taken after evacuation of the barium enema.

Transverse Colon. The transverse colon

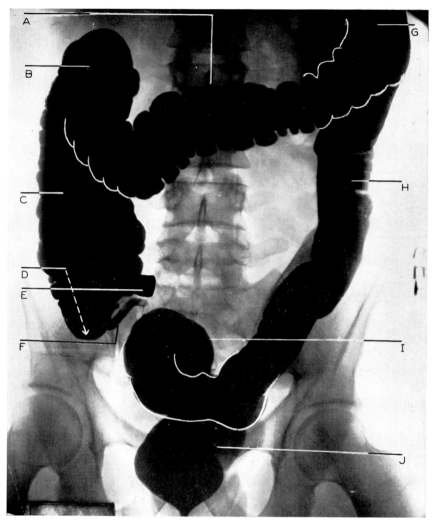

355

Normal colon.

A. Transverse colon
B. Hepatic flexure
C. Ascending colon
D. Cecum (from ileo-cecal sphincter to cecal pouch)
E. Ileum
F. Appendix

G. Splenic flexure
H. Descending colon
I. Sigmoid colon
J. Rectum (divided into upper and lower portions by the valves of Huston).

is surrounded by mesentery on all sides and hangs as a hammock suspended from the hepatic flexure on the right and the splenic flexure on the left, the latter being usually a little higher than the former. Also, not only is it higher but usually more fixed. It is believed that in visceroptosis one of the first signs is a downward displacement of the splenic flexure, so that it comes to lie on a lower level than its mate—the hepatic flexure. The transverse colon is freely mobile.

Splenic Flexure. The splenic flexure in the left upper quadrant of the abdomen is the junction of the transverse and descending colons.

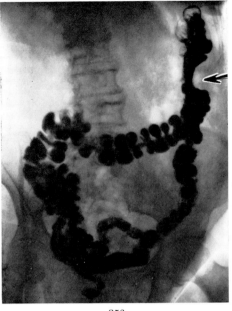

356

A normal indenture in the splenic flexure region.

It should be noted that the splenic flexure is found at a higher level in the abdomen than the hepatic flexure. The judgment as to the relative types of these flexures should be made when the colon is erected as a result of having been filled by a retrograde enema. A reversal in these heights (figs. 357, 358) is an important finding. Undue depression of the hepatic flexure as compared with the splenic flexure is also important and often finds its answer in either an enlarged liver or other regional mass pushing the hepatic flexure down.

A normal deformity in the splenic flexure may sometimes be produced by indirect pressure from the regional ribs (fig. 356).

Descending Colon. The bowel as it descends from the splenic flexure towards the sigmoid colon is usually narrowed to about two-thirds of its original width. Like the ascending colon, it is surrounded by mesentery on three sides, anteriorly, medially and laterally. Posteriorly it rests against the posterior abdominal wall. This too, like the ascending colon, maintains a moderate degree of mobility as determined on the fluoroscopic screen.

Pelvic or Sigmoid Colon. The "looped" part of the bowel from the descending colon to the rectum is called the pelvic or sigmoid colon. It is looped and has a long mesentery, thus being freely mobile. Of all portions of the colon, the length of the sigmoid loop is most varied. On occasion it may take one or two loops on the left side of the pelvis and then rise into the left iliac fossa, only to descend into the pelvis again at its junction with the rectum. Less frequently, it may be long enough to extend upwards to the left upper quadrant, even higher than the splenic flexure.

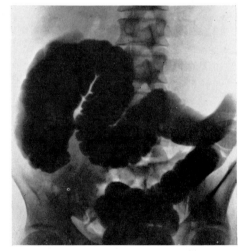

357

Question:

A retrograde enema has been done. The patient is supine and facing the examiner. What abnormalcy is seen?

Answer:

The relationship of the splenic and hepatic flexure is reversed, i.e., the splenic flexure should be higher than the hepatic flexure. In this case, the splenic flexure is lower, i.e., depressed. This may be produced by:

(1) Splenic enlargement.
(2) Retroperitoneal neoplasm within the region.
(3) Pancreatic cyst or tumor (tail of pancreas).

Comment: The depression in this case was produced by a cyst at the tail of the pancreas. (See fig. 358.)

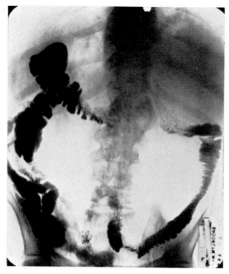

358

Question:

A retrograde enema has been performed. The patient is supine, facing the examiner. What abnormalcy is present?

Answer:

The splenic flexure is depressed (relative position of hepatic and splenic flexure reversed).

Comment: This depression was produced by retroperitoneal reticulum cell sarcoma. (See fig. 357.)

The Rectum. The rectum, starting at about the third sacral vertebra lies within the hollow of the sacrum and coccyx and ends at the anus. It is usually five to six inches long, being a little wider below and narrower above. The rectum is divided into upper and lower portions by the transverse valves of Houston. The upper of these two subdivisions probably acts as a reservoir whereas the lower is rather fixed and restricted and rarely contains fecal material. The upper portion is large and distensible.

NORMAL VARIATIONS

Redundant loops of bowel are a common finding in colon examinations. It should be remembered, however, that the barium enema method in the demonstration of redundancy of the colon is essentially an artificial procedure. Redundancy not actually present under normal conditions may be induced by the stretching and subsequent overlapping of the barium-filled loops of colon. Thus, after evacuating an enema, when the loops of bowel collapse, the true size of the various loops of bowel can better be gaged.

There are normal variations in the anatomy of the colon with which the examiner should become acquainted. Some of these are not too common; but if the observer understands these variations, he will be less apt, on encountering them, to consider them abnormal. For instance, the splenic flexure usually lying just beneath the left diaphragm, sometimes may be found only two or three inches above the crest of the left ileum. Also, it is entirely normal for the transverse colon to be so disposed within the abdomen that the configuration of the ascending, transverse and descending portions of the bowel together form an inverted U.

At times the hepatic flexure, which normally should lie beneath the liver may, when the colon is distended with barium, lie above the anterior surface of the liver in contact with the right diaphragm. Interposition of the colon between the liver and diaphragm has also been described.[3]

Varying positions of the cecum are commonly found in colon examinations. There are five varieties of undescended ceca,[4] all based on the embryology of the cecal descent. During development the cecum not only descends but, starting its development in the left abdomen, it rotates to the right abdomen. The anomalies as described depend upon the stage at which rotation and descent cease. There may be a failure of complete rotation and the cecum be found in the left upper quadrant. When descent is arrested and a little more rotation permitted, the cecum may be situated in the epigastrium or subhepatic region. The descent may be arrested, resulting in a high cecum, i.e., between the subhepatic region and its normal position in the right lower quadrant. The cecum may descend deep into the pelvis and it is then described as hyperdescent or low cecum.[5] A low cecum is diagnosed by finding the cecal tip below the horizontal line connecting the tops of both acetabula cavities. This relationship is observed with the patient in the prone position.

CONTOUR

The width of the lumen of the large bowel is greatest at the cecum and gradually lessens to the recto-sigmoid junction only to open into a terminal dilatation in the rectal ampulla. The colon is indented at intervals by haustra or sacculations. Distal to the left colic flexure the colon is relatively smooth, haustrations being much less marked. It would be interesting to dwell for a moment on how these haustral markings come about.

The taenia coli are three muscular bands arranged longitudinally on the outer surface of the colon, extending from the appendix to the rectum. The colon itself is much longer than these bands and so it must be "tucked in" or pleated at intervals to make it sufficiently short to fit under the taenia coli. It is these "tuck-ins" or "pleats" which form the haustral markings.

To summarize, these haustrations are largest in the cecum and ascending colon, most regularly formed in the transverse colon and gradually disappear as sigmoid is reached. These sacculations or haustral markings, according to Sabotta-McMurrich,[6] disappear when the longitudinal bands or taenia coli are removed.

MOBILITY AND FLEXIBILITY

These fundamental procedures are essentially the same as already described for fluoroscopy of the stomach. Within the colon, the mucous membrane pattern cannot receive the same "fluoroscopic" attention as it did within the gastric contours.

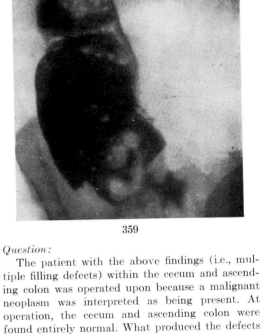

359

Question:

The patient with the above findings (i.e., multiple filling defects) within the cecum and ascending colon was operated upon because a malignant neoplasm was interpreted as being present. At operation, the cecum and ascending colon were found entirely normal. What produced the defects simulating malignancy?

Answer:

The patient was improperly prepared. Defects are produced by fecal residue. (See pp. 281, 282.)

Nevertheless, determining the mobility and flexibility of the various accessible coils is of extreme importance in helping to determine the presence of a lesion.

MUCOUS MEMBRANE PATTERN

The various indentures or haustral markings as found are not the mucous membrane pattern but are formed by all layers of the wall. However, after the expulsion of the barium enema, when the caliber of the lumen is so reduced that the inner walls are practically in contact, many mucous membrane folds form on the inner surface. These can be seen and are not present when the intestine is distended. These mucosal folds run irregularly and transversely. In the distal part of the colon they tend to run parallel with the long axis.

The pattern of the mucous membrane within the large bowel has been worked out. Fluoroscopically, however, it has not found great use. This is so chiefly because its pattern is best seen not when the bowel is distended with barium but after the opaque material has been evacuated. Some of the barium remains behind and coats the bowel wall. In the study of the formation of the various mucosal folds on the bowel wall, the detail and clarity of the radiographic film has proved superior to the fluoroscopic screen.

MOTILITY

The normal motility of opaque material given by mouth, or any food given by mouth, is variable. Barium given by mouth normally appears in the cecum from one to five hours later and may be seen in the rectum as long as seventy-two to ninety-six hours afterward. The bowel habitus of the individual should be inquired into before attempting to make any deductions. It is difficult to make any definite statements as regards the normal transit time within the colon.

The slower rhythmic waves within the colon are not detectable fluoroscopically and are seen only on serial roentgenograms. The rush peristalsis or mass peristalsis[7] described for the large bowel is also not important fluoroscopically. In this type of movement a 10 to 20 cm. segment of a colonic mass moves an average distance of 20 cm. at a time. Anti-peristalsis within the colon has also been described.[8, 9, 10]

It would not be amiss to discuss in a little more detail the waves that might be seen on the fluoroscopic screen.

Four types of wave have been described in the colon.[46] Types 1 and 3 are not de-

tectable fluoroscopically and thus will not be discussed. Type 2 and type 4 waves may be seen. Type 2 waves of the colon are seen as localized segmental contractions lasting 12–60 seconds. These are sometimes limited to individual haustra. Some observers believe that these waves may be coordinated to cause movement of colonic contents from one segment into the next distal segment.[65] Their main function is believed to be a churning and mixing movement which aids in the dehydration of the bowel contents.[66]

Type 4 peristaltic waves are strong, and usually arise just distal to the ileocecal valves or at the hepatic flexure. From these points, type 4 waves progress for varying distances. They usually stop in the vicinity of the splenic flexure or proximal descending colon. Type 4 peristaltic waves may sometimes continue along the entire length of the descending colon.[65] They are also known as mass peristalsis.

Although it has been said that little or no peristalsis occurs in the cecum, and that the cecum empties by overflowing, peristalsis is observed here and may continue distally along the colon.[67]

Anti-peristalsis within the colon has also been described.[68]

It has been found that mass peristalsis (or type 4 contraction) is almost always recognizable as an urge to move one's bowels.[46] In the administering of a barium enema, the pain which occurs when the region of the splenic flexure is reached or in the presence of the distention of the colon may be a manifestation of mass peristalsis. There are some individuals whose colon responds with marked increase in type 4 peristaltic waves. Since this is one of the earlier signs of ulcerative colitis,[68] this disease entity must be suspected in the presence of increased mass peristalsis. The mass peristalsis in these diseases decreases later, when the walls of the colon have become rigid.

Fluoroscopic examination of the large

bowel by barium enema does not usually concern itself with the emptying time. Perhaps the real value of examining the colon after administering barium from above, would be to know not when the bowel should be empty, but where the opaque material administered from above is held up. For example, if after twenty-four hours barium is seen in the mid-descending colon, the examiner should inquire as to why it is held up there and keep this in mind when performing a barium enema (fig. 375, p. 294). When, during the procedure, the opaque mixture reaches the blockaded region, the area can be given special attention by various palpatory manipulations and examined in various degrees of obliquity.

It should be stressed that when an obstructive lesion in the colon is suspected, a barium enema should be performed first, and if found normal, barium may next be given from above.

Fluoroscopic Methods of Examining the Colon

The *ingested meal* is not generally used since it does not fill the entire colon. By the time the opaque material taken by mouth reaches the large bowel, it is unequally distributed and does not fill the entire bowel satisfactorily.

BARIUM ENEMA

This is the usual method of examination of the colon and will be gone into in detail.[11, 12]

Position. Usually supine since it allows for manual palpation of the abdomen. The patient is also rotated into various angles so that all portions of the bowel are brought into view on the fluoroscopic screen.

Apparatus Necessary:
(1) An enema can capable of holding at least two quarts of mixture.*
(2) Stand to support it.
(3) Large bore rubber tubing which is

* Since it has been shown that feces and mucus from the rectum may pass into the tube and sometimes travel all the way back into the enema can, these alternate procedures are recommended[43]:
1. All equipment should be placed in an autoclave for each enema. This process is expensive and time-consuming and requires a sterilizer of sufficient size to accommodate an enema can.
2. A valve can be put in the tube or enema tip to prevent reflux. The valve must be sterilizable or of a cost to warrant disposal.
3. The most practical solution is an inexpensive, disposable enema container tube and tip.

interrupted by a glass connecting tube, the latter being used to observe the flow of barium.
(4) A stop-cock to control the flow.
(5) Rectal tube.
(6) Barium mixture. The usual barium mixture used for barium enema consists of barium sulfate suspended in water. The usual mix is approximately equal parts of barium mixture and water, two quarts of solution being used. The solution must be warm or brought up to body temperature. Two heaping teaspoons of tannic acid may be added to help the barium adhere to the bowel wall so that on the subsequent evacuation film the mucosal pattern will be more clearly delineated. The tannic acid is also helpful in securing good evacuation.[43] The mixture should be prepared in an electric mixer and should be free of lumps and have the consistency of heavy cream. Mixing should consume from ten to twenty minutes. No matter what mixture is used it is often wise to strain it into the enema can so as to remove all lumps which might prevent its ready flow through the tube.

Good results have been reported with administering Barotrast, Umbaryt, and liquid Micropaque.[43]

Preparation of Patient. The first step in preparation of the patient is adequate proctoscopic examination at least one day prior to barium enema administration.

For barium enema examination it is important to rid the large bowel of all fecal material. When present, feces may not only produce translucent areas simulating defects such as produced by tumors or polyps, but in addition the fecal material may actually cause an impediment to the progress of the barium as it flows into the bowel. The observer may become suspicious of an organic lesion when none actually exists (fig. 359).

The following is a good routine to adopt in order to have the patient properly cleansed:

A clear liquid diet is given for 36 hours prior to the examination. It begins with supper two nights before the examination. During this time, the patient should abstain from fats and dairy products. Toast, jelly, clear broth, tea are permitted.

Supper is forbidden the night before the examination. An increase in cecal residue has been observed when this meal is allowed. A light liquid breakfast, however, is permitted the morning of examination since this stimulates the gastro-colic reflex and thus helps evacuate and cleanse the colon. At about 7:00 P.M. the night prior to examination, a cathartic, usually one ounce of castor oil, is administered. This is to be followed by cleansing enemas the morning of the examination. The cleansing enemas should be administered with plain water. The patient should take these enemas at approximately half hourly intervals until the back flow is clean, that is, when no fecal material is returned.

Other types of enema commonly used are normal saline, as well as soapsuds enemas. Neither is recommended here. Normal saline has been found to interfere with the adherence of barium particles to the mucosa and thus be unsatisfactory for the subsequent evacuation and air contrast study.[13] Soapsuds enemas have been found to be too irritating.

If castor oil is contraindicated, the next best cathartic is Phenolphthalein (one to six grains). Dulcolax[44] or X-Prep[45] can also be used. Compound licorice powder is also effective. Saline cathartics such as epsom salts are not good because their hydragogue characteristics make them likely to retain too much fluid within the bowel. Adherence of barium to the bowel wall is then almost impossible. *It should be remembered that no cathartic or cleansing enema is to be given to a patient with ulcerative colitis or acute appendicitis.* If a cleansing enema must be given to a patient with ulcerative colitis, it should be administered under control, i.e., a physician being at hand and the procedure done with gentleness and care.

The patient should also be instructed as to how to take an enema. Fluid should be permitted to flow into the rectum and if cramping sensations are felt it is permissible for the tube to be pinched off for a moment until the cramp disappears. The fluid from the enema can should be allowed to flow until the patient feels it on the right side of the abdomen. Then the patient should lie on the right side for a moment before expelling the fluid. The last maneuver not only permits gas in the cecum and ascending colon to rise into the transverse colon so that it can be expelled but also assists in properly cleansing the right side consisting of ascending colon and cecum. The patient should be instructed that the enema be repeated until no solid matter is expelled.

Advice to Patient Prior to Actual Administration of Barium Enema. The patient should be warned to expect cramps and told to make every effort to retain the enema.

The patient should be told to advise the examiner of any undue pain. The most marked discomfort of the patient may occur as the barium reaches the middescending colon or above. Although this discomfort may occur when the colon is not distended, it is more frequently found with distention. It is also found in an enema when the time of administration is unduly prolonged. It is advised at this point that the tube be kept open and the enema container be lowered.[46] The patient will evacuate the bowel content into the container, thus relieving his discomfort. An advantage of this procedure is that the colon is allowed to empty itself of fecal material as well as any other interfering artefacts, i.e., castor oil. These substances will float in the barium containing mixture and will remain in the enema container while the colon is being refilled later on.

If the enema can is not used to siphon off the contrast media, an attempt should then be made to relieve this either by stopping the enema temporarily, rolling the patient from side to side, and occasionally merely asking the patient to take deep breaths. Words of encouragement on the part of the examiner are helpful.

The patient should be advised to give the examiner warning of feelings of back-leakage of barium past the tube.

Purpose of Maneuvers during Barium Enema. It is of course clearly understood that the main purpose is to discover any existing pathology by fluoroscopic examination during the administration of the barium enema. Yet, as the fluoroscopist is running the barium into the colon, he will perform various purposeful maneuvers (figs. 376–380, pp. 296–297).

First, he runs in only enough mixture to fill out each portion of bowel separately. He interrupts the flow when the rectum becomes filled, next when the entire sigmoid is filled, etc. If any irregularity or distortion is noted, films should be made before continuing the examination. He is aware that should he permit the entire bowel to fill at once, he will encounter great difficulty in separating and orienting one loop of bowel from another. He is also aware of the greater ease in examining one portion at a time. It is for this reason that he will also interrupt the flow when a loop

not commonly present is encountered—in other words, this additional loop is treated as if it were another portion of the bowel.

Next he is ever watchful for changes of *contour.* If an undue ballooning-out of any segment is seen he may suspect the flow of barium is encountering an obstruction with a damming back of opaque material and resulting distention. Or, if an area of narrowing is seen, he will observe its constancy and make every effort to prove its softness and lack of rigidity by distending it with opaque mixture. Should the area of narrowing not distend it may be taken as a clue to some constricting abnormality (figs. 360, 361). This technic of distending narrowed loops will be described below. If indeed a true obstruction is present, he will observe the junction between normal and abnormal and try to appraise whether it is abrupt as in carcinoma or changes gradually from the normal as in an inflammatory lesion (figs. 381 and 382, p. 298).

In observing the colonic contours he looks, too, for changes in profile suggesting diverticulosis or a serrated edge suggesting an inflammatory lesion, such as ulcerative colitis.

The *position* of the colonic loops is noted. Undue displacement or change of position is also noted (figs. 357, 358, pp. 277–278).

The rapidity with which the barium enters the colon is also noted—the observer being mindful of the rapid entry in colonic irritability and the general spasm associated with this condition.

Throughout this procedure the searching protected palpating hand is ever at work, separating one loop of bowel from another, finding sensitive or painful areas, and determining the mobility and flexibility of the various cells. Also, when a holdup occurs, the examiner will with gentle palpation try to overcome it, being always mindful that if the holdup is due to an organic lesion, it may be wiser not to allow too much of the barium beyond the lesion, since a great part may be retained.

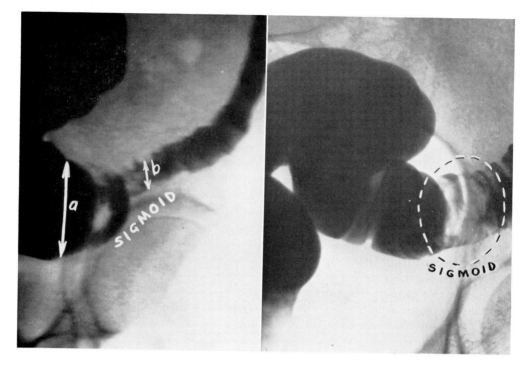

360

361

During fluoroscopy a sudden narrowing of caliber (compare arrow a with arrow b) should suggest that trouble may be present at the site of narrowing. (See fig. 361).

The barium in figure 360 has overcome the cause of the narrowing, which may have been a local spasm or sphincter causing temporary partial obstruction. (See sphincters, figure 367, page 288.

Actual Procedure. The patient is placed in a supine position on the fluoroscopic table. To make sure that the barium flow is free, the examiner will first run a small amount of barium out through the rectal tube. In order to avoid introducing gas via the enema, hold the tip horizontally or directed downwards during this flushing. If the tip is held upright, as the barium rises out of it, it may be replaced by air, and this then introduced into the rectum.[43] He then inserts the tube into the rectum for several inches. The enema can is suspended about two to three feet above the table top. Although special devices to hold the tube in place have been suggested, no special apparatus is really necessary. An intact anal sphincter is sufficient. In instances where

the tube is not retained firmly in position, the patient can be instructed to hold the tube in place himself with only minor inconvenience, or it may be held in position with adhesive tape. With infants and children, an assistant whose hand is protected by a lead glove should hold the tube in position.

The apparatus being checked and found in order, the pinch cock being ready, the examiner first makes a brief fluoroscopic survey of the entire abdomen, looking for opaque calculi or any undue gas distention. The chest, both diaphragmatic cusps, heart, and mediastinum are then quickly scanned.

Then, with the diaphragmatic shutters narrowed so that the examiner works with a small aperture, the mixture is permitted to flow slowly and its progress watched as it fills the colon. It is advisable to observe closely the head of the advancing column of opaque mixture. A splitting or division of the stream will suggest a polypoid lesion. When the rectum fills out the enema is stopped. A temporary delay is usually encountered at the recto-sigmoid juncture. This is normal and should not cause concern. The contours of the rectum are observed and the two portions above and below the valves of Houston delineated (fig. 355). The patient is rotated in various degrees of obliquity so that all of the rectal walls are observed in profile. (The examiner should do a rectal digital examination before discharging him.)

The pinch cock is then again opened and the barium permitted to flow into the sigmoid. When the entire sigmoid is filled out the flow is again interrupted. The patient is now turned into the right anterior oblique position (patient facing the examiner and the right shoulder brought forward). This is usually sufficient to "lay out" the entire sigmoid loop. On occasion when the sigmoid loop takes an unusual turn, the left anterior oblique is useful. It would be wise to turn every patient in both obliques. If spot film apparatus is available, when the sigmoid loop is laid out best, a spot roentgenogram should be taken.

The fluid is then permitted to travel upwards in the descending colon until the entire splenic flexure is filled out: The patient is again examined in various angles of obliquity so that the loops of bowel are not superimposed one on each other. Only by studying them in true profile without one segment overlapping the other can an adequate examination be performed (compare fig. 376 with fig. 377; see also figs. 378–380, pp. 296–297).

The pinch cock is again opened, the transverse colon and the hepatic flexure are next filled and studied with manual palpation and rotation in a similar manner to the previous portions of the bowel.

Finally, the ascending colon and cecum filled out, they, too, are palpated and determined as normal. The *terminal ileum* or *appendix*, when seen, can be used as an index to *cecal location* and *filling*.

Errors in diagnosing cecal disease can be minimized by being certain that the cecum is filled and by securing good mucosal spot film studied by compressing the cecum during the filled phase (figs. 362–366). It is not amiss at this point to stress that the cecum should also be compressed, and the mucosa studied after evacuation.

All accessible portions of the colon must be palpated and their mobility, flexibility and pliability demonstrated. Inaccessible portions of the bowel, such as the splenic and hepatic flexures when situated high up under the ribs, will often be reached by the palpating hand when the patient is asked to take a deep breath. Portions of bowel within the true pelvis which can not be palpated through the abdominal wall may often be palpated and manipulated per vaginum. The elicitation of tenderness or pain or the palpation of abdominal masses are important observations and their relationship to the mobility and flexibility of the adjacent bowel segments should be determined.

Helpful Hints:

1. A frequent finding during a barium enema examination is a *transient* segment of narrowing, commonly attributed to spasm, causing some delay to the flow. This transient segmental narrowing may not be spasm but may be the site of a colonic sphincter.[59-62] Usually these transient narrowings attributable to sphincters distend completely (often on repeat examinations), but occasionally they persist, in which event the knowledge of their presence and their relative smoothness are important points in differentiating them from organic colon dis-

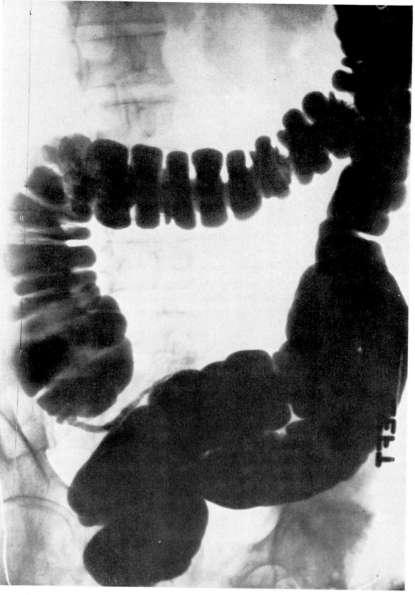

362

The cecum as seen on the full opaque study appears normal. (Cf. figs. 363–366.)

ease (fig. 367). Other functional causes of delay to the inflow of barium may be produced by a fold or turning of the bowel or by a localized spasm (type 2 peristalsis). Efforts to overcome this delay may be made by rotating the patient into different positions, thus eliminating the fold or turning of the bowel. By continuing the pres-

sure of the enema, the spasm may be overcome. Atrophine sulfate can be administered intramuscularly where the spasm is persistent. This type of delay is not unusual in the sigmoid flexure in the presence of diverticulitis.[46]

2. When the colon is being filled, if obstruction is present, no additional pressure

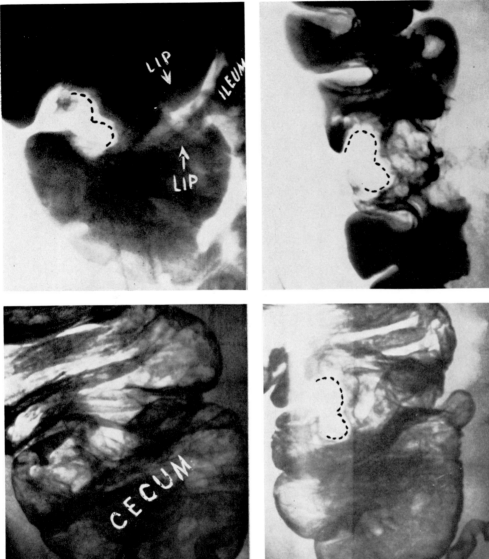

363

364

365

366

363

The same cecum as in figure 362, *compressed* behind the fluoroscopic screen, is laid out better and reveals a defect (dotted line).

365

Cecum distended with air appears normal.

364

The same cecum *compressed* during the evacuation study and spot filmed reveals the same defect as in figure 363.

366

Air-distended cecum *compressed* so that it is laid out better reveals the defect seen in figures 363 and 364.

Comment: In this patient, the air and barium filled cecum *without compression* appeared entirely normal. The compression study by better "laying out" the cecum revealed a defect. This proved to be neoplasm. This demonstrates the necessity for routine cecal compression.

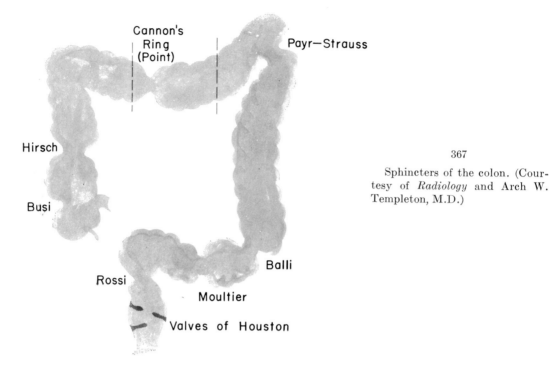

Cannon's
Ring
(Point)

Payr—Strauss

Hirsch

Busi

Rossi

Balli

Moultier

Valves of Houston

367

Sphincters of the colon. (Courtesy of *Radiology* and Arch W. Templeton, M.D.)

by means of elevating the enema can or manual palpation should be used. If any undue narrowing is encountered, there are various methods useful to prove that this constricted segment is abnormal. The examiner must determine whether it is *persistently* narrowed (thus pathological), or whether it possesses the ability to dilate (thus normal) (figs. 360–361). To ascertain whether the segment can dilate, the following maneuvers are used:

(a) Permit an additional inflow of barium. The additional barium may dilate the segment.

(b) *Gentle* palpation is necessary in an attempt to massage additional barium into the narrowed area with intent to dilate it.

(c) To take advantage of gravity, the patient can be so positioned that the narrowed loop is lower than the barium-filled loops above. This may cause barium to gravitate into and open such a segment of bowel.

3. In administering a barium enema a reflex of barium into the terminal ileum

may obscure the sigmoid flexure. When this occurs, it would be of advantage to empty the ileum when desired so as not to obscure the underlying portion of large bowel, especially if this latter is to be studied after evacuation. A physiologic method is to give the patient approximately 20–24 ounces of water as quickly as possible after the enema and repeat this in about 15 minutes. The evacuation studies should then be performed about 30 minutes later. The ingested water will stimulate the gastro-ilial reflex and empty the terminal ileum into the colon.[46]

4. The principle of interrupting the barium flow and going back to visualize different portions of the colon already opacified, is a useful maneuver.[47] First, it helps prevent overdistention. An overdistended bowel may obliterate small polyps and other lesions. Especially at a flexure or a localized turn in the bowel, the distended adjacent segments of the loop, in abutting one against the other, may obliterate a lesion (figs. 368, 369). In interrupting the

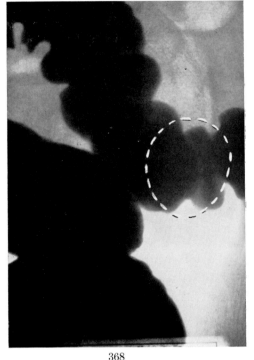

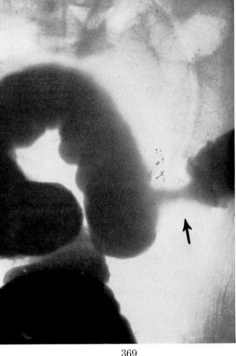

368

The sigmoid loop of the colon is well-filled and dilated with opaque material. Encircled region appears entirely normal.

369

The same patient in the *same position* reveals a lesion (arrow).

Question:

Why was it not seen in figure 368?

Answer:

A loop of intestine when *overfilled* will dilate and *overlap*, and thus may hide a lesion.

flow, the examiner secures an added advantage in that he need not divide his attention between the progress made at the head of the advancing column and the structures opacified behind. He is thus permitted more time and may exert greater care in studying and separating out as well as laying out the already opacified loops. The opacified segments thus positioned so that they are seen to the best advantage can be subjected to various degrees of pressure and spot filmed. Often this is the most important part of the entire enema.

During the periods of stoppage, the patient should be rotated in an effort not only to delineate the opacified segments more clearly, but to help the barium flow into further segments with minimal distention. As the segments become opacified, and when the examiner believes filling is adequate and not overdistended, spot films should be made. It is advised that no exposures should be made while the barium is flowing.[47] A polyp moving in the barium stream may escape detection.

5. When specific information regarding the rectum is sought, it is often better to examine the patient in the prone rather than the supine position since this may bring the sigmoid out of the pelvis.[1] To bring the cecum out of the pelvis, Gage[14] advises the patient to come for examination with the urinary bladder fully distended.

6. When inability to retain the enema is

encountered, the following should be considered:

(a) The flow of barium may be temporarily stopped. The patient should have the sympathy and encouragement of the examiner. A great deal of difficulty is often due to apprehension on the part of the patient and this can be avoided by gaining the confidence of the patient.

(b) Rotating the patient from side to side or asking him to turn over is often useful.

(c) The fluoroscopic procedure should be done quickly and efficiently. The average time for this procedure should be no longer than two minutes. Too much delay may not only be difficult for the patient but will also hinder in the production of good double contrast roentgenograms, if such are desired.

(d) If the patient is unable to retain the enema, a sponge rubber ball may be slipped over the edge of the enema tip and an assistant wearing a leaded glove inserts the tip into the rectum and presses the ball against the perineum. This maneuver has been described by Stevenson et al.[13] The pressure caused by the rubber ball elevates the levator ani muscles and prevents loss of fluid. This maneuver has also been found useful in patients with rectal tears.

(e) The Barden catheter has also been found useful. In the use of this as a barrier, the fluoroscopist must be extremely careful to avoid over-distention of the colon.

7. The examiner may on occasion experience difficulty in knowing exactly when the barium enema is completed as signified by a complete filling of the cecum. This can be determined when any one of the following is seen with assurance:

(a) Observing the round, pouch-like termination of the cecum being freely mobile, with the appendix hanging from it. Gentle massage of this area downward in the cecum should encourage complete filling in cases where undue spasm is encountered.

(b) Seeing the terminal ileum fill with barium signifies complete filling of the colon.

Employing these maneuvers the examiner may still lack assurance as to adequate cecal filling. When such is the case it is advised that the cecum be studied approximately five hours after the ingestion of barium mixture from above.

8. If the barium does not flow after the tube is inserted, the fluoroscopist should move the nozzle about since it may be pressing up against a fold of mucous membrane. If the flow is still not free an air lock may be present within the tube. By pinching the tube beneath the enema can with one hand and milking the mid-portion of the tube with the other hand, the air lock can be released. Finally, an improperly prepared barium mixture containing clumps may occlude the flow.

9. Every barium enema should be preceded by adequate proctoscopic and digital examination. Lesions in the rectum are often missed when barium enema alone is employed.

10. It has been recommended that the barium enema be administered cold, i.e., 41 degrees F. The advantages claimed are that the colder suspension will have a mild anesthetic affect, and with less hyperemia of the colon thus present, the colon would be less irritable. Further, the tonic contraction of the anal sphincter may be stimulated and hence contribute to the ease of retention.[49] Also, it is claimed that more gases are soluble with a cold than with a warm suspension and, therefore, there would be less tendency to bubble formation.

11. The Chassard-Lapine sitting position should be used whenever needed to "uncoil" superimposed segments.

12. These are some of the dangers in performing a barium enema: (a) A hazard reported is perforation of the colon. The improper use of enema tips[50] and balloons[51] is suggested as the underlying cause for such perforation. The injury is usually observed on the anterior wall of the rectum and is

more apt to occur in the presence of disease. A hard enema tip or proctoscope should be used with great care.

(b) It has been suggested that when large amounts of air are necessary to inflate the balloon to prevent evacuation of the enema, the rectum and recto-sigmoid should be fluoroscoped first with a deflated balloon in place, and examined for disease. In the absence of rectal disease, the balloon is next inflated up to 100 to 150 cc. of air. Next, 50 cc. increments are instilled until a point is reached at which the balloon (as observed fluoroscopically) prevents the passage of barium around it.[52, 53] The pressure applied by this method will be well within the range of safety. It is further recommended that with rectal pathology, the pressure in the balloon should be measured, and should never exceed 50 mm. of mercury.

(c) Patients with coronary artery disease or other disorders of the heart must be treated cautiously in performing air contrast examinations. It may be wise to forego air contrast on such patients. If the patient is aged, infirm or very uncomfortable after the air contrast examination, a tube may be placed into the rectum to remove the air into a water filled pail.

(d) Rupture of the bowel may occasionally result from too rapid air installation.[54] The technician should therefore introduce the air slowly, and discontinue the injection if the patient voices more than the usual complaint.

(e) Water intoxication during barium enema has been described as another cause of death.[55, 56] In order to avoid water intoxication where this danger exists especially where multiple enemas have to be given, also in suspected Hirschprung's Disease, normal saline should be used in place of tap water in preparing the barium suspension to be instilled.

(f) Death has followed the absorption of tannic acid from the intact bowel.[52] These cases were reported in children and came 8 days after the administration of the enema.

EVACUATION AND DOUBLE CONTRAST STUDY

Evacuation Study. The evacuation study is probably the most important part of a barium enema, and this, in the main, is a roentgenographic and not a fluoroscopic procedure. There are some examiners who recommend fluoroscopic palpation and observation at this time (figs. 370–375).

Double Contrast Enema. Additional material needed: (1) Air insufflator attachment to the rectal tip. (2) A ✳ 140 Barden Virden catheter.

The double contrast enema is useful in the roentgen examination of the large bowel. It should not be performed routinely. It is recommended in the main to demonstrate polyps, carcinomas and occasionally tuberculosis of the colon. It is also useful to uncover overlapping segments of the colon, especially in the sigmoid area.

In the performance of double contrast studies it is the purpose of the examiner to take advantage of the barium residue which coats the bowel wall. He neither wants the evacuation of the barium to be such as to remove all the residue nor to leave too much residue behind. Careful observation of the evacuation film must be made; air is not introduced until "just enough" barium has been left behind. If necessary it is advisable to overevacuate the barium rather than leave large residues. The examiner may attempt to siphon off excess barium by inserting the enema tube and lowering the enema can.[47] If overevacuation has taken place, the colon is then refilled with the barium mixture but the flow is stopped when the head of the opaque column reaches the splenic flexure. The patient is then quickly taken to the toilet and instructed to evacuate only enough to become comfortable. No more than one minute should be permitted for this. As soon as

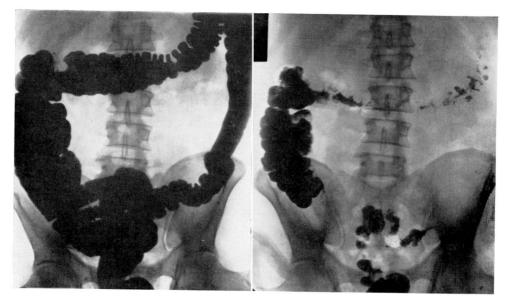

370

The colon studied by retrograde enema appears normal.

371

Evacuation study of figure 370. Barium appears to be held up at the hepatic flexure, i.e., the ascending colon and cecum do not empty well.

Question:

What are some of the factors to be sought for in an evacuation study?

Answer:

(1) The mucosal pattern: The mucosal pattern of the colon is often better seen during evacuation study. In this case, the study is not contributory.

(2) Defects: Defects present during the filled stage are re-evaluated. Defects not seen during the filled stage may sometimes appear in the evacuation study.

(3) Is there any suggestive obstruction to the outflow? I.e., is there a point behind which the barium appears to be held up and not evacuated?

In this evacuation study (fig. 371) the hepatic flexure appears to be a region which holds back the outflow of barium. The ascending colon and cecum do not appear to empty well. This is an apparent holdup point which may normally exist on an evacuation study and with no lesion present. This holdup point need not indicate a lesion, but is one of the signs noted during an evacuation study which should be suspect until proved normal. (See fig. 372.)

the patient returns to the fluoroscopic room, the insufflator is used to inflate the colon. The air is introduced under fluoroscopic control and its distribution is assisted by palpation and rotation of the patient.

One of the main causes of discomfort in air contrast examination is the rapid over-distention of the colon with air. The logical way to avoid this is by introducing the proper amount of air slowly. It has been shown recently that the use of carbon dioxide instead of air has resulted in absence of discomfort.[48]

Stereoscopic or single films can then be taken. This method has been described and found to give excellent results by Stevenson et al.[13]

Rules for Double Contrast Examination: A double contrast examination requires careful attention and the following details must be adhered to:

1. The colon must be thoroughly cleansed.

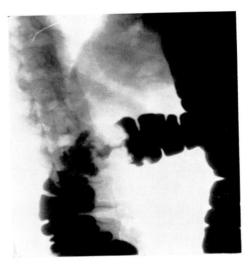

372

Same patient as in figures 370 and 371. The patient was refilled, and the hepatic flexure, subjected to further study, revealed in the deep oblique position a constricting carcinoma, which explains the "holding up" seen in figure 371.

Question:

Can such a holdup as shown in figure 371 always be relied upon to confirm the presence of a constricting lesion?

Answer:

No. See figures 373-374.

Comment: Although a constricting lesion is present at A (fig. 373), yet if such a lesion retains sufficient patency the barium may easily evacuate through the lesion. It is therefore obvious that a single sign can rarely be relied upon for a diagnosis. (Compare figs. 370-372.)

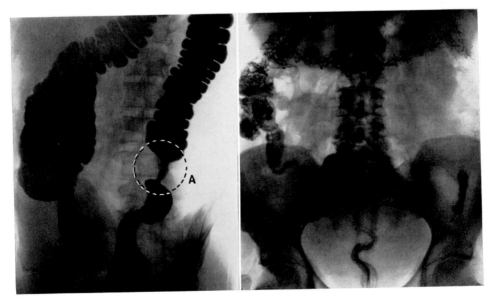

373

Retrograde enema reveals a constricting lesion at A (confirmed at surgery as carcinoma). See fig. 374.

374

An evacuation study of figure 373. Note there is *no* holdup of barium proximal to the lesion.

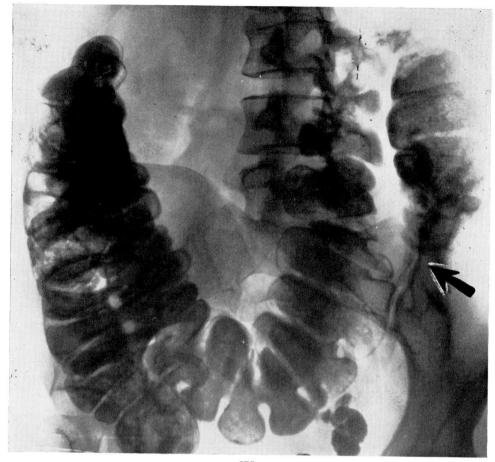

375

Question:

This is the 24-hour study of a barium meal taken during a gastrointestinal series. What are some of the factors to be sought in such a study?

Answer:

(1) The examiner should search for any lesion which may appear in the colon. It must be borne in mind that the barium given by mouth has been thinned out and that the colon is thus not well visualized. (For the colon, a retrograde enema is the study of choice.)

(2) The observer should further note any evidence of a holdup point, i.e., a point *beyond* which the barium appears not to pass readily, and *behind* which the barium appears to be held up.

Comment: In this study, note that the opaque column appears to be held up (arrow) in the descending colon. This site must be held suspect and properly studied. Subsequent retrograde enema revealed a constricting carcinoma.

2. The advice regarding the re-introduction of barium to the region of the splenic flexure must be followed with the purpose of having an even distribution of residue throughout the entire colon. To this end it may be necessary to run a small amount of barium in just below the splenic flexure and next introduce air as instructed above. Palpation and rotation of the patient will then assist materially in distributing the barium and air.

If too much barium has been retained and

the above procedures have been unsuccessful, the barium air contrast study should be delayed until the following day. The castor oil and the enema preparations are repeated and the patient is returned the following morning. The same technic of running barium to the splenic flexure is then performed.

3. Too much time must not be consumed between the administration of the barium enema and the subsequent taking of films.

4. Fictitious polyps may appear in contrast study and the nature of these has been investigated.[15] Mineral oil, castor oil and undigested animal fat can all cause these shadows. Vaseline from the enema tips may leave a residue in the rectum which can be carried up into the colon during the double contrast procedure, thus causing a fictitious polyp. Fictitious polyps can easily be formed by air insufflation through fluid barium suspension. Rapid introduction of air tends to less fictitious polyp formation.

Fictitious versus True Polyps.[15] Fictitious polyps are most common in the left half of the colon and tend to be near the center of the bowel. They normally change in size, shape or position when the patient is filmed in the prone and supine positions. Fictitious polyps normally have a very radiolucent center, while a neoplastic polyp will have a center of increased density. The only positive identification of a polyp is that on following examinations it maintains its position and contour. A slight positional change is likely only in the case of a pedunculated polyp.

Fluoroscopic Examination of the Pathological Colon

No definitive diagnosis can be made on a fluoroscopic screen. Perhaps the chief reasons for fluoroscopic examination of the colon are to determine the best position for the subsequent film examination and to know when the colon is filled. By preliminary visualization of the coils of large bowel on the fluoroscopic screen, the examiner is enabled to mark out in the darkened room on the patient's skin the exact location in which a suspicious lesion may be seen (figs. 376, 377). Then, turning on the light, the angle of obliquity the body of the patient makes with the *screen* is noted. The same factors are then used in making the radiographic film. All of this is facilitated when a spot filming device is available. The examining physician should rotate the patient so that each flexure or bend in the bowel is laid out in optimal fashion and immediately spot filmed. Certain portions of the colon, such as the cecum, should be compressed so that the various folds are not approximated, thereby possibly covering an underlying lesion (figs. 362–366).

Some other advantages the examiner can secure from the fluoroscopic examination which roentgenograms alone do not permit:

1. Palpation and separation of loops of bowel that overlie each other.

Vaginal examination while the colon is filled with barium is useful in separating masses in the pelvis from loops of bowel which produce compression and distention comparable to intraluminal defects. This maneuver is useful in helping to differentiate extreme pressure deformity from an intraluminal defect.[15a]

2. Determination of the mobility of various segments of the bowel, as well as their flexibility and pliability.

3. Discernment of any tender points and their relationship to any palpable masses or regions of suspected disease.

4. Observation of the barium flow so that the region presenting any suspicious holdup will be given greater attention in the subsequent radiographic film examination (figs. 360, 361).

5. Positioning of the patient to secure optimum visibility of certain regions or invaded segments of bowel.

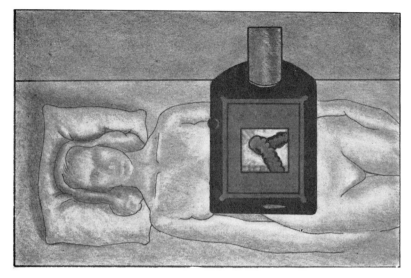

376

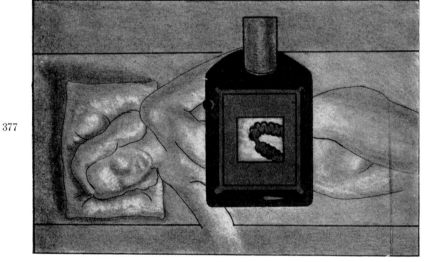

377

376

Question:

    1. Is the splenic flexure examined properly?
    2. Is the splenic flexure normal?

377

Answer:

    1. Because one loop of the flexure overlies the other, the examiner (in fig. 376) could not possibly see any existing pathology between the loops.

    2. With the patient properly rotated, the examiner looks in *between* the ascending and descending parts of the flexure and sees a neoplasm (region of narrowing).

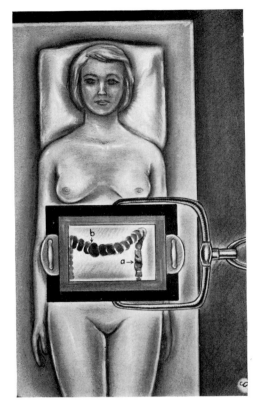

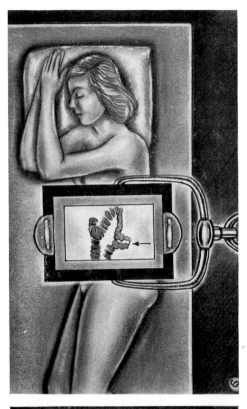

378

Is the colon normal at *a* and *b*?

379

A U-shaped loop might be located at *a*, and unless patient were rotated or the U-shaped loop separated manually, an underlying lesion would be missed.

380

A U-shaped loop may be located at *b*. Correct palpation and manipulation would separate the loops and permit visualization of the underlying lesion.

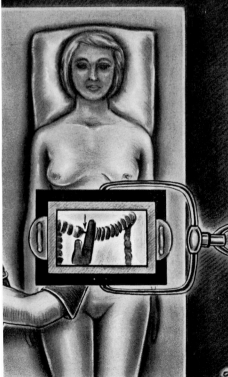

Execution of some of the following maneuvers in an attempt to distend suspiciously narrowed coils. (This is something no film examination can perform.)

(a) Placing the patient in such a position that the narrowed segment is at a lower level, thus permitting the barium to gravitate into it and dilate it.

(b) Continuing the flow of barium in the hope that the additional opaque mixture will distend the narrowed area.

(c) Massaging—*very gently*—some of the opaque mixture into the narrowed segment and so distending it.

The more important pathological deviations found in the large bowel and the manner in which the fluoroscopic screen may help in their identification will next be considered. The discussion will be directed into channels inquiring as to "contour," changes in barium flow and position. The grouping of the various illnesses will depend upon which of these—contour, alterations in flow, or position—is the predominant factor.

CHANGE IN CONTOUR

NARROWING

Narrowing of a section of bowel can occur in both malignancies and benign granulomas. The fluoroscopist, aware of the differential features distinguishing one from the other, can search for these on the fluoroscopic screen and find the best position in which they are demonstrated. He then

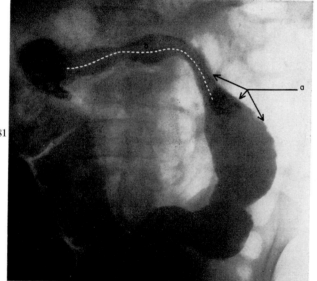

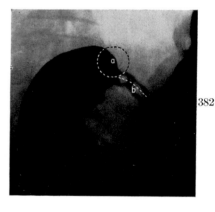

Question:

Regions of undue narrowing (b) are seen in both pictures. Which of the two is produced by a malignant neoplasm?

Answer:

381

1. "Change from normal to abnormal (a) *gradual.*
2. Length of lesion (b) comparatively long.

A lesion with the above characteristics is a benign lesion.

382

1. Change from normal to abnormal (a) *abrupt.*
2. Length of lesion (b) comparatively short.

A lesion with the above characteristics is a malignant lesion.

takes "spot" films of the involved region or, if this is not possible, he will note the exact angle the patient forms with the screen, which angle is then duplicated when conventional roentgenograms are taken.

Important differential features he seeks are:

(1) The precise area showing a "change" from the normal to the abnormal; an abrupt change from the uninvaded bowel to the invaded bowel speaks for malignancy. If the invaded region blends imperceptibly with the normal bowel, this speaks for benignity (fig. 381 compared with fig. 382).

(2) The length of the invaded area is helpful in reaching a diagnosis. If the invasion covers a short span of bowel, i.e. one inch, this speaks for malignancy. If several inches are involved, the process should probably be considered as benign (fig. 381 compared with fig. 382).

(3) A study of the mucous membrane pattern is helpful. When destroyed, the process is probably malignant. When intact, it is probably benign.

Carcinoma of the Colon. As the flow of barium is observed travelling in a retrograde fashion upwards from the rectum, an area of narrowing as caused by a malignancy may first manifest itself as a holdup to the flow (figs. 383, 384). With further accumulation of the opaque material, the segment of bowel immediately distal to the lesion will become dilated, and with this dilatation the hydrostatic pressure increases. When the obstructive process is overcome by the steady accumulation of opaque material, barium will be seen to flow through it. At this stage the examiner must observe the edge between the normal and the abnormal. The position of the patient should be so arranged that the change from the normal to the abnormal is seen at its greatest advantage (fig. 383).

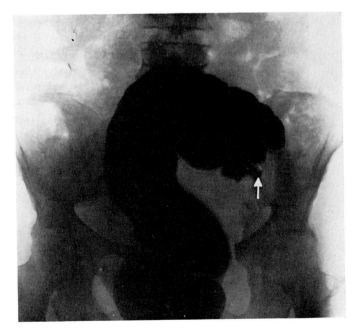

383

Barium permitted to flow into colon stopped at arrow. During fluoroscopy, the patient was so positioned as to demonstrate best the change from normal region of colon to abnormal region. Subsequent radiographs taken in this same position revealed the abrupt change from one to the other, thus enabling a diagnosis of cancer of the sigmoid to be made.

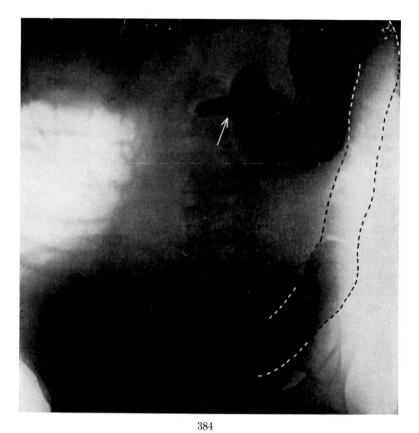

384

Question:

Before running barium into the colon the examiner was highly suspicious of an obstructive process. What aroused his suspicion?

Answer:

The undue gas distention of the bowel, as seen in the region of the cecum and ascending colon.

Comment: Observe *abrupt termination* of colon where barium flow was held up (arrow). This is indication of malignancy. (See figs. 381 and 382, p. 298.)

If possible, "spot films" should now be taken. If this is not possible the exact position of the patient should be noted, and as directed previously, roentgenograms should be taken in the same position.

With the further flow of barium, the exact *length* of the lesion should be determined and again the position of greatest advantage is utilized for filming.

The same process of observation is next made for the opposite end of the lesion, i.e., notation of whether the change from normal to abnormal is abrupt or gradual.

When the obstruction is marked, none of the barium will be seen passing through and into the segment of bowel containing the lesion. As previously directed, no undue pressure or force by either manipulative processes or by raising the height of the enema can should be employed. With careful observation and patience a thin stream of barium may be seen trickling into the invaded area. Filming of the observation when even only a trickle of barium enters is of great diagnostic help.

The fluoroscopist should be alert and watchful for fistulous tract formation. The actual area of communication may be traced fluoroscopically.

With the approach as outlined, a differ-

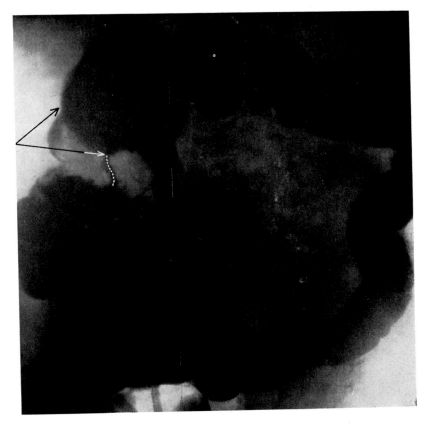

385

During the course of the barium enema the flow of barium was held up just beneath the hepatic flexure. The interruption was temporary and the entire colon soon filled out. Observe: (1) Abrupt change from normal to abnormal (between arrows). (2) Short extent of lesion (dotted line).

ential diagnosis of malignancy from other causes of narrowing will be facilitated. The ultimate conclusions are reached on the radiographic films. Some of the questions that must be answered before a final diagnosis is reached are:

a. Is the change from the normal to the abnormal abrupt? A positive answer speaks for malignancy (figs. 383, 384).

b. Is the area of involvement a short one? Again a positive answer speaks for malignancy (figs. 381, 382).

c. Do the radiographic films present evidence of mucosal destruction? A positive answer speaks for malignancy.

Inflammatory Granuloma. The invaded segment of bowel in granulomatous infil-

trations closely mimics the changes seen in carcinoma. Various *differential features* that should be searched for on the fluoroscopic screen and subsequently filmed are:

a. The change in contour from the normal to the abnormal must be noted. An inflammatory process of a benign nature involving the colon is more apt to fade imperceptibly into the uninvolved region.

b. The extent of the lesion is likely to be longer with an inflammatory lesion. Although the next two observations may often be evaluated on the fluoroscopic screen, detailed observation and confirmation require filming. Perhaps, as elsewhere, the fluoroscope serves only to determine the position which demonstrates the findings best.

c. Small sinus tracts and other diverticula in the region may serve to make the examiner suspicious of diverticulosis.

d. An intact mucosa is extremely helpful in determining the process as benign.

Miscellaneous Causes. Other abnormalities causing general as well as localized narrowing, including micro-colon, ulcerative colitis, strictures, should be approached fluoroscopically in the same manner as described above.

DILATATION

Abnormal collections of air within the bowel when visualized on the fluoroscopic screen (fig. 384) speak for dilatation of the involved segment. The fluoroscopist must be suspicious of some obstructing lesion immediately distal to the air-distended loops. When performing the barium enema and observing the retrograde ascent of the barium mixture, this must be kept in mind. Any lesion which either completely or partially obstructs the lumen of the bowel will tend to cause the proximal segments of the bowel to become dilated, i.e., carcinoma of the splenic flexure is apt to cause wide dilatation in the transverse, and ascending colon. A large collection of air localized to the cecum itself may be normal, but when *continuous* with air more distally, it should arouse suspicion of an obstructive process.

It should be pointed out that large collections of air within the large bowel are a prominent feature in the diagnosis of Hirschsprung's disease.

Another deformation of contour which is a protrusion from the bowel, such as a diverticulum, is also considered under dilatation.

Hirschsprung's Disease. Hirschsprung[16] first described this disease entity, and pointed out that although the dilatation is general throughout, the rectum itself is normal. In other cases the rectum also partakes in this process.

The fluoroscopist when specifically looking for Hirschsprung's disease may often content himself with observation of abnormal gas-distended loops, and confirm this finding on the roentgenogram. If a barium enema is next undertaken, the wide dilatation and elongation of the colon is seen. However, a functionally deficient segment of rectum or recto-sigmoid is sought.[57] This segment appears narrowed (figs. 386–387) and results from a congenital absence of ganglion cells from Auerbach's and Meissner's plexi. The process may often confine itself to the rectum or recto-sigmoid regions, but it can be more widespread. Immediately after the completion of the barium investigation, *it is important that evacuation by soap suds or water enema be undertaken.* This subsequent cleansing of the barium mixture is important because with the inability of the colon to evacuate its contents and the tendency of the barium to harden, serious consequences may ensue.[2]

The pattern, contour (absence of haustrations) and redundancy of colonic loops in normal infants may exactly simulate the colon of an infant with Hirschprung's disease. The examiner seeing the dilated colon should seek to find the *undilated normal* or *narrowed segment* diagnostic of Hirschsprung's Disease. *Another differential feature is the ability to evacuate the enema.* Normal infants have good contractions and good evacuation; infants with Hirschsprung's disease have deficient contractions and poor emptying power of the colon. Finally, the examiner will note that the child with Hirschsprung's Disease has a greater tolerance in receiving the barium than the normal infant.

Diverticulosis. Small grape-like herniations are often found in the large bowel (fig. 388). In the absence of any complicating inflammatory process they are relatively unimportant and the name applied to them is "diverticulosis." They may, on the other hand, "become the site of inflammatory disease"[17, 18, 19, 20] at which time

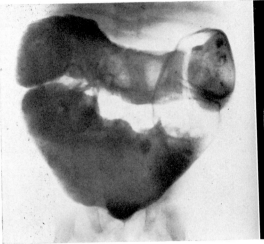

386   387

Question:

This is an *evacuation* study where Hirschprung's disease is sought. What clues are present
to suggest the diagnosis and how should it be
confirmed? (See fig. 387.)

Answer:

The poor evacuation in figure 386 is a clue suggesting Hirschprung's disease. It should be confirmed by suitable positioning and finding the
characteristically narrowed segment (arrow).

they are more properly termed diverticulitis. The bowel in the involved region becomes narrowed. Other differential features
between such a lesion and malignancy have
been discussed.

Occasionally, it may be difficult to determine the cause of a central grape-like
structure in the colon. No matter what degree of rotation is used, it cannot be
brought outside the colonic contour. The
examiner may hesitate to call it either a
polyp or diverticulum. A 24-hour film of
the abdomen may clear the dilemma. A
polyp will no longer appear present,
whereas a diverticulum is apt to retain
some of the opaque media and hence still
be visible.[47]

ALTERATIONS OF FLOW

The flow of the barium mixture as it
ascends can either be halted by an obstructive lesion, a carcinoma, or spasm, or the
flow may become more rapid, as in colitis.
The impediment to the free flow as caused
by carcinoma was described above. In this

section those diseases which may cause
other alterations in the barium flow will
be discussed.

Ulcerative Colitis. Ulcerative colitis is an
inflammation and possibly an infection of
the bowel wall associated with excavations
which are sometimes located in the superficial mucosa and sometimes deeper. One
of the main characteristics of this disease is
the speed with which the enema fills the
colon. The rigid pipe-like (fig. 389) walls
offer no resistance to the flow of barium
mixture and the opaque media flows from
the rectum to the cecum in a matter of
seconds. The young resident in radiology
observing the head of the barium column
is often surprised when, getting ready to
look for it in the sigmoid, he instead finds it
in the cecum. Because of the narrowing and
the accompanying irritability of the colon
the patient often finds it difficult to retain
the enema. (If the bowel is *wider* than
normal, i.e., a very early case, filling of
the colon may be slower.)

The contour of the bowel wall is so

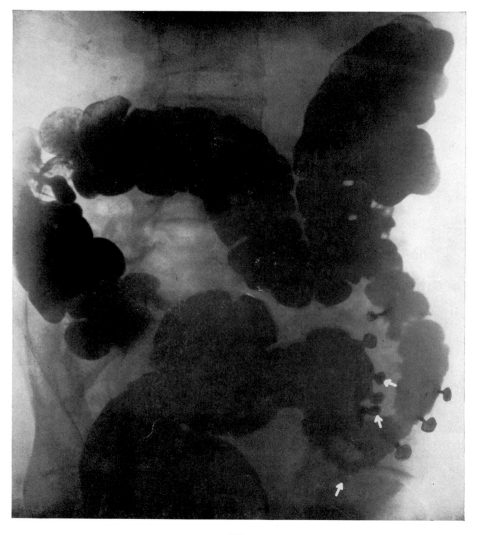

388

The "grape-like" shadows projecting from the bowel are characteristic of diverticulosis.

changed when the ulcer becomes deep enough that its margin is saw-toothed instead of smooth (fig. 390). This serrated margin caused by the ulceration is better seen on the radiographic film than on the fluoroscopic screen. The changes usually begin in the distal colon, sometimes in the rectum, and extend cephelad and rarely through the ileo-cecal valve into the ileum. The apparent depth of the ulcers may be increased by small polypoid elevation of the mucosa between the ulcers. Barium enema may not show this saw-toothed ap-

pearance but instead an abnormal smoothness of the wall, i.e., absence of haustra.[21] In advanced cases the wall of the intestine has a stiff pipe-like appearance, is shortened and is usually irritable.

In some cases with obvious ulceration, the haustral markings are preserved. This indicates that the inflammation is not deep enough in the wall or severe enough to interfere with the function of the tunica muscularis involved in the formation of the haustra.[22]

The ulcerative process may heal, leaving

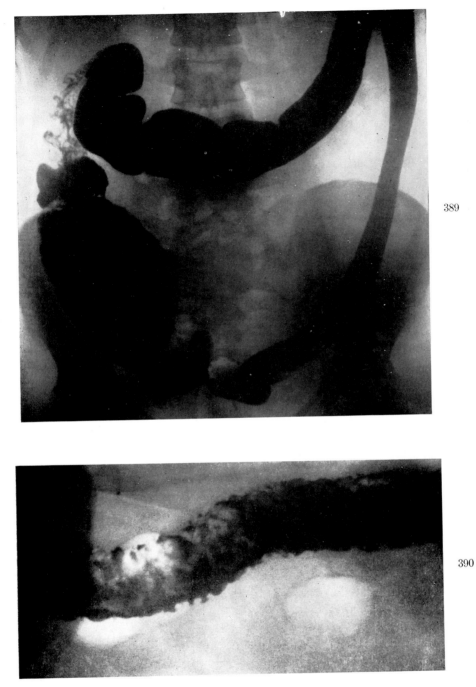

389

390

Ulcerative colitis at different stages.

389

Ulcerative colitis. Pipe stem colon. Descending and part of transverse colon are smooth and pipe-like. Note loss of normal haustration.

390

Saw-toothed appearance of ulcerative colitis.

irregular indentations in the barium shadow *indistinguishable from the appearance when the disease was active.*

A few words are indicated to describe the preparations of the patient in this disease. First, because of the diarrhea, it is likely that the colon is more or less cleansed of fecal contents. This makes preliminary cathartics and colonic irrigation unnecessary. Secondly, cathartics as well as enemas, if drastic, may cause the already weakened bowel to perforate. This is particularly true in the acute stage of the illness. These same factors should be kept in mind when barium is administered. Over-distention should be avoided and the entire procedure should be done slowly and

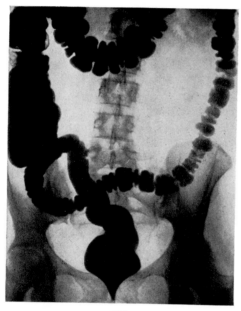

391

Question:

What is the normal width of the descending colon compared to the cecum?

Answer:

One-half to two-thirds of the cecal diameter usually equals the diameter of the descending colon.

Comment: In the figure above, the descending colon is less than the normal limits; this together with the increased haustral markings can be taken as evidence of a spastic descending colon.

carefully. Regarding air insufflation, further caution is also necessary, because of the danger of perforation.

Amebic Dysentery. Radiographically, the differential diagnosis between amebic colitis and idiopathic ulcerative colitis depends chiefly on the preponderating susceptibility of the cecum to become invaded by the ameba.[23, 24, 25, 26] These lesions occur in order of frequency in the cecum, ascending colon, sigmoid colon, and rectum. The balance of the colon, however, may also be involved.[2] In this disease, as in ulcerative colitis, alteration of the flow, the raggedness of the contours and the comparatively long extent of the lesion are important. The typical deformity sought for[26a] is a shortening and narrowing of the cecum and a patency of the ileo-cecal valve (as differentiated from tuberculosis, in which the terminal ileum is involved).

There are, however, no radiographic changes which make an accurate differential diagnosis of amebiasis possible. The diagnosis rests on the demonstration of ameba; radiographic examination serves to demonstrate the degree and distribution of the pathologic changes.

Spastic or Irritable Colon. The diagnosis of spastic colon is intimately bound up with the diagnosis of mucous colitis.

A spastic or irritable colon is a colon in which because of neurogenic influence there is a constant state of hypertonus. Normally, the descending colon and sigmoid when filled by a barium enema are usually about two-thirds of the width of the cecum and ascending colon. In a spastic or irritable colon the barium enema shows a relatively small-bored colon with fine haustral contractions (fig. 391) particularly exaggerated in the descending part of the large bowel. The width of the involved segment is markedly diminished, i.e., the descending colon, when involved, being less than two-thirds the width of the cecum.

When a barium enema is administered

in such a colon it rushes with great speed to the splenic flexure and usually with subsequent rapid filling of the entire large bowel. In some instances the narrowed distal colon relaxes as the rest of the colon fills. In others it remains narrowed. Also, as the barium enters the normal colon, the colon fills with the opaque material without contracting, or showing only slight changes in character during the procedure; whereas in spastic colon the haustral markings are more evident, clear cut and more numerous. The spasm may be so intense as to arrest completely the flow of opaque material. However, after a little while, this spasm usually relaxes without the aid of the palpating hand or raising the enema can, and the opaque mixture is again permitted passage. On occasion these spastic contractions of the colon may be so strong that the barium mixture instead of flowing towards the cecum is forced *caudad*, making it difficult for the patient to retain the barium and causing considerable discomfort and even pain. This irritability may be so great as not to permit filling the entire colon.

This hypertonicity is usually found in the sigmoid or descending colons, but not infrequently the entire colon may be so involved. When this is the case the distal colon has a changing contour and a great number of indentations into the barium shadow are usually seen.

The difference in caliber of the ascending and descending colon, although apparent on the fluoroscopic screen, is more readily seen on the radiographic film, especially the film taken twenty-four hours after the ingestion of barium mixture.

Sometimes the descending colon in such a condition appears narrow and long without any indentations or haustral markings.

This condition has been called irritable or spastic colon. It is a mechanism whereby the intestinal contents are delayed and it is usually associated, just as in carcinoma of the colon, with a history of alternating constipation and diarrhea. Tenderness may be present on pressure over the involved bowel.

Mucous Colitis. The borderline between the functional disorder called spastic or irritable colon and real mucous colitis is impossible to determine because in both conditions irritability is an important factor. In mucous colitis the changes in the barium enema are essentially those as seen with a spastic colon.[27] Perhaps in this illness the indentations are not as marked and instead one is apt to find a smoothened bowel contour. In mucous colitis, roentgenographic film examination after evacuation of the barium enema often shows two to three mucosal folds running parallel with the long axis in the descending colon, instead of the irregularly criss-cross folds which are characteristic of the mucosal pattern in this region. Crane[28] described a "string sign" associated with this illness. Bargen[29] demonstrated, however, that it may appear in any disease of the colon and therefore is considered of little consequence.

Tuberculosis. Tuberculosis as it invades the intestine is usually secondary to a Koch infection in the lungs.[30] When found in the large bowel, just as in amebic colitis, it usually starts within the cecum and travels upwards. It is rarely found in the distal sigmoid or rectum.

On the fluoroscopic screen the examiner should become suspicious of the existence of the lesion when in the presence of a suitable history he finds evidence of gaseous distention of the small bowel.

Perhaps the main characteristic of this lesion as observed on the fluoroscopic screen is the marked irritability of the involved colon. In the stage of superficial ulceration the fluoroscopist will find a marked inability to fill the cecum properly.[31, 32] At this stage the following sequence of events can be seen on the fluoroscopic screen[2]:

When the flow of barium reaches the

relaxed cecum it will momentarily fill out and the contour will be seen intact. However, the marked irritability of the invaded region will almost immediately cause a contraction of this part of the bowel with resultant expulsion of its contents. This alternate filling out of the cecum to be followed by spasm and emptying of this region is highly suggestive of tuberculosis. It has previously been suggested that when difficulty is encountered in filling the cecum properly, this area should be studied by the ingested meal method. The classic sign (Stierlin's)[31] of tuberculosis is an absence of a well filled cecal shadow, although the ileum and the part of the distal colon immediately above the cecum are filled (fig. 396, page 315).

Summary

The various inflammatory and irritable lesions of the colon as described do not permit diagosis fluoroscopically. The benign granulomas may closely simulate malignant infiltrations.[34] Moreover, the borderline between the the functional and organic in colitis is close and not distinct. In summary, it might be said that every patient with symptoms referrable to the colon must have the full benefit of the entire armamentarium of the physician including proctoscopic or sigmoidoscopic examinations, roentgenographic procedures, stool analysis and other procedures the examiner finds necessary.

PATHOLOGICAL ALTERATION OF POSITION

Lesions outside the bowel wall may produce various changes, including displacement, narrowing, and deformity. Extracolonic pressure may even cause a complete obstruction to the flow of barium. Actual invasion by a neighboring malignant process may simulate primary disease of the bowel.[35, 36] The full interpretive knowledge of the radiologist as well as clinician must be brought to bear in reaching a diagnosis.

Changes in the position of the colon as caused by "normal abnormalities" and benign processes can also be encountered. The sigmoid occasionally can be displaced high into the abdomen up to the hepatic flexure; at other times it can become elongated and redundant so as to form an additional one, two or three coils. The cecum also is subject to change of position and this is seen as cecum mobile, nondescent of the cecum, incomplete rotation, situs inversus and redundancy. Other causes of colonic displacement are hernia and adhesions.

When a change in position of the colon is observed, the examiner should determine whether the deviation is due to intrinsic colonic pathology or extrinsic pressure. The fluoroscopist observing the contours of the bowel wall, its flexibility and mobility and any alterations of flow, filming his findings in their optimum position, will receive invaluable aid in arriving at a diagnosis.

Adhesions

Perhaps one of these displacements, due to adhesions, deserves special mention. A description here will have a twofold value. First, it will serve as an exercise showing how the examiner should adjust his fluoroscopic maneuvers when a variation is encountered. Secondly, it will serve in demonstrating how the fluoroscopic procedure can offer help in arriving at a diagnosis of adhesions.

Various factors must be considered[37]: fixation of the adherent viscus; deformity of its contours; and obstruction to the onward pasage of the contents within the bowel.

Fixation. In order to demonstrate the first of these signs, fixation of the viscus, we must first assume that that portion of colon under discussion is accessible to the palpating hand, and in addition it must normally be mobile. The cecum lends itself admirably to such observation, especially when it is not low down in the pelvis. The patient lying supine, the palpating hand actually seeks it out and gently moves it

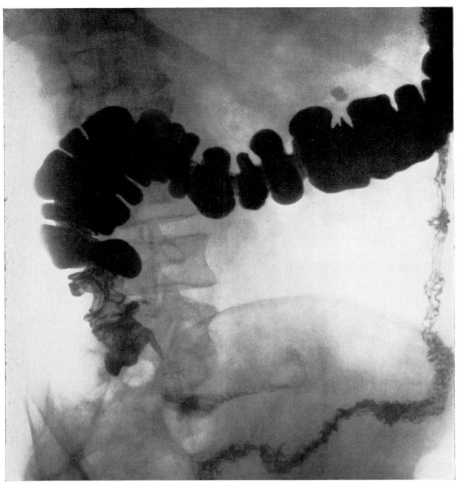

392

Question:

This is an evacuation study. The filled retrograde barium enema study was normal. The patient's main complaint was left upper quadrant pain. Is any abnormalcy present?

Answer:

In this evacuation study, a holdup of the barium column is seen in the region of the splenic flexure. The splenic flexure was reexamined and proved normal.

Question:

Can any *further* explanation be made for the patient's symptoms?

Answer:

An opaque calculus is seen in the left abdomen above the transverse colon. This proved to be a renal calculus and explained the patient's symptoms.

Comment: In any fluoroscopic and subsequent *film* study of the abdomen, the examiner must make certain that the *entire* field viewed is observed. The examination should not be confined *solely* to the organ in question. *Any* abnormalcies which appear must not be missed. As a guide to be certain nothing is missed, the examiner must ask himself three specific questions when he thus studies *any* abdomen:

(1) Calculi—are there renal, gallbladder or pancreatic stones present?
(2) Bones—are they normal?
(3) Soft tissues—are any masses present? Are the muscle planes in the *film* study normal? Are the other visceral shadows normal?

309

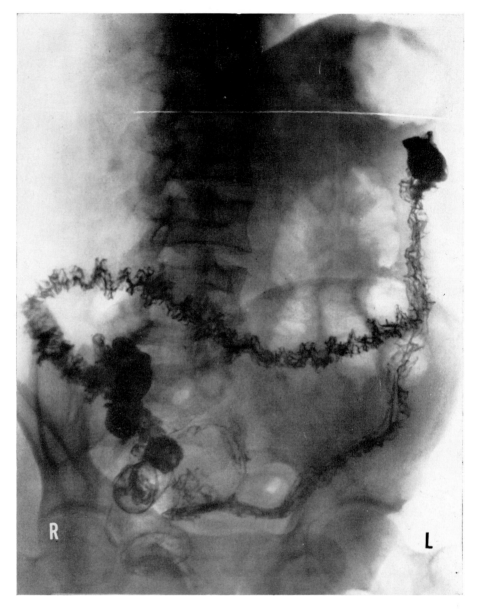

393

This patient presented a history of pain in the abdomen without true localization. A barium enema study was performed and found normal. This is the evacuation study.

Question:

Are any abnormalcies seen?

Answer:

An opaque calculus in the right upper quadrant proved to be a gallbladder calculus (see fig. 392).

about. Here as elsewhere, acquaintance and constant repetition of the normal is prerequisite before attempting to diagnose the abnormal. Segments such as the hepatic flexure or the splenic flexure, which may have little mobility and be located high up under the ribs, do not lend themselves as easily to fluoroscopic manipulation. The descending colon as well as parts of the pelvic or sigmoid colon can also be palpated and moved about behind the fluoroscopic screen, but the rectum and that part of the sigmoid colon placed too deeply in the pelvis can not so be examined. In the female, an attempt to palpate structures in the true pelvis can be made per vaginam.

Fixation must not be confused with the patient who, unrelaxed, holds his abdominal muscles rigid and thereby *prevents* the palpating hand from reaching the loops in question. The patient should be advised to hold his abdomen soft and relaxed, and the examination should be performed in as gentle a manner as possible. When muscular rigidity plays a part, changing the position of the patient may change the arrangements of the loops in question. In the presence of adhesions, however, changing the position of the patient will cause no separation of adherent parts. (See figs. 408–411, page 339.)

Deformity of Contours. The deformity of contour most typical of adhesions is an abrupt angulation. This angulation must be a real one, that is, it must be distinguished from a round bend. With manipulation behind the fluoroscopic screen the examiner may make this determination with some degree of certainty. The roentgenogram alone will leave him to wonder. Such an angulation is usually accompanied by some narrowing of the colonic lumen, which if marked produces the third sign or obstruction of the lumen.

Obstruction of the Lumen. This is manifested during the barium enema as a holdup to the flow of barium, and that part of the bowel already containing the opaque media, that is, distal to the obstruction, balloons widely. After sufficient dilatation some barium mixture may go through. The amount passing the obstruction is determined by how "tight" the narrowing caused by the obstruction is. Generally, it is not good procedure to force barium mixture beyond a true obstructive process. Often the barium mixture may become trapped and cause later difficulties.

It should definitely be understood that a diagnosis of adhesions should be shunned as far as possible except on clear evidence. It is a noncommittal diagnosis, one that seldom leads to operative interference except in very definite obstructive cases. It is still a regrettably common diagnosis on slender evidence and more often wrong than right.

(Further discussion of adhesions will be found in the concluding remarks of the next chapter, Intestinal Obstruction.)

MISCELLANEOUS DISEASES

Intussusception

When roentgenographic examination of an obstructive lesion is being considered it should be performed either by means of direct examination, (without contrast material) or by barium enema. Barium given by mouth may readily convert a partial obstruction to a complete obstruction.

It has already been pointed out that prior to injecting the opaque media the observer is to examine the abdomen grossly for either opaque shadows suggesting calculi, or loops of bowel unduly distended with air. When air-distended loops of bowel are present, the observer must consider this a valuable clue in reaching a diagnosis of obstruction. It is important that he be able to differentiate the air *normally present* in the bowel from air causing distention.[37a] When intussusception exists, the latter phenomenon will appear on the fluoroscopic screen.

In routine fashion the barium enema is next performed. The barium mixture can be visualized as it flows upward, filling out the colon. When the region of intussusception

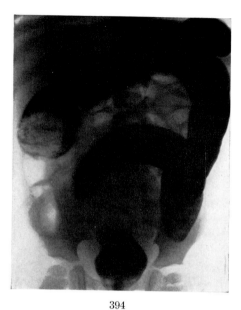

394

Question:

If no barium enema were performed, is there suggestive evidence in this picture of an obstruction?

Answer:

The various gas-filled loops in the region of the cecum and small bowel (i.e., bubbles of air) would suggest an obstructive process.

Question:

Is the configuration of the barium in the region of the hepatic flexure suggestive of an intussusception?

Answer:

Yes. Barium column starting in the rectum and terminating at the hepatic flexure ends in a concavity. This concavity is produced by the intussusceptum bulging into the barium.

Comment: The concavity as seen in the region of the hepatic flexure was first seen during fluoroscopy in the splenic area. It then suddenly slipped backward as if a barrel were pulled out of a syringe.

is encountered, the progress of the opaque media will be halted. The head of the barium flow will now reveal a characteristic concavity (fig. 394). This is produced by the telescoped proximal limb of the intussusception bulging into the barium mixture. Allowing more of the barium mixture to run in will cause a dilatation of the distal bowel.

As the pressure head is raised by additional entry of barium mixture, some of the opaque material may pass beyond the region of the concave defect. The spread now occurs in one of two ways. More commonly, the barium will travel proximally between the wall of the intussusceptum and the intussuscipiens. In such instances, the shadow on the fluoroscopic screen as well as on the radiographic film will show a "concertina" effect (fig. 395). Less frequently the barium may be seen as a fine stream entering the lumen of the intussusceptum. This rarely occurs since the edema of the intussusceptum hardly permits such entry.

Barium Enema Method of Reduction. In young children the introduction of the barium enema frequently has caused sufficient pressure to dislodge this proximal limb (intussusceptum). Such an occurrence may be seen during fluoroscopy and may be likened to a barrel pulled out of a syringe. The opaque material, after some holdup, suddenly rushes unhindered into the proximal gas-filled part of the colon like a stream filling an empty river bed (fig. 394). (When difficulty is encountered in producing this retrograde displacement of the intussusceptum and the examiner is desirous of such a result, it has been recommended that the enema can be raised up to two meters.[40])

The barium enema method of reduction of an intussusception seems to have suffered a hard fate in the English-speaking countries. In Scandinavia and France it has been otherwise. McLaren[38] explains it this way: (a) Good facilities for immediate examination and treatment by highly experienced radiologists, as in Sweden. (b) Educational campaigns aimed at earlier reference of the patient for adequate diagnosis and treatment. (c) A friendly attitude towards conservative procedures, especially the barium enema method. The barium enema method is particularly indicated during the first twelve hours, since damage to the bowel wall rarely occurs up to this time and every case is entitled to an attempt at

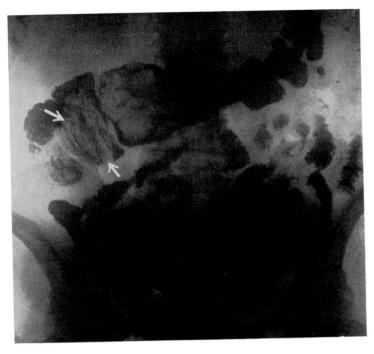

395

Barium entering between the walls of the intussusceptum and intussuscipiens produces a shadow which has been likened to a concertina (between arrows).

reposition.[58] Such an attempt has also been recommended at any time within the first twenty-four hours, but after passage of the twelfth hour, more care and gentleness should be used. After the first twelve hours, the enema can should never be raised above 150 cm.

Additional notes on the reduction of intus-susception with barium enema. Jens M. Nordentoft[40] advises and emphasizes the importance of correct pressure, i.e., two meters above the table top. The rectum should be occluded during this time. This writer also advises repeated injections and anesthesia are to be avoided. Williams[42] in 1940 maintained that a reduction can usually be obtained by brief anesthesia. Further experience, however, has shown that this measure is not necessary and that the same end can be achieved by re-peated enemas.

This retrograde displacement may be

further encouraged by gentle manual palpa-tion under fluoroscopic observation, pro-ducing gentle pressure from the area of obstruction proximally towards the ileum.

Having reduced the intussusception, the following criteria must be fulfilled in order that the examiner can be certain of the safety of the patient:

1. Films must always be taken to prove the fluoroscopic findings.

2. If a reduction of the intussusception is attained, fluoroscopic and radiographic ex-amination should also be made following the evacuation of the barium, since during the process of evacuation a recurrence of the intussusception may take place.

3. Hans Hellmer[39] made it a rule that the barium enema go up high into the small intestine before the reduction be pronounced complete. His experiences following this rule have been good.

4. Another criterion of success in this maneuver is the overcoming and unfolding

of the colonic defect as evidenced by the filling of its entire lumen. Even if reduction is complete, a certain amount of narrowing in the colonic lumen will be evident as a result of the residual edema of the colonic wall.

5. After fluoroscopic reduction the child must be kept under strict observation so that any evidence of early recurrence is immediately secured.

Objections have been raised towards treating a patient who has intussusception with a barium enema, used therapeutically. (a) It has been the experience of some examiners[40] that in children under two years of age, enema treatment is distinctly superior; whereas in older children its advantages are less marked. (b) Secondary operations on cases erroneously believed reduced carry considerable danger.[39] (c) Nordentoft points out that it is not possible to know how severely the large intestine was injured and that therefore the intestine may perforate under pressure of the enema, especially where it becomes necessary to raise the pressure by elevating the can. (d) Another criticism of the method is that often the cause of the intussusception is not determined by the roentgen method of reduction. (e) Hellmer[41] states that the individual physician should be advised against using this method without a trained staff and without a personal knowledge of the mechanism of the clinical picture and roentgenology of intussusception.

The Appendix

The appendix may be examined with opaque mixture given either by mouth or by barium enema. It is more often visualized when the barium is given from above and usually when so administered appears within the appendix in six to forty-eight hours after ingestion. According to Kerley, the Cambies technic is successful in visualizing the normal appendix in nearly 100 per cent of cases. This consists in giving a concentrated saline solution such as Mag.

Sulf. one to two drachms in 3 oz. of water by mouth three hours after the barium meal. The normal appendix projects from the medial and lower border of the pouch-like cecum and is approximately three to four inches long. A retro-cecal appendix usually projects upwards and may lie behind the cecum. It is better visualized when the cecum is not fully distended. A kinked appendix may be due to the type of mesentery supporting it or to adhesions. For valid evidence of kinking, the deformity should be constant at all times and be seen in all planes and positions. During successive examinations it must remain unchanged even by palpation.

When filled, the appendix is a tube-like structure which occasionally may be segmented. On palpation it moves when accessible, and the degree of mobility depends upon the length of its mesentery. Unless inflammatory changes exist, palpation should not ordinarily elicit pain. The optimum position for examination is supine since palpation and manipulation are much easier.

Acute Appendicitis. The roentgenologist should not be called upon to assist in the diagnosis of acute appendicitis.

Chronic Appendicitis. Chronic recurrent appendicitis is a common disease. Roentgenology is important in its differential diagnosis. In cases where the appendix is seen, a tender, fixed appendix can be taken as evidence of inflammatory change within it. Fluoroscopic study is essential in this case. The various fluoroscopic signs listed below should be considered as links in a chain leading to a diagnosis. No one of these findings is pathognomonic. Unfortunately, they are all susceptible to more than one interpretation. Any finding may be either a normal variation or a sign of a pathological condition. The probability of an abnormality or pathological process taking place within the appendix is in direct ratio to the number of these signs that the indi-

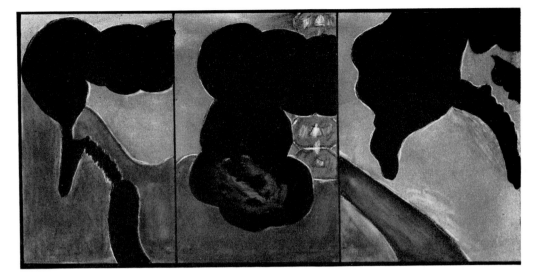

396	397	398

Cecal pathology.

Question:

Which of these pictures represents
  Tuberculosis?
  Carcinoma?
  Appendiceal abscess?

Answer:

396	397	398

1. Cecum spastic and difficult to fill.

2. Terminal ileum involved. The contour may be irregular.

Comment: This is a tuberculous cecum.

1. Cecum does not fill perfectly, due to presence of defects.

2. Terminal ileum not involved.

Comment: This is a carcinoma of the cecum.

1. Cecum relatively easy to fill.

2. Contour of terminal ileum smooth, but widely separated from the cecum.

Comment: This is an appendiceal abscess. The increased space between the cecum and terminal ileum is occupied by the abscess.

vidual case may present. The probability is further increased if on subsequent examinations these same signs recur and persist. In other words, constancy in any one of these signs is an important index that pathology may exist within the appendix.

Signs of pathology in the appendix may be listed as follows:

1. Pain or tenderness. Since the patient's subjective responses must be considered and ruled out as necessary, and since pain in the right lower quadrant may not be caused by the appendix, in cases when the appendix is seen after opacification by barium the examiner should move it about. He must be certain that with each new position of the appendix, tenderness is situated immediately over it. In the event that the appendix does not fill with opaque media (and is thus not visualized), the observer should move the cecum about, palpating its base, i.e., where the appendix is apt to be. Here, too, tenderness should shift with each new cecal position.

2. Fixation of the appendix. On rare occasions the appendix may normally be fixed because of a short mesoappendix. It sometimes requires fairly vigorous palpation to dislodge a normally mobile appendix, even though it is accessible. But with due regard to these limitations, a fixed appendix should suggest abnormalcy.

3. Non-filling of the appendix. At one time this was accepted as pathognomonic of chronic appendicitis. It was believed due to fibrotic stenosis of the lumen. The fallacy here is that a certain small percentage of normal appendices do not fill.

4. Segmentation of the opacified appendix may be normal and due to peristaltic contractions. If this is the case, the segmentation should change, and not remain in a constant or persistent pattern. But an area of dilatation and segmentation within the appendix, *when constant and persistent*, can be taken as a sign of an abnormal appendix.

5. Retention of barium in the appendix. Retention of barium in the appendix is of no significance if there is barium in the cecum or descending colon. It is of little significance at any time, even when present three or four days after ingestion, although possibly retention beyond one week may be evidence of some abnormality.

Appendiceal Abscess (fig. 398). A characteristic smooth defect may be seen in the cecal and adjacent ileal contours. This must be supplemented with adequate clinical history and findings.

EXAMINING THE ENTIRE FIELD

In the roentgen examination of any portion of the body, the examiner must make certain that he has seen the entire field presented to him. Because this examination may be time-consuming and especially when the examiner is not working with an image intensifier, the examination of the entire field under the fluoroscopic screen may prove cursory and inefficient. The spot films obtained during fluoroscopy and the subsequent *radiographic films* should be examined in their entirety. Whenever any *portion* of the abdomen or the *entire* abdomen is so examined, the examiner must make certain that he has seen the entire field presented to him. (figs. 392–393) In the abdomen, he should ask himself these *three specific questions:* (1) Are any calculi present in the field? This would include gallbladder, kidney and pancreatic stones. (2) Are any of the bony structures seen, i.e., lumber spine or lower ribs? Are they normal? (3) Are any of the visceral shadows present, e.g., kidney or liver? Are they normal? Are any other soft tissue shadows seen, e.g., psoas muscles?

Intestinal Obstruction

Fundamentals

THE IMPORTANCE of the radiologic examination in cases of intestinal obstruction cannot be minimized. In hospital routine, it has become one of the main forms of examination that the clinician uses in arriving at a diagnosis.

At the outset it should be pointed out that it is entirely possible for a patient to be apparently well, presenting very few symptoms, and yet be suffering from this condition. These asymptomatic periods may occur both at the *onset* of the illness or at an interval somewhat *after* the patient has already presented symptoms. If such symptoms-free patients are not subjected to radiographic examination, the consequences will indeed be serious. Strangulation and even death may occur. During these asymp-tomatic periods the condition may be progressing and becoming more grave. The value of the radiographic examination is not only to present evidence of the obstruction but to record progress of the condition. It bears repetition that almost complete *low small bowel mechanical obstruction* may exist for some days and yet the patient may present minimal or very few symptoms.[1] The fact that a patient has bowel movements does not exclude mechanical obstruction. The bowel distal to the lesion continues to evacuate its contents.

GENERAL PRINCIPLES OF EXAMINATION

When possible, the routine radiographic examination in cases of intestinal obstruction should include fluoroscopy, since the ability to see the intestinal movements is diagnostically important. Fluoroscopic examination should not be limited to the site of apparent pathology, i.e., the abdomen, *but should include a survey examination of the chest.* Although the seat of the patient's symptoms may appear to be below the diaphragm, the etiology may well be located in the chest. Important changes may be present within the thoracic cavity, which, when discovered, may be the clue necessary for the proper understanding of the abdominal distention.

For example, a pneumonic process with pleuritic involvement at the base of a lung may explain a bizarre clinical *abdominal* emergency. Lack of diaphragmatic movements on one side may lead directly to a diagnosis within the region which may explain the patient's symptoms. It may be an important link in the chain in reading the diagnosis. Or, finding the cardiac silhouette characteristic of rheumatic heart disease may be the clue which leads the examiner to a correct diagnosis of mesenteric embolization. The dividends which may be reaped by first examining the chest are indeed plentiful. These will be discussed presently.

Following the chest survey, the abdomen is next examined under direct fluoroscopic vision. Here, too, valuable information not seen on conventional films may be obtained. Not infrequently, paralytic ileus may not be distinguishable from obstructive ileus when conventional films alone are relied on. In cases of obstructive ileus, fluoroscopic visualization of the vigorous peristaltic waves of the distended intestinal coils, with an awareness that this degree of activity is absent in paralytic ileus, enables the examiner to reach a decision. Also of value in distinguishing large from small bowel is determining the mobility of the questioned segment as determined by fluoroscopic palpation. A loop of small bowel would be freely movable, whereas a segment of colon except for the sigmoid and transverse loop

would be fixed. Furthermore, careful palpation and manipulation during direct fluoroscopic vision may help establish the relationship of any intra-abdominal masses to the bowel, and may help locate the position of gas in the abdomen, as either extra- or intraluminal.

This section is not intended as a complete treatise on the topic, but rather attempts to give enough background to make the fluoroscopic examination more intelligible. As elsewhere, it is stressed that findings must usually be confirmed by conventional film examination. The ultimate diagnosis is eventually reached by integrating the film examination, fluoroscopic findings, and clinical and laboratory data.

PATHOGENESIS OF INTESTINAL OBSTRUCTION

Air Normally Present in the Small Bowel

Air is normally present in the *stomach* and *colon.* It is not generally found within the small intestine except for small amounts which may leak into the intestinal loops through the pyloric or ileocecal sphincters. Thus, finding an occasional air bubble within the duodenal bulb or terminal ileum is not considered abnormal.

In the main, air from the stomach passing into the small bowel is thoroughly mixed with the intestinal contents and becomes invisible. In this state it is propelled distally. If during its transit through the small intestine, it does not become absorbed, it reaches the colon and again becomes visible. Only a small amount of the air found in the colon results from intestinal putrefaction.

Aerophagic individuals may show a slight increase in the amount of small intestinal air. In them, an occasional scattered air-containing loop would not be an unusual finding. Also, in patients recumbent for a period of time, it is normal for air to accumulate and become visible within the small bowel. In infants, gas-containing small bowel loops are a normal finding.[2] When air is present in the small bowel and no true intestinal obstruction is present this is radiographically distinguishable in that the intestinal lumen is not ballooned or distended, the bowel wall is under no tension, and no fluid levels are present. It should be stressed that these air-containing loops are formless and shapeless and *not distended.*[3]

Physiologic Fluid Levels.

A. Gastric. Typically the level is found in the fundus and generally increases after food or drink.

B. Duodenal bulb and terminal ileum. Again the location is characteristic. Only a short loop of bowel is involved. *The intestine is not distended.*

C. Colonic flexures and sigmoid. Gas may be present, but because of the pulpy bowel content, generally no fluid levels are found. If an enema has been given, fluid levels may

appear. The false fluid levels will disappear in 2 to 4 hours if the patient is ambulatory and after a somewhat longer period of the patient is bedfast.

D. No enema should be given prior to examination for ileus. The retained fluid and air may create the false fluid levels described above.

Air Present with Intestinal Obstruction

In intestinal obstruction with ileus, air begins to accumulate within 1 to 3 hours after the onset of obstruction. This finding is often present before clinical signs of obstruction are clear.

The source of air causing the bowel to distend can be listed[5, 6] as: (1) Swallowed air, 68 per cent. (2) Diffusion from the blood, 22 per cent. (3) Resulting from digestive fermentation, 10 per cent.

Types of Ileus

Intestinal obstruction and ileus are not the same. Ileus is a coundition which follows obstruction. It is classified under two main headings. The obstruction may be of a mechanical nature. This is called *dynamic ileus* (often referred to as *obstructive* or *mechanical* ileus). The obstruction may be paralytic in origin, and is called *paralytic ileus.*

Within the *colon*, the most common cause for dynamic ileus is tumor. Other less frequent causes are intussusception, volvulus, and fecal concretions. Fecal concretions are generally found in the narrower part of the large bowel, i.e., the sigmoid portion.

The more usual causes for dynamic or *obstructive ileus* within the *small bowel* are[4]: (1) External hernia. (2) Adhesions and adhesive bands. (3) Intussusception. (4) Gall stone obstruction. (5) Volvulus. (6) Internal hernia. (7) Primary neoplasms.

This last does not include metastatic tumors which have spread throughout the peritoneal cavity, engaging the small bowel sufficiently to cause obstruction.

The more common causes for *paralytic ileus* are found within the various precipitating lesions capable of producing peritonitis, i.e., perforated ulcer, perforated appendices, postoperative cases with peritoneal trauma, etc. It may also be produced by such reflex phenomena as renal colic.

Paralytic ileus may result from pneumonia, spinal injury or hypoproteinemia. Protein depletion often exists with patients who have gastrointestinal disturbances. In patients with ileus, it may be aggravated by their inability to take food. Redistention of the intestine along the Miller-Abbott tube may often be due to a hypoproteinemia.[4]

Vascular disease will be discussed as a separate group.

DYNAMIC (MECHANICAL, OBSTRUCTIVE) ILEUS

Dilated air-distended bowel, containing fluid levels, may be seen fluoroscopically. Most dramatic and important however, is the visualizing of active peristalsis and the spilling of bowel contents from one limb of a loop into another. These will be discussed below. First an explanation for these phenomena.

In cases of mechanical obstruction resulting in dynamic ileus, a true barrier exists. In the gradual development of a constrictive lesion, the intestine compensates for the obstruction by dilating proximally to the lesion. At this stage the intestinal lumen is widened, but not distended, i.e., the wall is not ballooned or stretched. Ileus is not yet present. A point is reached where physiologic compensation is no longer possible and decompensation results. While the constriction was gradual, the intestine adapted itself well to the slowly developing dilatation, but when the point of decompensation is reached, the intestine becomes distended, the walls ballooned and stretched. Fluid then gradually accumulates in the intestinal coils proximal to the lesion. The air traversing the gastrointestinal tract, mixed within the intestinal contents, comes out of solution and becomes visible.

Soon after the onset of intestinal obstruction, the distended loops contain much fluid and a relatively small amount of gas. As the condition progresses, the relative amounts change and more gas accumulates.

Increased activity and hyperperistalsis becomes evident in the intestine proximal to the obstruction. This is an effort on the part of the bowel to overcome the obstructive lesion. The increased peristaltic activity above the obstruction brings the accumulated fluid and gas in sufficient quantity to produce distention *first in the region just above the block*. In cases of small bowel obstruction, ultimately the distention may progress in a retrograde fashion all the way back to the duodenum. In cases of large bowel obstruction, the distention starting in the distal colon, i.e., in the region of the lesion, may terminate in the cecum. In the presence of an incompetent ileo-cecal sphincter, gas may next leak into the small bowel, making it dilated and distended.

Thus the dilatation in large and small bowel obstruction becomes progressive, and the degree of obstruction can often be gaged by the amount of air and liquid dammed back behind the obstruction.

It should be pointed out that in obstruction of the sigmoid or rectal portions of the large bowel, the proximal sigmoid and descending portions of the bowel are relatively slowly distended. The thinner walled cecum and ascending colon, on the other hand, are greatly expanded. At times, the distended cecum may be distinguished by a fluid level and its free mobility.

Dynamic Ileus Resulting from Small Bowel Obstruction and Associated with Gas in the Colon

With obstruction in the small bowel, increased peristaltic activity is present not only within the loops of the intestine proximal to the lesion but also in the gastrointestinal tract distal to the lesion, i.e., in both the large and small bowel. The hyperperistalsis makes for a general tendency towards evacuation. *This would explain the presence of bowel movement although intestinal obstruction is present.*

While increased air distention is taking place proximal to the lesion, the air distal to the lesion becomes diminished in amount. *Often in small bowel obstruction, the colon may be completely emptied of its air.* At least two factors are responsible for this important observation. Normally, the air in the colon is derived from that transported to it via the small bowel. After the small bowel becomes obstructed, the gas fails to arrive in sufficient amounts, and air in the colon thus becomes diminished. Also, as a result of the obstruction in the small bowel, peristaltic activity increases, which expels the air *previously* present in the colon. Yet, although the absence of air in the colon, *in presence of ileus*, is indicative of small bowel obstruction, a number of cases *retain* at least *small amounts* of gas within the large bowel. This *retained* colonic air is *not* generally associated with fluid levels.

Dynamic Ileus Associated with Decrease of, Small Amounts of, or Absence of Intestinal Gas.

Gas accumulation is not *necessarily* proof of the severity of the obstruction. We have seen above that obstruction associated with ileus evidences itself by air accumulation within the bowel. It has been pointed out that the progress and degree of obstruction can be gaged by observing the increasing accumulation of air and the number of air-distended loops. It should, however, be noted that in small bowel obstruction of *increasing duration*, the ratio of gaseous to fluid content eventually decreases until at the end of 7 to 8 days no apparent gas may be present within the small bowel.[4]

Obstruction high up in the jejunum may, from its inception be associated with *little* or *no small bowel gas accumulation*. This lack may be the result of ready access of the gas back into the stomach and subsequent regurgitation and vomiting of this air.

In true strangulating obstructions too, only a minimal amount of gas accumulates. This is the most dangerous of small bowel obstructions and because of this minimal gas accumulation the diagnosis is most difficult.

DYNAMIC ILEUS AND PARALYTIC ILEUS MIXED

If the mechanical obstruction is unrelieved, strangulation of the bowel eventually may occur and this is followed by gangrene. At this time, there is marked prostration and development of a shock-like state with profound toxicity. Mechanical obstruction at this stage changes. The obdomen becomes silent. Whatever the cause, whether gangrene or perforation of the bowel, etc., involvement of the peritoneum means that a paralytic type of ileus becomes mixed with the mechanical.

PARALYTIC (ADYNAMIC) ILEUS

Paralytic or adynamic ileus can be looked upon as a reflex or inhibition type of ileus.[7]

The intestinal tract is innervated by the sympathetic and parasympathetic nervous systems. Normally, intestinal peristalsis produces a constant change in the shape of the villi lining the bowel, and this change provides new surfaces for absorption.

Stimulation of the sympathetic or inhibition of the parasympathetic results in cessation of peristaltic activity. With cessation of peristalsis, no new villi surfaces are exposed. The result is diminished absorption. With lack of absorption, the gas is no longer held in solution and becomes visible. Since the nerve supply within the small and large bowel is the same, gas accumulating with paralytic ileus will be seen scattered *throughout* the gastrointestinal tract, i.e., *colon and small intestine, and in the same relative proportions*.

A few words are indicated to describe the gas distention in paralytic ileus. Reflex distention of the bowel may vary from a few distended segments to distention of the entire gut. General distention is the more important form. As described, it is possible for gas to be in the colon in the presence of mechanical obstruction of the small bowel, yet the simultaneous presence of gas in the large *and* small bowel should suggest a paralytic type of ileus. When peritonitis is the cause of the paralytic ileus, certain other characteristic findings appear. The free fluid in the abdominal cavity separates the distended intestinal loops, widening the spaces between them. When fibrinous adhesions form, these loops appear fixed even when the patient's posture changes.

ILEUS ASSOCIATED WITH VASCULAR ABDOMINAL CATASTROPHES

Vascular abdominal catastrophes may be classified into *retroperitoneal lesions* and *interperitoneal lesions*.[9]

1. Retroperitoneal vascular accidents.

A. Abdominal aorta (aneurysm, embolus, and thrombosis).

B. Splenic vessels (splenic vein thrombosis, ruptured spleen).

C. Renal vessels (thrombosis or embolus).

2. Intraperitoneal accidents. These involve vessels lying between the layers of peritoneum.

A. Arterial-mesenteric embolus.

B. Venous mesenteric thrombosis.

C. Intestinal strangulations.

The result of a mesenteric vascular occlusion is closely similar to that of intestinal obstruction. Stasis of the intestinal contents takes place. Hemorrhage and infarction occur. When evidence of gas distention within the bowel, i.e., ileus, is present, the examiner must always consider the possibility of a vascular disturbance as a possible etiology.

Roentgenologic and Fluoroscopic Procedure

Whenever possible, the patient should be brought to the x-ray department. If his condition permits, films of the abdomen should be taken in the right and left lateral decubitus, prone, and erect positions. A chest film should also be made.

With the patient on the x-ray table and the foot rest in position, the table is tilted vertically so that the patient comes to rest in the erect position. When the condition of the patient does not permit such a full shift, the table should be brought as nearly erect as he can tolerate.

After the necessary filming, the patient is fluoroscoped.

These *preliminary* examinations do not employ contrast media.

CHEST EXAMINATION

The fluoroscopic examination starts with a survey of the chest. (The reader is referred to Chapter II for a fuller discussion of this examination.) Systematically and quickly the *lung parenchyma, pleural cavity* (for fluid), *diaphragms, mediastinum* and *heart shadows* are examined. The examiner must be mindful that lesions present within the chest may be either secondary to the intra-abdominal disease, or, in some cases, the primary etiology for the subdiaphragmatic findings. When pleural effusion is suspected and not clearly seen, the patient should be examined for fluid when in the erect position. He should be turned into an oblique plane in order to expose the posterior costophrenic sinus. The right oblique may be used when the right side is in question, and the left oblique for the left side (see figs. 60, 61, p. 49). The fluid may then be seen obscuring the posterior costophrenic sinus. It is often more clearly seen in expiration than in inspiration. If doubt remains, the patient may be tilted directly toward the side in question. The clouding by the fluid will then be more evident. The costophrenic sinus will be seen to clear somewhat if the patient is next tilted to the opposite side.

The diaphragmatic movements are observed. The examiner should be mindful that inflammatory processes adjacent to the diaphragm tend to inhibit diaphragmatic movements more or less completely.[7] The side on which the movements are diminished or absent would indicate the side of the lesion.

Diffuse peritonitis or pancreatitis inhibits movements bilaterally.

Intestinal obstruction and increased abdominal distention raise both sides of the diaphragm. The diaphragmatic movements, however, remain within normal limits for an extended period of time. In the presence of *severe* distention, the diaphragms may become completely paralyzed,[7] but this is generally due to complicating peritonitis.

The cardiac shadow should also be studied. Careful study of the heart and mediastinal shadow may yield valuable clues explaining the abdominal findings. The size and shape of the heart should be noted. The cardiac pulsations should be observed. If a segment of the heart reveals absent or contrapulsile pulsations, coronary thrombosis as a cause should be suspected. If the heart is triangular or mitral in contour, a valvular lesion should cause the examiner to be mindful of embolus within the mesenteric vessels. Cardiac decompensation may be responsible for secondary congestion within the abdominal vessels, with resultant severe gas distention.

ABDOMINAL EXAMINATION WITHOUT CONTRAST MEDIA

The screen is next lowered and the abdomen examined. Recognizing the increased air-filled loops is important. Herein lies the main clue to the existence of an ileus, either paralytic or dynamic. It is important to train oneself to be able to identify the early air-filled loops.

Air-Distended Bowel

Air-distended bowel is recognizable in that the involved loops of bowel are not merely air containing, but actually *distended*, i.e., ballooned, and its walls put on the stretch.

The large bowel may be recognized by its peripheral position. Under direct fluoroscopic vision, its relative immobility in the ascending and descending portions can be determined. The haustra, when seen, generally do not completely cross the bowel lumen, i.e., from top to bottom. They interdigitate.

The small bowel may be recognized by its central position. As opposed to the relatively fixed character of the colon, the small bowel's freedom of mobility may be determined under direct fluoroscopic vision. The Kerkring folds cross the bowel lumen from top to bottom, simulating accordion folds

(figs. 399, 400). When seen in their length, the distended small bowel loops may present pictures of elongated air-filled cross-hatched sacs with sharp turns, often called "hair pin" loops. When seen in cross section, they are chiefly round. But when one loop abuts on the other, they may appear "squared off."[3] By the continued accumulation of air proximal to an obstructive lesion, a "layering" of distended loops one upon the other next takes place.

Gas distention does not obliterate the mucosal folds in the *jejunum* which are seen as striations in the gas-filled loops (figs. 399, 400). Under the same conditions, the mucosal folds in the *ileum* disappear. The large bowel loops tend to become smooth, but the inter-digitating haustral markings persist.

Under direct fluoroscopic vision, the palpating hand may push the intraluminal gas in various directions thereby visualizing different sections of involved bowel. The newly visualized section may present a more characteristic appearance and thereby render its identification easier.

Here as elsewhere, no amount of descriptive material is as valuable as actually reviewing various films revealing these findings and seizing every opportunity to fluoroscopically examine patients who may demonstrate the same.

Fluid Levels

As described above, where possible the fluid and air-distended bowel loops should be viewed with the patient in the upright position. With the patient so arranged, the air rises above the fluid to present fluid levels. In dynamic ileus with increasing distention in the small bowel, the loops erect themselves and become inverted and "U" shaped in appearance (figs. 399, 400). (See discussion of physiologic fluid levels earlier in this chapter.)

With paralytic ileus, fluid levels in the erect position are less numerous and frequent than with dynamic ileus.[30]

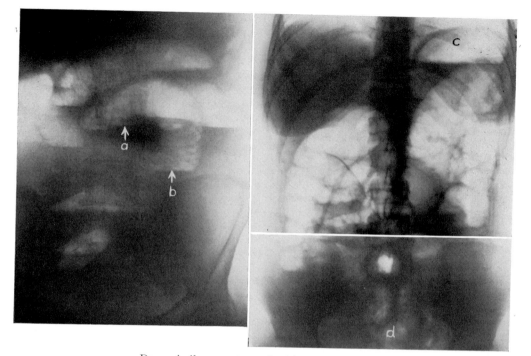

Dynamic ileus contrasted with paralytic ileus.

399

Dynamic ileus.

1. Fluid in inverted U-shaped loop (*a*, *b*) spilling from one limb of the U into the other produces unequal heights *a*, *b* of fluid levels in each limb.
2. Coil-like appearance of Kerkring folds.
3. In erect position, air-filled loops have a tendency to rise, fluid-filled loops tend to fall. Note greater density below as compared with air-filled loops above. (Cf. *c*, 400.)
4. No air present in stomach or rectum.
5. Degree of activity great.
6. More numerous fluid levels.

400

Paralytic ileus.

1. Inverted U shaped loops, without the unequal fluid levels seen in figure 399.
2. No real coil-like appearance of Kerkring folds.
3. Paralytic ileus unassociated with peritoneal fluid. Shows no greater density below, as in figure 399.
4. Air present in stomach (*c*) and rectum (*d*) (composite film). Small and large bowel distended.
5. Degree of activity small.
6. Less numerous fluid levels.

Peristalsis

Fluoroscopically the findings are dramatic. In dynamic ileus, the examiner may observe a great deal of bowel unrest and increased peristaltic activity. In the small bowel, the peristaltic waves in their effort to overcome the obstruction tend to push the intestinal contents from one limb of the inverted U-shaped loop to the other. The fluid as it is being spilled from one limb of the loop into the other has been likened to water spurting from a small fountain.[7] *Uneven*

fluid levels, resulting from lessening the fluid content in one side of the limb and simultaneously increasing the content in the other limb, are characteristic of this process. *Thus, existence of fluid levels at different heights in either limb of an inverted U-shaped loop is an almost certain indication of mechanical obstruction* (figs. 399, 400).

In the large bowel, when the condition of the patient permits, shaking the patient will visibly move these fluid levels, which may be seen on the fluoroscopic screen.[8]

Differentiating Paralytic from Dynamic Ileus (figs. 399, 400)

We may recapitulate and enlarge on the foregoing differential diagnostic points, then, as follows:

1. It is of vital importance to distinguish between the intestinal distention produced by paralytic ileus and that by obstructive (dynamic) ileus, and it is here that fluoroscopic examination may be particularly helpful. When the patient is able to stand, he is examined fluoroscopically in the erect position. The bowel unrest, peristalsis and changing fluid levels, so that the contents from one limb of a U-shaped loop may be seen poured into the other limb, are pathognomonic of dynamic ileus. It must, however, be remembered that at the onset of intestinal obstruction, the increased peristalsis responsible for the spillage of the air-fluid contents may not be of sufficient vigor so that the changing levels may be almost invisible. The examiner must also be aware that *temporary periods* of inhibition of intestinal movements may occur some hours after the onset of the attack. In such cases, after an interval the movements may be expected to start anew. Re-examination, therefore, should be undertaken whenever obstructive ileus is suspected and the fluoroscopic findings are indeterminate.

In cases of paralytic ileus, air fluid levels are also present, but because peristalsis is relatively absent, they are relatively immobile. The main movement imparted to them is the rising and falling of the loops with respiration.

2. Paralytic ileus associated with peritonitis and free peritoneal fluid reveals a wider separation of the gas-distended intestinal loops because of the fluid present between the loops. And when adhesions form, the involved segments appear immobile, fluoroscopically, and will not change position although the patient changes posture. Also, with the general relaxation within the *entire* gastro-intestinal tract that takes place in paralytic ileus, air becomes apparent within the fundus of the *stomach* and the *rectum*. In dynamic ileus, very little air is seen in the fundus of the stomach and is absent in the rectum (compare figs. 399 and 400).

VASCULAR ABDOMINAL CATASTROPHES

Acute Arterial Mesenteric Embolus

This is a dramatic abdominal catastrophe. The patient clinically presents acute abdominal pain, shock, rapid pulse rate and a fall in blood pressure. Blood-stained diarrhea may be present, to be followed by constipation. Abdominal distention appears. Initially there may be increased peristaltic activity but this gives way to a paralytic type of ileus. Fluid and gas collect in the dilated bowel loops. Clinically, a valuable clue to this type of occlusion is the severe degree of collapse and abdominal pain which is out of all proportion to the degree of radiographic evidence of obstruction. The presence of bloody stools is also important.

The superior mesenteric artery is the blood vessel most frequently involved. The entire small bowel and colon up to the splenic flexure is affected. Gas distention is present within these sections and cannot be distinguished from other types of ileus.

Fluoroscopic and Radiographic Sings. Early, increased peristaltic activity may be seen within the small bowel. This is later followed by a decrease in the motor activity.

The small bowel becomes distended with fluid levels. This may appear in 3 to 5 hours after embolism. The fluid levels tend to be relatively small and behind the fluoroscopic screen they are relatively immobile.

When the colon is involved the abrupt termination at the splenic flexure is present. This would simulate an obstructive lesion at that point. If a barium enema is performed, the opaque media will be seen to flow *through* the area of apparent obstruction into the air-containing portion of the colon.[10]

Mesenteric Venous Thrombosis

Mesenteric venous thrombosis does not present as acute an abdominal catastrophe. None of the dramatic picture of acute arterial embolus is present. Rather, the patient is of the age group which frequently gives a history of previous vascular accidents.

Fluoroscopic and Radiologic Signs. No great gas distention is present. Slight increase of gas and fluid may appear in the affected portion of the bowel. It is seldom sufficient to make a diagnosis.

Roentgenologic Management of Intestinal Obstruction with Contrast Media and Intubation

LARGE BOWEL

Further Examination with Contrast Media. In certain cases, study with contrast media becomes necessary. If a large bowel obstruction is most likely, the barium enema examination is indicated in order to establish a definite diagnosis. The large bowel examination should also be first performed in those instances where it is impossible to decide whether the obstruction is in the large or small bowel. If the lesion is not discovered within the colon, the obstruction must obviously exist in the small intestine.

The study of the large bowel by barium enema has been described in Chapter VII. It should be pointed out that fluoroscopic demonstration of the lesion depends upon visualization of the stenotic site and the interruption of the free flow of barium at the site of pathology. As the opaque media ascends and opacifies the more distal unobstructed portions of the colon, the flow is smooth and a normal degree of filling first takes place. When the stenotic site is reached, the flow ceases and the unobstructed portion of the colon previously filled in normal fashion next becomes dilated and ballooned, owing to the inability of increasing amounts of barium suspension to pass. Some of the opaque media may be seen trickling into and outlining the stenotic site. Spot films should be immediately taken. It is important that the pathologic region should not be hidden from the examiner by filling of the colon beyond the site of the lesion (figs. 378–380, p. 297). This situation is not uncommon, and the examiner should be on the watch for it. The nearer a lesion is situated to the rectum, the more evident is the ballooning and dilatation of the over-filled portions of the colon *distal* to the lesion. Lesions in the sigmoid and rectum are especially prone to overfill the uninvolved lumen and cause the patient to evacuate during the barium enema administration.

SMALL BOWEL

INTRODUCTION

When the obstruction is not present in the large bowel, the small bowel is next studied. Administering the barium by mouth is contraindicated in large bowel obstruction, since a partially obstructed lesion may thus be converted into one that is completely obstructed. In the small bowel, this danger is not generally apt to occur. Although small amounts of barium may be given orally in acute small bowel obstruction,[12] the method of choice employs the long intestinal tube.[12-15]

Origin and Development of the Tube

Unlike most other methods of examination, the use of the long type of intestinal tube is not confined to diagnosis but is used therapeutically as well.

The Miller-Abbott tube originally was described for use in physiologic experiments.

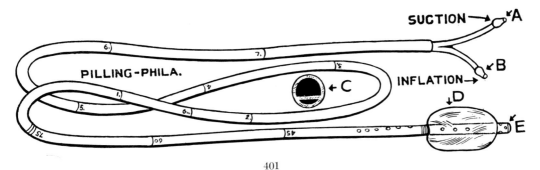

401

The Miller-Abbott tube.

Two requirements were necessary. First, after the tube's passage, it would have to be self propellent. Second, it would have to be capable of carrying liquid down to the intestine, as well as removing intestinal contents when necessary. Hence, a double-channeled tube was employed. One channel led to a tube which contained, at its distal end, perforations through which intestinal contents were aspirated and material injected back down the intestine. The other channel led to an inflatable rubber balloon at the distal end. The inflatable bag would act as a bolus of food, stimulating the intestine and thereby propelling the tube through the bowel.

It became desirable to work with isolated walled off segments. For this, a triple lumen tube was devised. Here two balloons were spaced about 30 cm. apart, each of which could be inflated separately through two of three channels. With both balloons distended, a small segment of bowel would be blocked off at its proximal and distal ends. That segment of the tube lying between these two balloons was perforated and connected into the third channel, allowing withdrawal or injection of various materials.

With these use of suction as an adjunct in the treatment of intestinal obstruction, the Miller-Abbott tube found its place in therapy.[6, 13-16]

Description of Miller-Abbott Double-Lumen Tube (fig. 401)

The channels of the Miller-Abbott double-lumen tube are of unequal size (C in fig. 401 represents a cross section of this tube). The larger lumen represents the tubing concerned with suction (A). The smaller lumen (B) ends just above the metal tip (E), with several small holes placed in the tubing immediately proximal to this connection. Air which may be injected through the smaller lumen is collected in a thin rubber bag or balloon, made of a finger cot or a condom (D). This balloon is attached between the metal tip and the most distal suction aperture by means of silk thread. The proximal end of the tube is Y-shaped with one limb of the Y connecting with the suction side and the other with the balloon side. The tube recommended here is No. 18 F, with an over-all diameter of 6 mm. and walls approximately 1 mm. in thickness.

Indications for Use

Therapeutically, the main indication for the of the Miller-Abbott tube is for the relief of distention in intestinal obstruction.

Diagnostically, its main indication is in conditions where the lumen of the bowel is so completely obstructed as to make a barium meal dangerous, and yet, a diagnosis, at least as to site of the obstruction, imperative. By injecting a small amount of opaque media down the tube to the region of holdup, a reasonable attempt at a diagnosis can be made. This will be described in greater detail in the discussion of Stage IV, below.

According to indications, the tube finds its chief use in patients with dynamic ileus and those with adynamic ileus.[17, 18] Where operative interference is contemplated, it also affords time to replace needed fluids, salt, plasma, and protein.

The tube has also been used for diagnostic purposes in cases other than obstruction. In obscure small bowel lesions where the diagnosis cannot be confirmed by more conventional methods, the tube may be passed to the suspected site of pathology. If blood is aspirated at this point, the suspicion can reasonably be deemed to be confirmed. The balloon may then be used as an artificial obstruction. The opaque media can next be injected, permitting detailed study of any desired area in the small intestine (termed a "segmental survey"). In some instances where double contrast has proved desirable, air may be injected through the tube after the introduction of barium.

Advantages

Use of the long intestinal tube yields important benefits. In cases of ileus, the fluid- and air-distended obstructed small bowel is in dire need of an outlet. This is supplied by the long intestinal tube. As the intestine is thus decompressed, the circulation is improved, the smooth muscle regains its tone, peristalsis returns, and nutrition may be resumed. While decompression of the bowel and the restoration of the electrolytic balance is taking place, sufficient time is allowed to prepare for operation, where indicated, thereby converting a surgical emergency into an elective procedure. With the patient in better condition and the bowel no longer distended, the technical work of the surgeon becomes easier. After the operation, if the tube is left in place the suture lines are protected.

Role of the Radiologist

Because of the important role the fluoroscope and roentgenogram play in passing, next following, and finally helping to decide upon the removal of the long intestinal tube, it is necessary that the individual in charge of its management be well trained in both the necessary fluoroscopic procedure and film interpretation. For this reason it becomes evident that the radiologist should be in charge of the Miller-Abbott tube. He in turn must actively cooperate with the surgeon and internist.

At the outset, the original diagnosis of intestinal obstruction and distention must be confirmed by him. The diagnosis made, it is he, because of his training with fluoroscopy and various roentgen methods, who should next be in charge of inserting the tube. After successful passage through the pylorus, and into the duodenum, he next follows the forward progress of the tube through the bowel. Eventually, when the forward progress of the tube ceases and a lesion is reached, he may inject barium down through the tube, coating the lesion and attempting to arrive at a diagnosis. Even after the cause of obstruction has been identified, further requirements are made of him. He must keep the surgeon and internist constantly informed as to the extent of distention, the progress of decompression, and the position of the tube. His obligations do not cease until the tube is finally removed.

General Principles of Intubation[5, 19, 20]

Intubation methods vary to some degree with the different types of tubes, and with different operators, but all have certain broad principles in common. Use of the long intestinal tube may be divided into four stages:

  (1) Nose to pylorus.
  (2) Pylorus to destination.
  (3) Diagnostic procedures at destination.
  (4) Withdrawal of tube.

These will be described in detail in the following sections.

Precautions

It should be emphasized that the actual performance of the procedure should be learned by the side of an experienced worker. The conditions dealt with are of an emergent character. They are not static. They are rapidly progressive, and the life of the patient may be at stake if the beginner unsuccessfully attempts to pass the tube.

A further general note of caution should be observed. A single individual should be assigned to the management of the tube, and should be held responsible. The method is time-consuming and difficult, and as already implied, requires active cooperation between the roentgenologist, surgeon and internist.

Before the tube is used, certain specific precautions should be observed:

The rubber tubing should not be soft and limp. It should maintain a certain degree of stiffness. Improper cleansing and sterilization tend to soften the rubber. All connections should be tight and all lumina unobstructed.

The balloon should not be too small when inflated. A small balloon has been found to curl the tip of the tube. Neither should the balloon be too large, since it can obstruct by overlapping the suction tip.

The silk that binds the balloon to the tube should be tied tightly, but care should be taken thereby not to obstruct the lumen.

After the balloon is attached, it should be inflated under water and tested for leaks. The suction side should again be tested for patency. It is also important at this point, to test the ability of the balloon to deflate. The tube connecting the balloon may be constricted by the thread holding the balloon. If the constriction is valvular, permitting entry of air into the balloon but not deflation, dangerous distention of the balloon may occur. When performing such tests, the same amount of air should be taken out of the balloon as put in. It is important that the lumina leading to the outside of the tube be labeled. Injecting liquid into the balloon by mistake is obviously dangerous and may make withdrawal impossible.

STAGE I. FROM NOSE THROUGH PYLORIC SPHINCTER

Because the fluoroscope can play so significant a role in the passage of the tube down the esophagus and into the stomach, and also because it is so useful in managing the passage of the tube through the pyloric sphincter, it would be well for the procedure to be started on the fluoroscopic table. Administration of fluids by venoclysis or hypodermoclysis may be started immediately as the patient is brought to the table and thereafter continued without interruption. The tip of the tube is lubricated. The rubber bag at its end is neatly folded back on itself. The tube is next passed via the nose through the esophagus and into the stomach.

With the tube positioned within the antral region of the stomach, the stomach should be emptied of its contents. This can be done with a large syringe inserted in the larger opening of the tube. During this time the tip of the tube may pass through the pyloric sphincter. When no further material can be withdrawn, *continuous* suction drainage should be connected to the suction side of the tube. Periodically the patient is fluoroscoped and, if necessary, attempts can be made to pass the tube through the pyloric sphincter.

Technical Aids

1. *Facilitating passage of the tube from nose through cardiac sphincter.* Local anesthesia may be applied to the larger nostril when necessary. The tube is then slowly fed through the nose. Passage down the esophagus to the stomach may be facilitated by having the patient suck some small pieces of ice.

2. *Emptying the stomach.* In dealing with obstructions of some duration, it is not always possible to empty the stomach completely. Reflux back into the stomach from the obstructed small bowel may be a complicating factor. In order to empty the

stomach in such cases it may be useful to have the patient lie on his left side. Suction should be continuous except to detach the tube once or twice each hour and wash the stomach with 50 to 100 cc. of warm water. As a result the stomach becomes deflated, regains its tone and peristalsis starts anew.

3. *Passage of the tube from cardiac sphincter to pyloric end of stomach* (figs. 402–407). With the tip of the tube within the stomach air bubble and coming to rest immediately beneath the cardiac sphincter, further passage of the tube within the gastric lumen may be observed fluoroscopically.

With the stomach in an empty state, the tube is slowly fed and the tip observed traveling towards the pyloric antrum. The direction from the cardiac sphincter towards the pyloric sphincter is *caudad* and to the patient's *right*. Any movement of the tube in the direction opposite—that is, away from the cardiac sphincter either *upwards* or towards the patient's *left* should immediately place the examiner on his guard that the tube may be following an improper course (figs. 402–405). He should, however, be mindful that in some instances the tube

could curl softly upwards and then run to the right along the greater curvature of the stomach to the pyloric end. A safe rule would be that any time the tip of the tube directs itself either upwards or to the left, the examiner should pull the tube back to the cardiac sphincter and start anew.

The examiner should bear in mind that visual proof that the tip of the tube is at the pyloric end of the stomach is secured when it is seen to have crossed the patient's spine and come to lie slightly to the *right of the spine*. The pyloric portion of the stomach is most often directed *posteriorly*, and thus visualization of the tip of the tube directed posteriorly, i.e., towards the spine, would be further assurance of its correct positioning at the pyloric end of the stomach. To visualize this fluoroscopically, the patient should be rotated so that his right side is down, and in this position (the right lateral decubitus) the image on the fluoroscopic screen will reveal if the tube is directed *posteriorly* (fig. 405).

4. *Passage through the pyloric sphincter.* The examiner may attempt under direct fluoroscopic vision to pass the tube through

---

402

The tip of the tube is observed pointing *upward* and toward the patient's *left*. With correct technic it should point towards the pyloric sphincter, which is caudad (*downward*) and to the patient's *right*. In this case further progress of the tube would be in the wrong direction, and passage through the sphincter would be difficult if not impossible.

404

The tube, misdirected as in figures 402, 403, is withdrawn and is now shown redirected in the proper direction. The tip is here seen to have reached the region of the pyloric sphincter. This is determined because the tip lies to the right of the spine (see text). The patient is in the supine position.

406

The tip of the tube, as it travels into the second or descending portion of the duodenal sweep, should continue to travel on the right side of the spine, but in a downward or caudad direction.

403

The tube, pointing in the wrong direction, with continued feeding, becomes curled in the stomach.

405

To make certain that the tip is passing *through the pylorus and into the duodenum*, the patient should be rotated into the lateral positon and the tip of the tube should be seen traveling posteriorly towards the spine. The first portion of the duodenum points in this backward direction.

407

The further passage of the tube completes the duodenal sweep and crosses back to the left side of the spine.

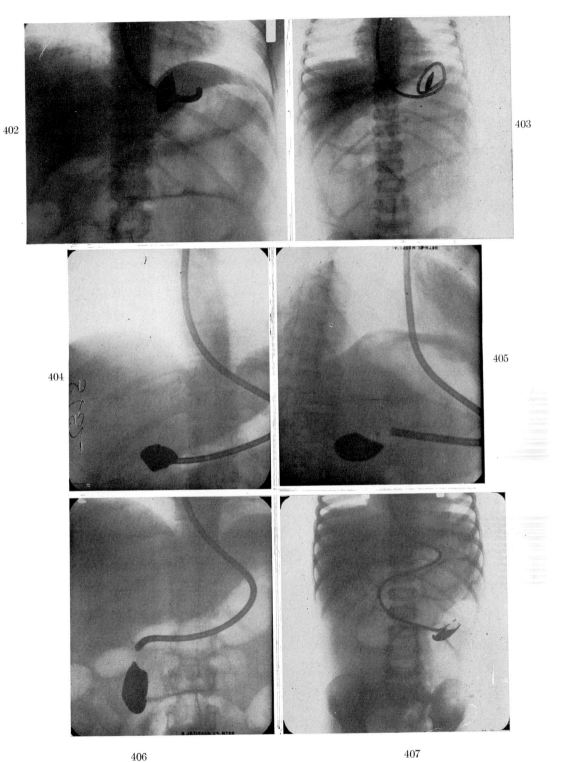

Passage of the tube through the pyloric sphincter.

(See legend, opposite page)

the pyloric sphincter. With the stomach empty, the tip of the tube should be pushed through the pylorus. The balloon, of course, at this point would be in a deflated state.

If difficulty is encountered in guiding the tube to its proper location at the pyloric end of the stomach, the aid of gravity may be enlisted by placing the patient with his right side down. In this position the pylorus is low and dependent and gravity will help carry the tip of the tube downwards towards the pyloric sphincter.

5. *Waiting for the tube to pass through the sphincter and aiding its passage.* If the tube does not readily pass through the sphincter, the patient is allowed to remain on the table, lying with his right side down, the tube still inserted. The examiner should then fluoroscope the patient again in three-quarters of an hour. With the stomach empty, and its tone regained, if the tip of the tube was properly located in the pyloric region, the stomach contractions may have carried the tube through into the duodenum. Some slack must be provided in order to allow the tube to travel. Several centimeters of slack tubing may be taped to the patient's forehead above its entrance at the nostril. A few centimeters of this slack tubing are swallowed during this waiting period, swallowing being assisted by either sucking a small piece of ice or sipping a small amount of water.

If upon inspection the tube has still not passed into the duodenum, an attempt may be made to pass the tube through the sphincter with the aid of direct fluoroscopic visualization and manipulation. Although in the main, having the patient lie on his right side is recommended, placing the patient in other positions, either prone, Trendelenberg, or erect may now be useful.

In most patients the tube will pass through the pyloric sphincter within 4 to 6 hours. It has taken as much as 48 hours. During this interval before the tube passes through the sphincter, the suction should be temporarily turned off and the stomach washed with 50 to 100 cc. of warm water. This should be done as previously directed approximately once each hour.

While waiting for the tube to pass, the examiner should *periodically* check the position of the tube and make certain it lies within the pyloric region, so that the tip may be in position to maneuver itself into the duodenum when gastric peristalsis is present.

If, during the *periodic* inspections, the tip of the tube is not within the gastric antrum, or, having arrived at the antrum, it becomes directed away from the pyloric sphincter (i.e., curled in an upwards direction, or curled or kinked on itself within the stomach) it should be pulled back to the cardiac sphincter. The examiner may inflate the balloon and pull the tube gently outward, recognizing that the sphincter is reached when he feels the characteristic tug of the distended balloon as it is pulled against the cardiac sphincter. This is confirmed under direct fluoroscopic vision. The subsequent re-passage of the tube from the cardiac sphincter to the pyloric end of the stomach is as described above, i.e., *downwards and to the right.*

When necessary, gastric peristalsis may be stimulated by having the patient drink a glass of warm water. A liquid which is more to the patient's liking may be more effective.

Before passing to the next stage, a word of caution is advisable. When fluoroscopy is to play an important role in the handling of the long intestinal tube, an accurate record should be kept of the radiation received by patient and examiner. (See the danger of over-radiation, and precautionary measures, Chapter I.)

STAGE II. PROGRESS OF THE TUBE FROM PYLORIC SPHINCTER TO DESTINATION

Determining Position of Tube in the Duodenum

With the apparent passage of the tip of the tube through the pyloric sphincter it is important to determine its position in the duodenum before the tube makes further progress.

An understanding of the normal anatomy of the duodenum and the duodenal sweep is necessary in order to correctly visualize the course of the tube within the region. (Variations in the duodenal sweep are described on page 179 and in figs. 233–236.)

The first portion of the duodenum continues the backward direction initiated within the pyloric region of the stomach (fig. 405). Except in obese individuals or patients with hypertonic stomachs, the junction of the first and second parts of the duodenum is at the posterior abdominal wall, i.e., immediately to the right of the spine and in the same plane as the spine (figs. 404, 405). In the obese patient, this junction is also in the posterior abdomen and to the right of the spine, but in a plane *anterior* to the spine.

To prove the position of the tube as within the first portion of the duodenum, the tube, as seen in the frontal position, should be slightly to the right of the spine (fig. 404); that is, it has passed through the pylorus, which lies to the right of the spine. Next, the patient is rotated into a lateral position so that he is lying with his right side down. The tip of the tube should now be seen directed posteriorly and approaching the spine (fig. 405).

The descending or second portion of the duodenum next travels downwards to the right of the spine. In normal and long, thin individuals, the second or descending portion of the duodenum is behind the peritoneum and, resting on the posterior abdominal wall, travels downward in line with the spine. In stocky patients it also travels down to the right of the spine, but in a plane slightly anterior to the spinal column.

To determine whether the tip of the tube is within the second or descending portion of the duodenum, in the frontal position it is again seen slightly to the right of the spine but directed *downwards* (fig. 406).

With the patient in the lateral position, his right side down, the tube will be either in the same plane as the spine or slightly anterior to it.

Another method useful in determining whether the tube is in the duodenum is to aspirate some of the contents and test their reaction. If the secretions are bile-tinged, and the reaction alkaline, the tube may be assumed to be within the duodenum. An acid reaction would indicate that the tube is still within the stomach. Regurgitation of alkaline- or bile-stained secretions from the duodenum into the stomach should be borne in mind.

Also useful for determining the position of the tube is to inflate the balloon with 20 to 30 cc. of air. The expanding balloon would meet the resistance of the duodenal walls and this would be transmitted to the examiner as a resistance in the plunger of the hand syringe.

Technical Aids in Final Progress of Tube[21]

It might be said that once the tip of the tube reaches the third portion of the duodenum its forward progress is almost automatic. With the maintenance of suction and periodic lavage the intestinal contents are removed and distention of successive loops diminished. In cases of simple mechanical obstruction, the tube may be in the terminal ileum, if this be the location of the lesion, in 12 to 36 hours or less. The progress of the tube in adynamic ileus is slower. In this condition, several days may be required until the tip of the tube reaches the cecum. During this process the patient becomes progressively more comfortable and is permitted food. The food must be of the type that will not obstruct the tube. It should also help to keep the serum protein and electrolytic balance intact. Factors concerned in the second stage:

1. *Provision of tube slack.* The progress of the tube may become quite rapid and sufficient loose tubing must be provided. From 8 to 10 inches of tubing is left slack

and fastened to the forehead or cheek. A slight excess may be present in the stomach. The exact length of tubing which should be passed into the stomach during any period is difficult to determine. The role of the examiner should be to make certain that not enough slack is present in the stomach to allow knotting or prolapse of an extra loop through the pylorus. The forward progress of the tube can be stopped should this occur. Frequent x-ray films and fluoroscopic observation are useful in making this determination. In general, the tube should be passed into the stomach at approximately the same rate as it is passing out through the pyloric sphincter. By this method it is hoped that not enough tubing accumulates to prolapse or knot. Approximately six inches of tubing may be introduced every hour or two, depending on the patient's peristalsis. The forward progress of the tube is in proportion to the rate and strength of peristalsis within the bowel, the tip advancing in this way until the obstructing lesion is encountered. At this point, forward progress ceases. In the absence of small bowel obstruction, the tube will pass into the cecum and colon.

Some reefing of the intestine on the tube may be expected as the tube progressively passes through the small bowel loops. Excessive reefing, however, is undesirable.

2. *The inflated balloon, suction, drainage, feeding, electrolytic balance.* Since satisfactory progress of the tube depends upon the maintenance of the balloon in an inflated state, it is important that the balloon be frequently tested for leaks. Periodically, air should be withdrawn and next reinjected. The amount withdrawn should be the same as when the balloon was last inflated. It is recommended that 20 to 40 cc. of air be used, the exact amount depending up on the width of the bowel lumen that the balloon is in. With continuous progress of the tube suction drainage is maintained. It would be wise to keep accurate records of the amount of drainage since this is an index of fluid and chlorides lost. These must be replaced.

Once the tip of the tube has passed the duodenum, mouth feeding may commence. Feeding should have electrolytic balance, vitamins and protein replacements as its aim. Foods, given orally, should thus be given with the necessary amount of salt and only such foods given so that the residue can be removed by suction and not block the tube. A low residue diet should be used. A satisfactory diet is suggested by Noer and Johnston.[22]

3. *Determining progress of deflation of gas distended loops.* As a result of the continuous suction taking place while the tube makes progress through the small bowel, a diminution in both the number of gas distended loops as well as narrowing of the caliber of the gas dilated loops occurs. This can be appraised by roentgen ray examination performed at least once over 24 hours.

In the absence of complicating factors, when the tip of the tube is believed to be arrested at the obstructing lesion, gaseous distention should progressively become less until no longer present. If distention persists, and no complications have arisen and it is known that the suction has been effective up to the point of arrest, then it must be assumed that the tip of the tube had not yet reached the obstructing lesion and failure to progress is probably due to some reflex disturbance, deflation of the balloon, etc. It may be that the tip of the tube had reached one point of obstruction and yet one or more other obstructions are present more distally. The distention may also be due to complicating factors such as peritonitis.

A loop of bowel obstructed at both ends such as occurs in the presence of a volvulus, would remain distended since the decompression tube could not enter into the loop. The balance of the distended small bowel would, however, become deflated.

If after the tube is arrested and the bowel is apparently decompressed, should distention recur, the tube should be pulled back to a level immediately above the site of distention and permitted on its way again, consultation with the surgeon and internist being made. Possible causes would include peritonitis, hypoproteinemia or hypovitaminosis.

It should be further noted that although satisfactory deflation of the small bowel may occur, yet the gas distention in the large bowel which may exist concurrently cannot be handled in the same way. Even with the tube within the cecum the large bowel fails to deflate. This is probably due to the character of the cecal contents, i.e. being too thick to pass upwards through the tube. *Deflation of the small intestine does not deflate the large bowel.*

4. *Determining the progress of the tube.* The progress of the tube should be observed by fluoroscoping the patient and by taking films. This should be performed at least once daily.

In rare instances the progress of the tube may be so slow that the examiner may believe that an obstruction is reached. In cases of paralytic ileus, it may take several days for the tube to reach its destination in the cecum.

Should the tip of the tube become arrested before the cecum is reached, this would suggest an obstructive lesion involving the small bowel. This, however, does not exclude a concurrent lesion more distally. In the event that a definite decision regarding large bowel obstruction cannot be made, a barium enema of the colon bowel may be advisable.

Figiel claims that coiling of the tube in the small intestine should be regarded as absolute evidence of obstruction,[31] even though previous studies of the small bowel were regarded as normal. The coiling occurs, he explains, because the leading end of the tube reaches the point of obstruction, and further progress is prevented. The continued peristaltic activity in the small bowel carries additional tubing into the obstructed area, thus, forcing the leading end of the tube to turn backwards on itself. As more tubing enters the area of obstruction, coiling of the tube will start.

5. *Determining arrest of the tube.* In order to determine whether the tube is advancing or not, various observations are useful. (1) The amount of slack left from the patient's nose to the forehead is observed. When no additional tubing is drawn into the nose, that would tend to indicate the forward progress of the tube had stopped. (2) Should the examiner now attempt to gently push more of the tube into the stomach and intestine, regurgitation of the tube out of the nose is apt to occur. (3) Estimating the length of the tube on the film is also useful in determining the arrest of its forward progress. Unchanged length on consecutive studies would indicate no advancement.

Reefing of the bowel onto the tube should, however, be borne in mind.

In summary, if observation suggests arrest of the forward progress of the tube, confirmation may be secured by the injection of opaque suspension. This will be described in Stage III. Also, sharp angulation and fixation of a loop of small intestine adjacent to a colonic lesion may result in false stoppage of the tube. In the case of colonic lesion, a reflex spastic obstruction of the terminal ileum may occur.

Stage III. Injection of Barium

When the observer believes that the forward progress of the tube has stopped, opaque material may be injected. An attempt is thereby made to determine, first, whether a point of obstruction has been reached, and second, when possible, the nature of the obstructing lesion. If possible the injection of the material should be performed on the fluoroscopic table.

Before the barium is injected, the balloon must first be deflated. This is done in order to permit the barium to pass distal to the balloon and by coming into contact with the lesion, outline it. Thin barium mixture, 50 to 100 cc., is injected through the tube. Should the opaque material not advance, although the balloon is deflated, an attempt should be made to stimulate intestinal peristalsis by alternately inflating and deflating the balloon. As peristalsis returns, the opaque material is then propelled to the narrow segment ahead of the tube tip. Experience then shows that no small bowel obstruction is complete in the strict sense of the word.

In the presence of an obstructive lesion, search is made for the lesion when the opaque media arrives at the pathologic site. Some of the characteristics of the lesions are outlined below. The fluoroscopic skill of the examiner now comes into play.

The opaque media may collect in a mass at the site of the lesion, or regurgitate backward along the intestine. Regionally, hyperperistalsis and general increased activity may be seen fluoroscopically.[23] Films made at later intervals reveal some barium to have passed beyond the obstructed lesion.

In order to bring the lesion into profile, fluoroscopically, the region must be carefully and gently manipulated, overlapping loops displaced, and the patient properly positioned. Films should be taken to confirm the fluoroscopic findings. Graduated compression of the opacified loops may aid in demonstrating abnormalities in the mucosal pattern, but, again, film examination must confirm the finding.

Some of the possible findings[23] which may be outlined by the barium are:

1. *Is the tube tip in the cecum?* It is usually possible to tell whether the tube tip has entered the cecum or not. When doubt arises, injection of barium suspension clears the dilemma. The mucosal pattern and the outline of the pouchlike cecum are then observed.

2. *Obstruction produced by adhesion.* An adhesion produces a short, narrow kink in the intestine. The mucosal pattern within the region appears normal.

3. *Strangulation.* Strangulation causes congestion and edema of the wall. As a result, the mucosal folds are flattened, widened and occasionally obliterated. It may be impossible to distinguish this from inflammation.

4. *Inflammation.* Inflammation involving the intestine intrinsically causes partial obliteration and coarsening of the mucosal folds within this narrowed region. If a short narrow segment is involved, such inflammation is difficult to distinguish from tumor, since in both instances the mucous membrane may be destroyed. (See fig. 321D, page 236.)

5. *Malignant tumor.* A malignant tumor, by invading the mucous membrane, distorts or obliterates the mucosal pattern. (See fig. 321E, page 237).

In cases of paralytic ileus, the barium injected into the small bowel will slowly pass to the cecum.

Factors Involved in Stage III

1. In small bowel obstruction, the question may arise as to the advisability of administering barium by mouth for diagnostic purposes. As described above, barium can be used in small amounts, but it is not recommended here when the long intestinal tube is not concurrently used. Some disadvantages of its use may be listed. The opaque material may become sufficiently diluted by the fluid in the small bowel as to lose diagnostic detail. Also, peristalsis in the dilated obstructed small intestine *may* not be sufficient to materially propel the barium solution down through the various loops of bowel. Finally, especially if *large bowel obstruction has not been excluded*, barium must not be given by mouth. Not only may this convert a partial obstruction in the colon into a complete obstruction, but in subsequent surgery the barium at the site would interfere with proper surgical technique.

2. However, although not recommended, the injection of barium in the presence of small bowel obstruction has produced no deleterious effects within the small bowel itself. It seems that within these loops the barium remains in a more or less fluid state and the obstruction itself is not really complete.[21, 24]

Observations at the Time of the Barium Injection

1. It should be remembered that a considerable part of the small intestine proximal to the point of obstruction is probably telescoped upon the tube. As a result, when the balloon is deflated, a considerable portion of this telescoped bowel may migrate distally carrying the lesion with it. The false impression may be gotten that no obstruction exists. The opaque media will be seen to travel distal to where the balloon was situated and the point of obstruction thus is often found some distance ahead of the tip of the tube.

2. Fluoroscopic observations are made with the aid of palpation. The patient's position should be changed in order to help the barium advance. Spot films should be made.

In some instances barium is seen to advance only as the patient is rotated. When this occurs, suspicion of a kink should arise.

3. In some cases, while barium is seen to pass a point of incomplete obstruction, distention of a loop immediately proximal to the lesion will persist. This is apt to occur when the obstruction is of long standing and the lumen permanently widened.

4. The segment of bowel distal to the obstructed lesion should be of normal width. When this is not the case, the possibility of a more distal lesion should be considered. This is especially the case if fluid and gas are present beyond the point of obstruction. Under these conditions, further observation by films and fluoroscopy should be continued until the opaque media has had a chance to reach the obstructed lesion. If the distance is great, the barium may become sufficiently diluted as to lose its diagnostic value.

5. When the examination is completed, where desired, barium remaining proximal to the lesion may be removed by suction and irrigation.

In summary, it should be borne in mind that the barium injection is useful in determining the presence or absence of a lesion. Although in many instances the demonstration of sharp angulation of the bowel with incomplete obstruction is suggestive of adhesions, yet often the exact nature of the obstructing lesion may not be demonstrated.

STAGE IV. REMOVAL OF THE TUBE[25]

Before the tube is removed, the cause for the obstruction should be dealt with. Intestinal tonus and peristaltic activity must be restored. The patient must be able to take food with the tube clamped off. A useful procedure is to clamp the suction tube for about 3 to 4 hours at a time 4 times daily and observe whether the distention recurs. Employing this technique, mild partial obstructions may be overlooked.

The use of roentgen methods of examination makes the determination as to the removal of the tube more exact. The cause of the obstruction having been dealt with, a thin barium mixture is injected. The suction is turned off and the tube clamped. Periodic inspection of the opaque media within the abdomen is made. At 5 hours the progress of the barium mixture is observed. Although each case should be individualized the possible findings at this time are:

1. With complete obstruction distal to the tube, the barium will collect in a pool at the site of the lesion. The cause of the obstruction has not been dealt with and needs further treatment. The tube is not removed. Where so desired, the opaque media may be removed with either suction or irrigated with normal saline through the tube.

2. With partial obstruction, some puddling will appear at the site of the lesion, but some barium will also pass through. Further observation, the condition of the patient permitting, is made every few hours. At 24 hours, barium will still be present at the site of the lesion, but a small quantity of barium will also be present distal to it and in the colon. In the presence of partial obstruction the tube is not yet ready to be removed.

3. In those cases where the tube is ready to be removed, direct fluoroscopic observation during the passage of the opaque media, will reveal no hold-ups. Observation in 5 hours will usually demonstrate conclusive evidence of marked barium deposits distal to the apparent site of the lesion, i.e., in the cecum or colon.

4. In cases of doubt, the patient should be kept under close observation. *The 24-hour observation is important.* For example, an occasional case of post-operative stomal edema may reveal at the 5 hour study some hold-up at the site of the anastomosis with a thin streaking of barium in the colon. At 24 hours, large amounts of barium will be seen in the colon.

Care should be exercised in removing the tube. The balloon should be deflated and the withdrawal should be slow. Reverse intussusception may be a complication. During withdrawal the position of the tube and the possible presence of kinks and knots should be checked fluoroscopically. If at any time during withdrawal, difficulty is encountered, further fluoroscopic observation should be made immediately.

COMPLICATIONS

1. Pain and soreness of the nose, throat, larynx and ear are common. Anesthetic sprays, chewing gum, sucking lozenges or small sips of water are helpful.

2. As a result of feeding the tubing too rapidly or sometimes with excessive gagging or retching, knots may form in the tube. If left alone they may untie themselves within the stomach. This complication can be seen fluoroscopically. If it does not correct itself the tube should be withdrawn.

3. A particle of food may obstruct the lumen of the aspirating tube. Washing the tube by carefully injecting water and again aspirating may successfully clear it. If this maneuver is not successful, the tube should be withdrawn until the particle is outside the nose. It can then be milked out.

4. A complication to be avoided by proper care is the injection of any liquid into the lumen connected with the balloon. The balloon distended with fluid could not be aspirated or withdrawn and surgical withdrawal may become necessary.

5. The entire tube may be swallowed. This is usually harmless. In the majority of cases the tube will pass by rectum. Transit time may vary from 4 hours to 29 days.[26]

6. Continuous pressure of the tube in one region of the small intestine has caused perforation of the bowel.[27] Prolonged intubation should be accompanied by frequent roentgenographic and fluoroscopic check-ups. When necessary, the tube may be withdrawn for short distances, and reinserted after a day.

7. The greatest trouble in the use of the tube is delay in the passage through the pylorus. This has been facilitated by substituting mercury for the air within the balloon.[28] Magnetic alloys have also been applied to the tip of the tube, and with the aid of a magnet, the tip of the tube led through the pylorus.[29]

ADHESIONS

Abdominal adhesions are one of the more common causes for either partial or complete intestinal obstruction. They follow inflammatory diseases, occur postoperatively, and may follow abdominal trauma. Congenital bands (see below) produce similar changes.

The adhesive process may exist between loops of bowel, neighboring bowel and adjacent viscera. They may also be present between intestinal loops and the abdominal wall. In the presence of small bowel adhesions, the examiner is unable to manually separate one loop of the bowel from another. When intestinal segments are bound to either a viscus or abdominal wall, no amount of maneuvering, or palpation can separate them (figs. 408–411). An important maneuver in the diagnosis of adhesions, then, is to *prove an inability to separate the adherent parts.*

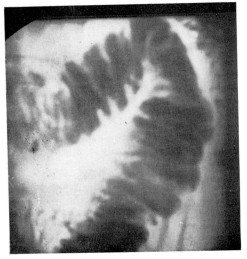

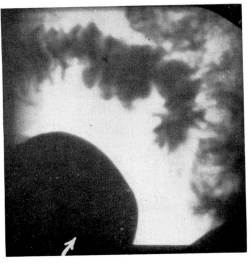

408

Adhesions are suspected in this loop of bowel.

409

Palpation distorts and displaces the limbs of the loop. The distortion and displacement are normally consistent with the direction of the force applied. The palpating finger (arrow) thus shows that adhesions are not present. (Cf. figs. 410, 411.)

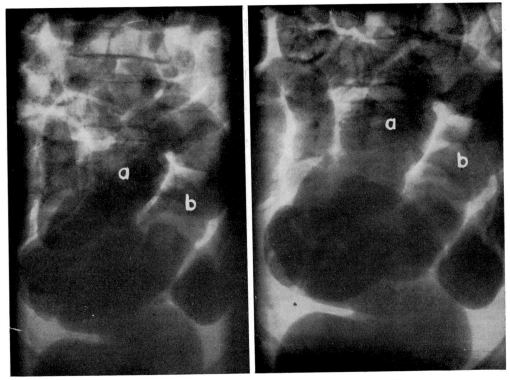

410

Loops of bowel *a* and *b* are suspected of being bound by adhesions.

411

Graduated compression and manipulation could not change the relative positions of the loops, thus confirming the presence of adhesions. (Cf. figs. 408, 409.) Upon changing the patient's posture, these loops still remain immobile and in their same relative positions.

Radiographic Findings. Adhesions reveal themselves as short constricted segments produced by kinks or twists in the bowel. The mucous membrane pattern is normal. Adhesions may be present, yet cause no symptoms. Examination should take place *only during symptom-producing periods.* When symptoms appear, partial or complete obstruction is present.

A more extensive discussion of adhesions will be found on pages 308–311.

BANDS

The most common site for abnormal bands of the membranes are the duodenum, ileum, cecum and ascending colon. Most of them are found in the ileo-cecal region. They are found at any age, and are frequently found in adults. The condition seems to be more common in the female sex. Valuable information is found by fluoroscopic examination, which permits a study of the fixation or mobility of the organs, and their movements under pressure and during respiration. The examination is made in the erect and recumbent positions. Visualization of the bands and membranes is not possible, but their presence is suggested by (1) impairment of mobility because of fixation, (2) displacement of the involved segment, (3) adherence of bowel loops so that there is difficulty in separating them and (4) stages and varying degrees of obstruction.

The Gallbladder

Fundamentals

ANATOMY (Fig. 412)

THE GALLBLADDER is a sac-like pear-shaped structure located beneath the liver, above the hepatic flexure of the colon and to the right side of the first portion of the duodenum. It consists of a fundus, a body, infundibulum, neck and cystic duct (fig. 412). The cystic duct and the hepatic duct combine to form the common bile duct, which normally enters the duodenum at the sphincter of Oddi. It should be borne in mind that occasionally the common duct and the pancreatic duct open into a duodenal diverticulum.[15] This variation, recognized, should not be a cause for confusion.

The gallbladder, when filled with dye, appears as a homogeneous, smooth, pear-shaped shadow. (However, in the erect position this homogeneity presents a layered effect, as seen in figure 413.) In the main, this homogeneous appearance indicates a gallbladder without structural defect. Nevertheless, as will be described below, papillomata, polyps, calculi, and other pathological lesions may be so engulfed in the opaque media that they are not visible in conventional studies. Special technics, both fluoroscopic and radiographic, are necessary to demonstrate such "inundated" pathology. Further, before a decision as to normalcy of the gallbladder can be made, contraction of the sac after taking a fatty meal must be appraised, a procedure to be described in the next section of this chapter.

Shape. Generally, the gallbladder appears as pear-shaped. Its shape, however, may vary with the individual habitus. In the hypersthenic individual it is normally more rounded, whereas in the asthenic it tends to be elongated and narrowed.

Position. In the hypersthenic individual the gallbladder is usually found higher in the abdomen, located more laterally under the costal arch and disposed in a more or less horizontal fashion.

In asthenic individuals, it is usually closer to the spine, parallel to the spine and on occasion may even be projected on to the shadow of the spine. It may be located deep down in the pelvis (fig. 414). It has been found in the left side of the abdomen.[17, 18]

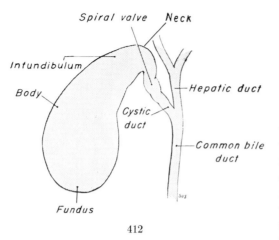

412

Anatomy of the gallbladder and its ducts.

Rarely, the gallbladder may be absent.[19]

Size. The gallbladder is about the size of a large hen egg.

In hypersthenic individuals it may appear smaller and rounder. This *apparent* size, however, may often be caused by foreshortening. What actually is seen, is the rounded fundus of the gallbladder directed towards the examiner, while the infundibular apical portion is hidden behind the rounded fundus. Turning the patient into the oblique position behind the fluoroscopic screen will reveal the pear-shaped sac in profile (figs. 415, 416) and give a truer picture of the size.

In asthenic individuals, the gallbladder may be somewhat elongated.

The gallbladder's size is further influenced by its tone, the atonic gallbladder hanging low and being of greater dimension.

It may be enlarged as a result of obstruction of the common duct.

Finally, its roentgenologic size may also vary with the period of examination, depending upon the degree of filling with the dye.

Contour. The gallbladder is normally extremely smooth, with no real indentures or irregularities. Irregularity of contour should

suggest abnormality. Adhesions do not produce any considerable degree of irregularity.[3] The phrygian or bilocular gallbladder may be considered a normal variant.

Mobility. This may be estimated by changing the position of the patient. By simultaneously opacifying the stomach and the gallbladder, and manipulating both these organs while the patient is behind the fluoroscopic screen, the examiner is able to determine fixation or adhesions of either in regard to the other. In similar fashion, fixation and adhesions of the gallbladder to the opacified hepatic flexure may also be determined fluoroscopically.

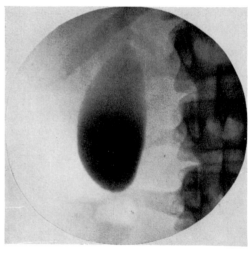

413

The normal opacified gallbladder is commonly described as a homogeneous shadow.

Question:

This patient is examined in the *erect* position. The shadow of the gallbladder is not homogeneous, being denser at the fundus. Is this gallbladder normal?

Answer:

There is lack of homogeneity, i.e., a layering effect is seen. The normal opacified gallbladder in the *erect* position reveals that the heavier bile constituents have settled to the bottom, while the lighter constituents remain above. This is normal.

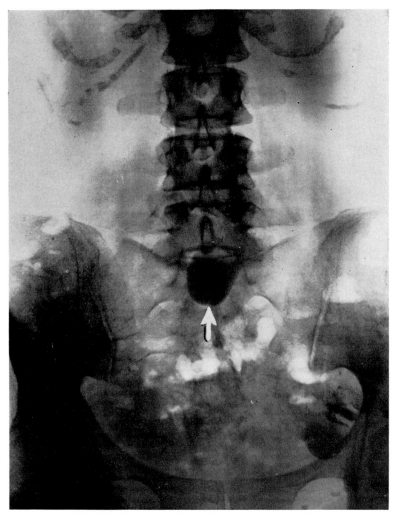

414

The gallbladder is commonly expected to be situated in the right upper quadrant.

Question:

Is the gallbladder in its "normal" position?

Answer:

In asthenic individuals, *absence* of the gallbladder in the right upper quadrant is within normal limits. In these individuals it is not unusual for the gallbladder to be situated deep in the pelvis, overlapping the spine.

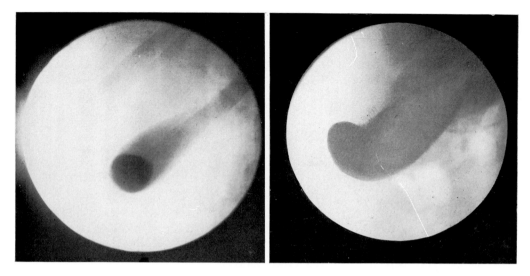

415

Is a gallstone present in the fundus of the gall-bladder? (see fig. 416).

416

Under direct fluoroscopic vision, rotating the patient, the apparent density seen in figure 415 is found to be produced by a kink in the fundus, and overlap of the kinked portion on the body of the gallbladder.

Fluoroscopic Procedures in the Normal

POSITIONING IN GALLBLADDER FLUOROSCOPY AND RADIOGRAPHY

Fluoroscopic Aids (Figs. 417–420)

The fluoroscopic procedure is a valuable adjunct in the radiographic examination of the gallbladder. Prior to filming, *direct fluoroscopic visualization* of the gallbladder will enable the patient to be so arranged in each of the positions desired for radiography that regional confusing shadows (i.e., gas, fecal material, or spine) may be rotated out of the field.

The value of spot filming the gallbladder during direct fluoroscopic visualization should be stressed. Filming at this time is valuable because of the maneuvers available to the examiner during direct fluoroscopic observation not otherwise obtainable. Thus, the examiner by graduated compression of the gallbladder is enabled to manually thin

the overlying opaque media, thereby causing underlying obscure shadows to be made visible. Gas and occasional fecal shadows may also be displaced manually or with a pressure cone.

Fluoroscopic Examination with the Patient in the Erect Position

Various positions for fluoroscoping and filming of the gallbladder are available. These include prone, supine, oblique and right lateral decubitus. Special mention will be made of the upright position (a subject to be enlarged upon further in the section on "Negative Shadows within the Gall-bladder").

With the patient standing and facing the examiner, the gallbladder sac is anteriorly located and separated from the fluoroscopic screen by the anterior abdominal wall. In this position, the gallbladder lends itself admirably to palpation and manipulation. In

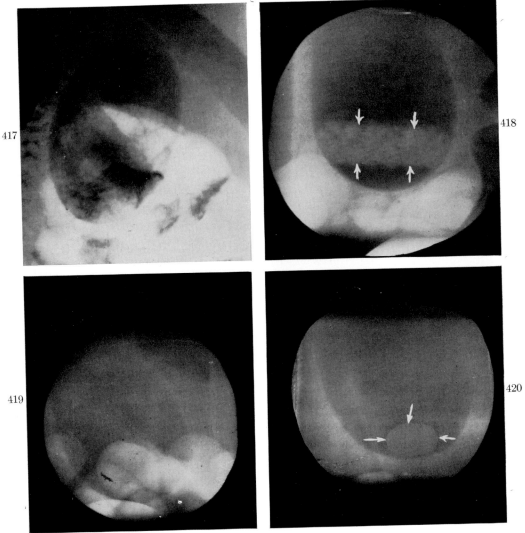

417

Overlying gas shadows may cause difficulty in appraising pathology within the gallbladder.

418

Under direct fluoroscopic vision, the patient in the erect position is rotated until the overlying confusing shadows are thrown free of the gallbladder. Compression and spot films in this position reveal the presence of a layer of calculi.

419

Again, gallbladder pathology, is hidden by overlapping confusing shadows.

420

The patient in the erect position, under direct fluoroscopic vision, is rotated so that confusing shadows are no longer present. The gallbladder is compressed, and spot films taken reveal a solitary calculus in the fundus of the gallbladder.

the occasional case where regional shadows are confusing, such palpation and manipu- lation overcomes the difficulty. If gas bubbles are the source of confusion, the air-filled colon drops below the region of the gallbladder and any distended intestinal loops or stomach can be gently pushed aside by the pressure cone or the palpating hand. These maneuvers leave the gallbladder area clear for inspection and subsequent spot filming. Confusing shadows from calcifying chondral cartilage may be differentiated by asking the patient to breathe. Any structure in the rib cartilage will move *up* with inspiration, whereas any structure in the gallbladder is pushed *down* during inspiration by the descending diaphragm.

According to the "law of the circle" (described in the chapter on Chest, p. 19ff) with the patient erect, *posteriorly* placed opaque renal calculi when located fluoroscopically *will rotate in the same direction as the spine*, whereas shadows within the gallbladder, being *anterior*, will rotate in the same direction as the *anterior abdominal wall*.

The erect position is also useful in helping make visible small stones, papillomata, and polyps when not clearly seen. The rationale is described presently in the section on "Negative Shadows within the Gallbladder."

In occasional cases, the mobility of negative defects within the confines of the gallbladder must be determined in order to establish a diagnosis. Thus, a negative defect produced by a gallstone is expected to be freely mobile. A similar defect produced by a polyp or papilloma is fixed. Tests for mobility include not only changing the patient from the prone to erect positions, but manipulating the gallbladder during fluoroscopy and proving the mobility or immobility of the shadow in question by immediate spot filming.[15]

It should be re-emphasized that when negative defects within the gallbladder are tested by changing the position of the patient to observe a possible shift, 5 to 10 minutes should be permitted after the patient stands for this rearrangement to occur.

CHOLECYSTOGRAPHY

Rationale

Certain drugs, because they can be excreted by the liver, are useful in hepatic function tests. Mixed with bile such a drug subsequently enters the gallbladder. When they are opaque to the x-ray, they can be used to visualize the gallbladder. Such drugs are today commercially available as Telepaque, Orabilex and Oragraphin.

Technic of Examination

Cholecystography has been performed by both oral and intravenous routes.

Oral Cholecystography

Oral cholecystography may be divided into five stages: 1. Preparation. 2. Direct examination of abdomen before the administration of contrast material. 3. Administration of contrast material. 4. Examination after the administration of contrast material. 5. Examination with contrast material and fatty meal.

1. *Preparation.* In preparing the patient for cholecystography the aim is to rid the abdomen of confusing shadows, such as fecal material or gas, which might otherwise interfere with the gallbladder examination either before or after opacification. A suitable laxative for such preparation should be mild, so as not to excite gas formation. Cascara sagrada fulfills this requirement and should be given for 2 days *prior* to preliminary filming (Stage 2). Enemas are generally not given when oral cholecystography is done.

Where preliminary filming (i.e., before opacification of the gallbladder) or filming after administration of contrast material to opacify the gallbladder reveals confusing fecal shadows, an enema may be given. When enemas are given, it is important to be aware of the air which may be injected at the same time.

2. *Direct Examination of the Abdomen before Administration of Contrast Material.* The patient, as described in the preceding

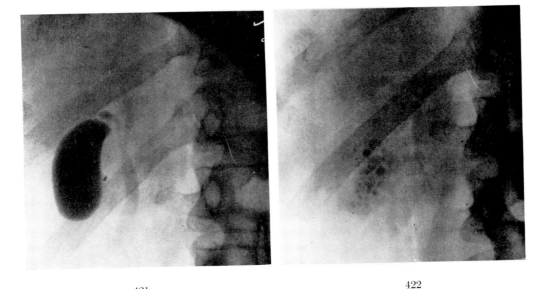

421   422

Question:

   The gallbladder here is homogeneous and without defect. Can calculi still be present?

Answer:

   This is the same patient examined without contrast material. Calculi are present.

Comment: Occasionally the examiner may take a "short cut" and content himself with examining the gallbladder after dye has been given. The gallbladder should always be examined both *before* and *after* the administration of contrast material. The opaque material may enter the gallbladder and blot out calculi and thus render the shadow homogeneous. Without a preliminary film wherein no dye was given, the stones would have been missed.

section, having been cleansed by a laxative taken for the two previous days, a film of the abdomen is taken *before* the gallbladder is opacified. This examination may demonstrate opaque gallstones, abnormal renal shadows, masses in the abdomen, bony involvements, undue gas or fecal shadows, etc. (figs. 421, 422).

   3. *Administration of Contrast Material.* After the above-mentioned film is taken, the patient's gallbladder is next opacified. Drugs in common use today are, as already noted, Telepaque and Oragraphin. Such a dye should be administered enough in advance that films of the gallbladder can be conveniently taken 10 to 18 hours afterwards. The average dose of these preparations is approximately 1 tablet for each 25 lbs. of body weight. It is recommended that at no time should the dose exceed 12 tablets.

   Varying technics of administration have

been used. However, a satisfactory method has been to take a full dose at approximately 4 o'clock in the afternoon and to have the same amount administered a second time at 8:00 P.M., examination next being performed the following morning at 9:00 A.M.

   At each of these times the tablets are taken 1 every 5 minutes until the total required amount has been completed. A non-fatty meal at the same time may help the patient swallow the pills. After the second set of pills has been taken (8 P.M.) the patient should be instructed not to have any further food and to appear at the office at the required time the next morning.

   Other methods of dye administration vary from one complete dose of the dye one day prior to the examination, to fractional methods wherein the patient receives divided doses of dye on two days prior to examination.[4, 5] The theory of this interrupted technic is that some of the dye passing from the liver to the gallbladder finds its way into the intestines, from which it is reabsorbed into the blood stream and again carried to the liver. If the timing is such that additional dye given by mouth and absorbed from the intestines into the blood stream meets with the reabsorbed dye, the result is said to be fortification and better gallbladder visualization.

Further differences of opinion exist as to whether a fatty meal should be given prior to the oral administration of contrast material. Since dye entering a gallbladder already full of concentrated bile would become diluted it seems wise to first rid the gallbladder sac of this obstacle. A fatty meal, taken about 6 hours prior to administration of contrast material, performs this function, and is especially indicated in patients on a fat-free diet who recently have not adequately emptied the gallbladder.

4. *Examination after the Administration of Contrast Material.* Films should be taken, as recommended in texts on roentgenology, in the prone, oblique, right lateral decubitus and erect positions. This immediate filming may be completed at one time. Because optimum visualization occurs 10 to 18 hours following oral administration of dye, filming at hourly or 2-hourly intervals has also been recommended.

It is intended here to emphasize the fluoroscopic aid that may be secured.

In any of the positions employed, it is advantageous for the patient *first* to be fluoroscoped and the opacified gallbladder located. When clearly seen and free of overlapping gas or other confusing shadows (e.g., spine), it can be spot filmed. Further, the positioning of the patient for the subsequent conventional film examination would correspond to that degree of obliquity determined as optimum during direct fluoroscopic visualization (figs. 417–420).

Further discussion of fluoroscopic findings and technics will be dealt with below.

5. *Examination with Contrast Material and Fatty Meal.* The gallbladder having been visualized as homogeneous and smooth, a fatty meal is next administered. The meal recommended consists of two eggs and a glass of milk (eggnog). Other fatty meals have been used, but that recommended here has been found to be more certain to contract the gallbladder in a relatively short period of time. It is important that whatever mixture is used be palatable. The patient may be fluoroscoped and films taken 30 minutes after drinking it.

The purpose of the fatty meal is twofold. *First*, it is essential to observe shrinking of the gallbladder shadow during its *contraction phase*. This gives some clue as to its function. *Secondly*, while small stones and papillomata are occasionally missed because they are hidden by large amounts of opaque material, the gallbladder in its contraction phase partially empties and leaves a lessened amount of dye to overlie these shadows. With diminution in the amount of overlying opaque media, the *underlying gallstones, etc., may more easily be seen*[6] (figs. 423, 424, page 354).

As described below, when the contracted gallbladder is examined *fluoroscopically*, graduated compression is a further valuable aid in thinning the overlying media. It should, however, be emphasized that *excessive pressure* may not only rid the region pressed upon of all of its dye, thereby making it invisible, but may also *push the possible underlying calculus out of the field.*

Contraction Phase: Within one-half hour after the above recommended fatty meal, the normal gallbladder may exhibit about 50 per cent diminution in size. Others may fail to empty for hours. Delayed emptying of the gallbladder may especially occur if the patient is starved or has been living primarily on carbohydrates. Functional derangements, too, such as spasm of the sphincter of Oddi, may play a role in delayed emptying, although organic disease be absent.

In pancreatic disease, the common duct may be encroached upon by an enlarged or edematous pancreas, with resultant poor emptying of a well opacified gallbladder.

Biliary dyskinesia is a condition associated with poor emptying. It is manifested by a gallbladder which fills well and reveals good opacification but fails to contract after a fatty meal.

Intravenous Cholecystography (Cholangiography)

The intravenous method of cholecystography has been somewhat facilitated by employing Cholografin. The oral method is, however, simpler, easier, more acceptable to patients and less hazardous.

Nevertheless, in selected cases, by employing intravenous methods, radiographic impressions of the gallbladder have been obtained in a significant percentage of cases which failed to opacify with oral media. This is a supplementary method. It gives no information regarding the function of the gallbladder and it indicates patency of the cystic duct.[20] For practical purposes, its main use is for visualization of the biliary ducts in postcholecystectomized patients. It is contraindicated in the presence of fever (cholangiitis or hepatitis) or in the presence of combined hepatic and urinary disease. It is seldom successful in jaundice.

For this method to be efficient, fluid intake should be restricted for a day prior to the examination. The dye will visualize with greater concentration when the patient is relatively dehydrated. Food should be withheld after midnight of the day of examination.

Before use of Cholografin the patient should be tested for sensitivity. One-tenth milliliter should be administered intradermally, or two drops instilled on the conjunctiva. If a positive response results, it should become evident within ten to fifteen minutes and appear as either a wheal or an inflammatory reaction on the conjunctiva. Further testing, especially where a history of allergy is obtained, may be done by injecting small amounts intravenously (fractions of milliliter), with the patient observed for approximately ten minutes for any untoward reaction.

Assuming no sensitivity, Cholografin should be injected slowly, allowing about 10 minutes for the complete administration. During the injection the patient should be observed for untoward reaction, such as warmth, flushing, nausea and vomiting. Although these side effects are usually transitory, Adrenalin should be available, should these reactions become unduly exaggerated and the patient may even go into shock. The usual dose of the dye is 40 cc. In thin patients, 20 cc. may be adequate.

Biliary Radical Examination

To visualize the bilary radicals, films are taken from 10 to 40 minutes after injection, although the time varies with liver function. The study of the common duct should be continued up to two hours. It requires from two to three hours for the gallbladder to become visualized although faint concentrations of dye may be seen as early as half an hour. Where the liver is damaged, the drug will be excreted through the kidneys.

When the sphincter of Oddi is patulous, dye may run quickly into the duodenum and poor visualization may result. This may be prevented by administration of a dose of morphine.

Further, slowed dye entering into the duodenum and collecting in the bulb, may be mistakenly interpreted as a gallbladder sac. This may be cleared up by giving the patient a drink of water; thus, the dye is washed from the duodenum.

In the presence of jaundice, or where good visualization is not obtained, better filling has been described as being obtained by injecting 250 cc. of 30 per cent glucose with 20 units of regular insulin intravenously prior to the injection of the dye.[20a]

Gallbladder Examination

The technic for examination of the *gallbladder* after intravenous dye administration is the same as described for oral cholecystography, i.e., including fluoroscopic positioning, administration of fatty meal, etc., when the gallbladder becomes visible.

The advantage of the intravenus method

is that the bile ducts may be visualized. Also a gallbladder which may fail to visualize with the oral study may occasionally be seen when studied intravenously. Thus it has been used as an aid in differential diagnosis between acute pancreatitis and cholecystitis. If the common duct and gallbladder should be visualized after their failure to be visualized by the oral method, pancreatitis may be the underlying diagnosis.

If, after total nonvisualization by the oral method, the common duct becomes visualized by the intravenus method but the gallbladder is not seen, this would indicate cystic duct obstruction. If the common duct measures more than 1.5 cm. in its greatest diameter, some degree of obstruction is suggested. A time-density relationship is also useful in diagnosing obstructive mechanisms in the common duct where no dilatation may be present. A dye concentration greater at 2 hours than at 1 hour would be suggestive of an obstructive mechanism.[21]

Stratification of the dye in the gallbladder has been described.[25] It is produced by the slow miscibility of the Cholografin with the bile. In the early stages of gallbladder filling, mixing of the dye and bile is not complete. The portion of bile mixed with the Cholografin may layer out and form a separate level from the bile. In the prone position this may simulate a ring calculus.[26] Being aware of these features, the examiner should take films after further mixing, as well as after a fatty meal. The layering effect will disappear when adequate mixing takes place.

CHOLANGIOGRAPHY

Cholangiography consists of injecting opaque material in order to fill the ducts, and also gallbladder if the latter is present. The injection takes place either through an existing biliary fistula or through T tubes during or after operation.

Opacification of the common duct and biliary radicals after operative removal of the gallbladder is important in determining their patency, residual calculi, undue spasm and stricture.

The injection of the opaque material is made under direct fluoroscopic vision. Overfilling of the common duct and biliary radicals may thus be avoided, and also an attempt can be made to prevent opaque material entering and traveling into the pancreatic duct.

TECHNIC

The actual technic first requires the drainage of the available secretion within the ducts. This can be performed by syringe withdrawal or the T tube draining freely into a hand basin. Approximately 15 to 20 cc. of Diodrast or Neo-Iopax is injected until the common duct and biliary system are filled. The contrast material should be heated to body temperature prior to injection. Overfilling and entry into the duct of Wirsung should be avoided. Filming then takes place at 5 minute intervals over a period of 20 to 30 minutes, and the entry of the opaque material into the duodenum is observed.

In the diagnosis of calculus formation, it is important to bear in mind that no additional entry of air should accompany injection of the opaque material, since small air bubbles may simulate gallstones.

Prior to cholangiography, any drugs which may cause spasm of the sphincter of Oddi (e.g., morphine) should be avoided.

The Pathologic Gallbladder

DEFECTIVE VISUALIZATION AFTER ORAL CHOLECYSTOGRAPHY

Poorly Visualized Gallbladder

Poor visualization of the dye within the gallbladder should be cause for suspicion although the cause may be an inadequate amount of contrast material entering the gallbladder and not a diseased gallbladder. Dye first entering the gallbladder is poorly visualized because it is diluted by the various bile components. Normally the wall of the gallbladder reverses this dilution by absorbing water thus concentrating the dye and affording visualization. A poorly visualized gallbladder shadow should, therefore, suggest pathology of the gallbladder wall. The examiner must be certain, however, that the patient in preparing for the gallbladder examination has faithfully followed all of his instructions. It should be emphasized that normal gallbladders may at times be poorly visualized.

When poor visualization is obtained, further attempts at visualizing the gallbladder should be performed with the aim of subsequent better dye concentration. If necessary, the intravenous route as described above should be used.

Complete failure in visualization of the gallbladder after repeated examination is an important sign of gallbladder disease.

Nonvisualized Gallbladder

How Dye Makes the Gallbladder Visible. Nonvisualization of the gallbladder generally indicates a diseased gallbladder. It has been stated[7] that 80 to 90 per cent of nonvisualized gallbladders are associated with stones, and perhaps an even larger proportion with gross disease. To obviate nonvisualization in gallbladders that are not diseased, it is wise to review the basic physiology and possible sources of error.

Oral cholecystography entails the passage of a contrast medium from the mouth through the stomach and into the small bowel. It is absorbed from the small intestine and carried by an intact portal circulation to the liver. Next, mixed with the bile, it passes from the liver cells into the various biliary radicals and eventually into the common duct. Entry into the duodenum is prevented by the tonicity of the sphincter of Oddi. The bile-laden dye is stored within the common and hepatic ducts until the pressure is raised to about 70 mm. of water, at which time it is forced through the cystic duct and into the gallbladder. Within the gallbladder the dye becomes concentrated through the absorption of water by the gallbladder wall, thus resulting in better radiographic and fluoroscopic visualization.[8]

Factors Accounting for Nonvisualization. Failure to visualize the gallbladder may result from interference at any stage of the above mentioned mechanism. It may include improper intake of dye, obstruction preventing entry of the dye into the small bowel, any mechanism causing inadequate absorption of the dye through the wall of the small intestine, liver dysfunction which fails to excrete the dye adequately, a sphincter of Oddi which does not permit sufficient increase of intracholedochal pressure, and obstruction within the cystic duct preventing entry of the dye into the gallbladder. Finally, even though the contrast material does enter the gallbladder sac, nonvisualization may result because of inadequate dye concentration; this is a dysfunction of the gallbladder wall itself.

The foregoing factors may be considered in a sequential fashion.

1. Factors Considered during Preparation: Fat in the diet must be considered when nonvisualization of the gallbladder occurs. It should be borne in mind that a fatty meal taken during preparation with the dye

is slow to evacuate the stomach, and motility may further be slowed if the stomach is of the hypotonic or atonic type. Such a fatty meal, although given prior to intake of the dye, may cause the gallbladder to contract and empty during that phase when it should be filling with dye. Thus, nonvisualization may result.

On the other hand, as pointed out, a gallbladder filled with concentrated bile may not permit adequate entry of the fresh bile-laden dye, or even if entry is permitted, improper or nonvisualization may result from dye *dilution*.[9, 10] Such a prior accumulation of thick, concentrated bile within the gallbladder is likely to occur in subjects who have been on a prolonged fat-free diet. On this type of diet, the gallbladder would not have emptied satisfactorily for prolonged periods of time.

2. Intake of Dye: It is important to question the patient regarding *vomiting* or *diarrhea*. Vomiting all or part of the pills will of course result in inadequate intake. Diarrhea, because of its possible association with rapid transit of the opaque material through the intestine, may not allow sufficient time for absorption of the pills.

3. Obstruction to Dye Passage and Absorption: Since absorption of the dye takes place within the small intestine, any obstructive phenomena in the esophagus, stomach or pylorus, either functional or organic, may interfere with the opaque material reaching the small intestine. Absorption through the bowel wall and entry into the liver also entails an intact portal circulation, with no disease or deficiency in absorption present in the bowel itself. Pancreatic disease may likewise result in failure of absorption.

4. Excretion from Liver: Diseases of the liver may prevent the dye from entering into the choledochal system.

The administration of dye in the presence of jaundice is innocuous, but under such circumstances the gallbladder is unlikely to be visualized. If, however, in the presence of jaundice, the gallbladder fills and empties, the lesion producing the jaundice may be within the liver (hepatitis).[13]

Assuming, however, that the dye has passed through the liver and an intact choledochal system, it may be prevented from entry into the gallbladder by cystic duct obstruction. Further, a gallbladder full of stones, mucus or pus may also prevent the dye from entering the sac.

5. Factors within the Common Duct Interfering with Visualization: It is important that the patient report for examination in a fasting state. It is in *a fasting state* that the sphincter of Oddi is closed and the bile pressure permitted to build up. It has been pointed out that an intracholedochal pressure of about 70 mm. of water is necessary before the bile-laden dye may be forced through the cystic duct into the gallbladder. This also implies normal tonicity of the sphincter of Oddi. Further, a disease process (e.g., tumor of the sphincter of Oddi) or obstructions within the hepatic or common duct may interfere with the passage of dye and result in nonvisualization of the gallbladder.

6. Factors within the Gallbladder Wall Itself Preventing Adequate Visualization: As pointed out above, a diseased gallbladder wall with either acute or chronic inflammation, etc., will not concentrate the dye. The result is inadequate or nonvisualization of the gallbladder.

7. Hydrochloric Acid Abnormality: In individuals with *hyperchlorhydria*, the gallbladder may contract and empty itself prematurely.[11] This may result in nonvisualization. *Achlorhydria*, on the other hand, may result in atonicity of the duodenum with consequent decrease in intradochal pressure; i.e., the bile-laden dye is permitted to run freely down the duct into the duodenum without ever entering the gallbladder.[8, 12, 13]

As a general rule it should be stated that before determining any gallbladder as abnormal because of nonvisualization, a repeat examination—after new preparation with contrast material—should always be done. The gallbladder may now be visualized and may prove entirely normal.

Special Causes of Nonvisualization. Since there are special circumstances which have nothing to do with the foregoing sequential consideration of nonvisualization, they are considered separately.

1. Nonvisualization may result from previous gallbladder removal, its congenital absence, or its location in other than the usual position. It should be emphasized again, however, that a repeat examination will often make manifest a previously non-visualized gallbladder shadow. It should be remembered too, that in rare instances failure to visualize the gallbladder in the right upper quadrant may be owing to its location on the left side.[17, 18]

2. In obese individuals, finding the gallbladder shadow may be difficult. In these instances it is often advisable to give the patient a few ounces of barium solution and opacify the duodenal bulb. The gallbladder is expected to be located immediately to the right of the bulb.

3. Olsson has demonstrated that in lactating mothers, nonvisualization of the gallbladder may be caused by excretion of the dye in the milk.[14]

4. In acute abdominal disease—especially with peritoneal irritation—the normal gallbladder may inexplicably fail to concentrate the dye. Failure to visualize the normal gallbladder for as long as 12 weeks after an attack of acute pancreatitis has been described.[20a]

5. Nonvisualization of the gallbladder may also rarely be present as a result of diabetes and hyperthyroidism.[25a]

NEGATIVE SHADOWS WITHIN THE GALLBLADDER

Definition. A negative shadow within the dye-filled gallbladder may be defined as an area within its contours which fails to fill with dye. It is less dense than the surrounding opaque media and therefore radiolucent. Thus, a negative shadow within the confines of the gallbladder appears as a "hole" or space within its borders. (See negative defect of the stomach, page 153 and fig. 184.) The appearance of a number of negative shadows would render a "Swiss cheese" pattern.

Uncovering Negative Defects. Calculi, papillomata, polypi and malignant tumors may cause negative shadows within the gallbladder. It should be borne in mind however, that an apparently well filled gallbladder, homogeneous in appearance (i.e., without visible negative shadows), may, in a small percentage of cases, also contain stones, papillomata, polyps, etc. (figs. 423, 424). Understanding why these are not seen explains the maneuvers necessary to make them visible.

Two difficulties are present: first, the smallness of their individual size; secondly, the large amount and density of the overlying dye, inundating and obscuring them. To overcome the first obstacle, the examiner attempts to concentrate the many small negative defects into *one larger, more visible mass.* To overcome the second obstacle, the examiner seeks to *diminish the amount or thin* the overlying opaque media.

Both of these aims may be achieved by examining the patient in the erect position, after a fatty meal, with the aid of graded compression. The examination should be performed behind the fluoroscopic screen. Under direct visualization the patient is arranged in the optimum position; i.e., underlying and overlying shadows are rotated out of the field. The gallbladder shadow is compressed and spot films are taken (figs. 423–424).

The erect position after a fatty meal and with graded compression has the following advantages:

1. With the patient in the prone position, calculi if present will be dispersed over the broad roentgenographic aspect of the gallbladder (the broad side of the sac acting as

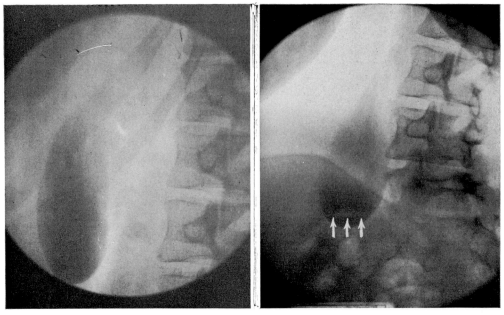

423

424

This gallbladder contains calculi.

Question:

Why are the calculi not seen?

Answer:

With the patient in the *prone* position, as here, the calculi in the path of the x-ray beam are *dispersed* and difficult to see. Also in the prone position the dye overlies and helps hide the gallstones.

Question:

Why does the same gallbladder now present evidence of calculi?

Answer:

1. In the erect position, the calculi *layer out* and in such a manner present a *concentrated*, more opaque shadow to the x-ray beam.

2. Graded compression applied after some of the overlying dye has emptied (as a result of the contraction after the fatty meal) also helps visualize the stones.

the gravitational base in this position) and will thus be difficult to visualize. With the patient in the erect position, however, the gallbladder elongates, and if calculi are present they will either sink "en masse" to the narrower true base of the gallbladder or, depending on their specific gravity, float in layer formation. Thus, the individual *smaller defects*, drawing closer together, become concentrated in a more solid mass, and hence they form a larger, more easily visible defect (figs. 423, 424). Also, the cumulative effect of the stones as a single large cluster or layer, acting as a "larger mass," will push aside or displace a greater amount of the opaque media. This displacement of dye is instrumental in producing

some thinning of the overlying opaque material (figs. 423, 424).

2. The advantage of performing this maneuver after a *fatty meal* is twofold. First, the fatty meal causes the gallbladder to contract and partially empty. With the diminution of dye resulting from partial emptying, the obscuring overlying dye becomes thinned. Secondly, the gallbladder in contracting helps in the formation of the "larger single mass" by contracting and drawing the stones closer together.

3. Behind the fluoroscopic screen the examiner himself may thin the overlying dye by graduated compression. In employing this last maneuver it is important to remember that *excessive* pressure may not

only displace all of the dye but also push the underlying stones out of the field.

Finally, with the gallbladder properly positioned to avoid overlying confusing shadows, the patient in the erect position after a fatty meal, and the proper degree of pressure applied, spot films should be taken to confirm the findings (figs. 417–420, p. 345).

DIFFERENTIAL DIAGNOSIS OF NEGATIVE DEFECTS

Differentiation of Negative Defects

Negative defects may be produced by papillomata, polyps, gallstones and malignant tumors. In differentiating stones from polyps, papillomata, or malignant tumors, it should be borne in mind that *calculi are freely* mobile and change position with change in the patient's position. The layering effect, or falling of calculi to the fundus of the gallbladder when the patient is in the erect position, has been described above. In this connection, however, it should be remembered that in rare cases, gallstones may apparently become adherent to the mucosa and be unaffected by change in the position of the patient. This situation can be confused with polyp formation, and radiographic differentiation is usually impossible. Further, 5 to 10 minutes must be allowed for the "mobile" calculi to rearrange themselves when the patient is changed from the prone to the erect position.

Benign tumors of the gallbladder are diagnosed by the appearance of an oval, more or less smooth negative defect within the opaque gallbladder. They are usually small, the diameter being less than 0.5 cm. Although in most cases single, they may occasionally be multiple. Important signs differentiating multiple negative defects from calculi are the *unchanging position* of these defects and their usual *marginal location.* They are best seen through the thin layer technic described above.

In differentiating a *benign* from a *ma-*lignant tumor, the immobility is not helpful. The irregularity of the malignant defect is the important sign. It should be borne in mind that a gallbladder sufficiently destroyed by malignant disease may not be visualized after dye administration. In a series of 12 malignant gallbladders only in 2 cases was the gallbladder successfully opacified. Both of these revealed poor concentration and no filling defects.[22] In fact, a filling defect in malignant disease of the gallbladder has been described by some as rare.[23, 24] Occasionally a gallbladder may at first concentrate the dye properly in the presence of a malignant tumor, but because of the rigid character of portions of the muscular wall, contraction after the fatty meal may be interfered with. If an irregular negative defect is suspected of being a tumor, and is constant in appearance, even with change in the patient's position, failure of contraction after the fatty meal may be explained by infiltration of the gallbladder wall.

Associated changes which the examiner should seek in order to confirm the presence of malignant disease of the gallbladder might include a mass in the right upper quadrant. The mass may displace the stomach and duodenum to the left and downwards. Pressure defects might thus be expected in the superior aspect of the duodenal bulb and the anterior aspect of the descending duodenum. A pressure defect might also be expected on the anterior portion of the pyloric antrum extending down to involve the greater curvature of the stomach.

In distinguishing a carcinoma of the gallbladder from carcinoma of the head of the pancreas, the latter may show pressure defects on the inferior aspect of the duodenal bulb and medial aspect of the descending duodenum (fig. 283). Pressure on the posterior antrum may also be present.

Gas Shadows Differentiated from Negative Defects

Gas in the region of the gallbladder may overlie the gallbladder sac and not only obliterate underlying pathology but often be so located as to appear as numerous negative defects within the gallbladder confines, simulating calculi within the sac. With the patient in the erect position, the gallbladder may be found fluoroscopically; the patient is then rotated into various positions until the overlying gas shadows are *thrown free of the gallbladder.* Manual manipulation of the opacified gallbladder is also useful in separating its shadow from confusing regional gas shadows. Spot filming should confirm the findings (figs. 417–420, p. 345).

Pitressin is useful in ridding the patient of gas but is contradindicated in hypertensive patients because of the change in blood pressure which may occur. It is administered subcutaneously, 0.5 cc. being injected one to two hours before the examination. This dose may be repeated without harmful effect in half an hour.

CALCIUM CARBONATE GALLBLADDER

The calcium carbonate gallbladder is usually smaller than normal. It is associated with severe chronic cholecystitis. The calcium carbonate may be deposited in the gallbladder wall, producing a calcified gallbladder. This is seen fluoroscopically as "egg shell" calcified plaques in the wall. The calcium carbonate may also be present as a pasty or putty-like mass within the gallbladder lumen. Fluoroscopically or on films, this presents an opacified gallbladder before dye administration, and has been called "limey gallbladder."

The value of *preliminary* filming should be stressed. The gallbladder containing calcium carbonate is opaque and may not be differentiated from the dye-filled gallbladder. Confusion is avoidable, then, by examining the gallbladder region for opaque shadows *before* opaque media is given.

Bibliography

Chapter I—Basic Concepts: Mechanics, Protection, and Dark Adaptation

1. STEVENSON, C. A., AND LEDDY, E. T.: The Dangers of Reducing Fractures under the Roentgenoscope and Methods of Protection against Them. Am. J. Roentgenol. 37: 70–82, 1937.
2. Excessive X-Radiation Exposures during Roentgenography and Roentgenoscopy. War Department Technical Bulletin—TB Med. 62. Washington, War Dept., July 1, 1944.
3. HENNY, GEORGE C., AND CHAMBERLAIN, W. EDWARD: Roentgenography: Fluoroscopy. In: Glasser, Otto: Medical Physics, Vol. 1. Chicago, Year Book Publishers, 1944, p. 1295.
4. UHLMANN, ERIC.: Significance in Management of Radiation Injuries. Radiology 38: 445–452, 1942.
5. SAUNDERS, T. S., AND MONTGOMERY, H.: Chronic Roentgen and Radium Dermatitis. J.A.M.A. 110: 23–28, 1938.
6. LEDDY, E. T., AND RIGOS, F. J.: Radiodermatitis among Physicians. Am. J. Roentgenol. 45: 696–700, 1941.
7. GLASSER, O., QUIMBY, E., TAYLOR, L., AND WEATHERWAX, J.: Physiological Foundations of Radiology. New York, P. B. Hoeber, Inc., 1944. p. 151.
8. BRAESTRUP, C. G.: X-Ray Protection in Diagnostic Radiology. Radiology 38: 207–216, 1942.
9. COWING, R. F., AND SPALDING, C. K.: A Survey of Scattered Radiation from Fluoroscopic Units in 15 Institutions. Radiology 53: 569–574, 1949.
10. DE VOE, S. J., AND CORNEY, B. A.: X-Ray Injuries, the Preventable Occupational Hazard. New York State J. Med. 482: 1601–1602, 1948.
11. KIRKLIN, B. R.: Roentgenoscopic Examination of Stomach and Duodenum. Radiology 26: 537, 1936.
12. Medical X-ray Protection. U. S. Dept. of Commerce, National Bureau of Standards. Handbook 41, p. 1–42, March, 1949.
13. GARLAND, L. H.: X-Ray Burns Resulting from Fluoroscopy of Gastro-intestinal Tract. J.A.M.A. 129: 419–422, 1945.
14. CHAMBERLAIN, W. E.: Fluoroscopes and Fluoroscopy. (Carman Lecture.) Radiology 38: 207–216, 1942.
15. Keleket: Manual of Directions and Warnings.
16. MORGAN, R. H.: Physical Problems of Fluoroscopy and Spot Film Radiography. Radiology 52: 786–795, 1949.
17. TURNER, A. E.: The Use of the X-Ray Fluoroscope and the Dangers Associated with its Operation. X-Ray Technician 16: 161–164, 1945.
18. LEDDY, E. T.: The Dangers of Roentgenoscopy: Summary and Recommendations. Am. J. Roentgenol. 38: 924–927, 1937.
19. ZOETHOUT, W. D.: Physiological Optics, ed. 3. Chicago, Professional Press, 1939.
20. NEWELL, P. R.: The Photopic Fluoroscope. Am. J. Roentgenol. 51: 414–415, 1946.
21. HARVEY, R. A.: A Rapid Dark Adaptation Test. Radiology 38: 353–359, 1942.
22. COLTMAN, J. W.: Fluoroscopic Image Brightening by Electronic Means. Radiology 51: 359–367, 1948.
23. MOON, R. J.: Amplifying and Intensifying Fluoroscopic Images by Means of a Scanning X-ray Tube. Science 112: 389–395, 1950.
24. MORGAN, R. H., AND STURM, R. E.: The Johns Hopkins Fluoroscopic Screen Intensifier. Radiology 57: 556–560, 1951.
25. HODGES, P. C., AND STAGGS, L.: Electronic Amplification of the Roentgenoscopic Image. Am. J. Roentgenol. 66: 705–710, 1951.
26. STURM, R. E., AND MORGAN, R. H.: Screen Intensification Systems and Their Limitations. Am. J. Roentgenol. 62: 617–634, 1949.
27. TEVES, M. C., AND TOL, T.: Electronic Intensification of Fluoroscopic Images. Phillips Tech. Rev. 14: No. 2 (Aug.), 1952.
28. MORGAN, R. H.: Screen Intensification: A Review of Past and Present Research with an Analysis of Future Development. Am. J. Roentgenol. 75: 69–76, 1956.
29. GORSON, R. O., LIEBERMAN, J., AND GREEN, M.: A Limited Survey of Radiation Exposure from Medical Fluoroscopes. Radiology 73: 898–910, 1959.
30. RIEBEL, F. A.: Efficiency of Red Goggles. Am. J. Roentgenol. 70: 827–830, 1953.
31. DUKE-ELDER, W. S.: Text Book of Opthalmology. Vol. I. St. Louis, C. V. Mosby Co., 1933, p. 903.
32. SOUTHHALL, J. P. C.: Introduction to Physiological Optics. New York and London, Oxford University Press, 1937, p. 268.
33. RIEBEL, F. A.: Use of the Eyes in X-ray Diagnosis. Radiology 70: 252–257, 1958.
34. CHANTRAINE, H.: Vitamin A und Durchleuchtungssehen. Rontgenblaetter. 12: 91–93, March 1959.
35. CAPP, P. M., AND SPACH, M. S.: Dosimetry during Cineradiography and Other Specialized Radiographic Diagnostic Procedures. Radiology 78: 744–750, 1962.

Chapter II—Examination of the Chest

1. RABIN, COLEMAN: Personal communication.
2. GOLDEN, R.: Diagnostic Roentgenology, Vol. 1. New York, T. Nelson & Sons, 1948.
3. WESTERMARK, N.: Roentgen Studies of Lungs and Heart. Minneapolis, University of Minnesota Press, 1948.
4. ROBBINS, L. L. Idiopathic Pulmonary Fibrosis: Roentgenologic Findings. Radiology 51: 439–467, 1948.
5. SGALITZES, MAX: Roentgenological Examination of the Power of Resistance of the Tracheal Wall. Am. J. Roentgenol. 56: 355–360, 1946.
6. EPSTEIN, B. S.: Diaphragmatic Changes Incident to Hepatic Neoplasms. Am. J. Roentgenol. 82: 114–119, 1959.

Chapter III—Examination of the Heart

1. FRIEDBERG, C. K.: Diseases of the Heart. Philadelphia, W. B. Saunders & Co., 1949, p. 19.
2. PILLMORE, G. U.: Clinical Radiology, Vol. 1. Philadelphia, F. A. Davis Co., 1946, p. 10.
2a. ZDANSKY, E.: Roentgen Diagnosis of the Heart and Great Vessels. New York, Grune & Stratton, 1953.
3. PARKINSON, J.: J. Lancet 1: 1391–1399, 1936.
4. SCHWEDEL, J. B.: Clinical Roentgenology of the Heart. In: Annals of Roentgenology. New York, P. B. Hoeber, Inc., 1946.
5. ROESLER, H.: Clinical Roentgenology of the Cardiovascular System. Springfield, Ill. Charles C Thomas, 1937.
6. KIRCH, E.: Herzkraeftigung und echte Herzhypertrophie durch Sport. Ztschr. f. Kreislaufforsch. 28: 893, 1936.
7. STROUD, WM. D.: Diagnosis and Treatment of Cardiovascular Disease, Vol. 1. Philadelphia, F. A. Davis Co., 1945, p. 772.
8. WILSON, M. G.: Rheumatic Fever. New York, Commonwealth Fund, 1940, p. 401–411.
9. WILSON, M. G.: Radioscopic Studies of the Heart in Children; roentgenologic criteria of cardiac enlargement, size of angle of clearance of left ventricle, as criterion of ventricular enlargement. Am. J. Dis. Child. 47: 751, 1934.
10. STEELE, J. M., JR., AND PATERSON, R.: Distortion of the Bronchi by Left Auricular Enlargement. Am. Heart J. 4: 692–707, 1929.
11. KING, T. W.: Observations on Abdominal Tumors and Intumescence: Illustrated by Cases of Ovarian Disease. Guys Hospital Rep. 3: 178, 1838.
12. ROESLER, H., AND WEISS, K.: Ueber die Veraenderung des Oesophagusverlaufes durch den vergroesserten linken Vorhof. Fortschr. a. d. Geb. d. Roentgenstr. 33: 717, 1925.
13. EVANS, W.: Great Britain Medical Research Council. Spec. Rep. Ser. U. 208, London, 18: 43, 1936.
14. UNGERLEIDER, H. E.: Cardiac Enlargement. Radiology 48: 129–142. 1947.
15. HODGES, P. C., AND EYSTER, J. A. E.: Estimation of Transverse Cardiac Diameter in Man. Arch. Int. Med. 37: 707, 1926.
16. UNDERLEIDER, H. E., AND CLARK, C. P.: A Study of the Transverse Diameter of the Heart Silhouette with Prediction Table Based on the Teleoroentgenogram. Am. Heart J. 17: 92, 1939.
17. COMEAU, W. J., AND WHITE, P. D.: A Critical Analysis of Standard Methods of Estimating Heart Size from Roentgen Measurements. Am. J. Roentgenol. 47: 665, 1942.
18. SHERMAN, C. F., AND DUCEZ, E. F.: Cardiac Mensuration. Am. J. Roentgenol. 5: 439–443, 1944.
19. SUSSMAN, M. L., AND GRISHMAN, A.: A Discussion of Angiocardiography and Angiography. In: Advances in Internal Medicine. New York, Interscience Publishers, 1947.
20. TAUSSIG, HELEN B.: Congenital Malformations of the Heart. New York, Commonwealth Fund, 1947, pp. 44, 45.
21. WOLF, L.: Acute Pericarditis with Special Reference to Changes in Heart Size. New England J. Med. 229: 423–431, 1943.
21a. NEUHAUSER, E. B. D.: Am. J. Roentgenol. 56: 1, 1946.
22. BARNES, A. R., AND BURCHELL, H. B.: Acute Pericarditis Simulating Acute Coronary Occlusion. Am. Heart J. 23: 247–269, 1942.
23. BROWN, S., AND MCCARTHY, J. E.: A Study of the Esophagus in Relation to Heart, Aorta and Thoracic Cage. Radiology 24: 131, 1935.
24. STUMPF, P., ET AL.: Roentgenkymographische Bewegungslehre innerer Organe. Leipzig, Geo. Thieme, 1936.
25. ARENDT, J.: Radiological Difference between Pericardial Effusion and Cardiac Dilatation. Radiology 50: 44–51, 1948.
26. UNGERLEIDER, HENRY E.: Personal communication.
27. WILLIAMS, R. G., AND STEINBERG, I.: The Value of Angiocardiography in Establishing

the Diagnosis of Pericarditis with Effusion. Am. J. Roentgenol. *61:* 41–44, 1949.

28. N. Y. Heart Association Nomenclature and Criteria for Diagnosis of Disease of the Heart, 1939, p. 85.

29. Esser, C.: Über das kymographische Verhalten der Herzspitze bei Ausgesprochener Dilatation. Fortschr. a. d. Geb. d. Roentgenstrahlen *52:* 213, 1935.

30. Master, A. M., Gubner, R., Dack, S., Jaffe, H. L.: The Diagnosis of Coronary Occlusion and Myocardial Infarction by Fluoroscopic Examination. Am. Heart J. *20:* 475, 1940.

31. Sosman, M. C.: Curable Heart Disease. Radiology *41:* 351, 1943.

32. Kerley, P.: A Textbook of X-Ray Diagnosis by British Authors. London, H. K. Lewis, 1938.

33. Sussman, M. L.: Section on Congenital Heart Disease. In: Pillmore, G. U.: Clinical Radiology, Vol. 1, Chap. IV. Philadelphia, F. A. Davis Co., 1946.

34. Taussig, H., Railsback, O. C., and Dock, W.: Erosion of the Ribs to Stenosis of the Isthmus of the Aorta. Radiology *12:* 58–62, 1929.

35. Batt, H. D.: Wandering of the Retrocardiac Esophagus: A Pitfall in the Diagnosis of Left Atrial Enlargement. Radiology *74:* 588–592, 1960.

36. Viamonte, M., Jr.: CO_2 Angiocardiography. Am. J. Roentgenol. *88:* 31–37, 1962.

37. Stauffer, H. M., Durant, T. M., and Oppenheimer, M. J.: Gas Embolism: Roentgenologic Considerations, Including Experimental Use of CO_2 as Intracardiac Arrest Material. Radiology *66:* 686–692, 1956.

38. Mellins, H. Z., Kottmeier, P., and Kiely, B.: Radiologic Signs of Pericardial Effusion. Radiology *73:* 9–17, 1959.

39. Golden, R.: Pericardial Effusion on Lateral Roentgenogram: Preliminary Report. Presented at the Annual Meeting of the American Roentgen Ray Society, St. Louis, Mo., Sept. 1950.

40. Steinberg, I., von Gal, H. V., and Finby, N.: Roentgen Diagnosis of Pericardial Effusion: New Angiocardiographic Observations. Am. J. Roentgenol. *79:* 321–322, 1958.

41. Keats, T. E., and Mart, J. M.: False Paradoxic Movement of the Posterior Wall of the Left Ventricle Simulating Myocardial Aneurysm. Radiology *78:* 381–387, 1962.

42. Sayman, M. I.: A New Sign in the Diagnosis of Cardiac Aneurysm and Myocardial Infarction. Radiology *67:* 242–246, 1956.

43. Lester, R. G., Gedgaudas, E., and Rigler, L. G.: Method of Radiologic Diagnosis of Congenital Heart Disease in Children. J.A.M.A. *166:* 439–443, 1958.

Chapter IV—Examination of the Pharynx, Hypopharynx and Esophagus

1. Evans, W.: The Course of the Esophagus in Health and Disease of the Heart and Great Vessels. No. 208, Medical Research Council, 1936.

2. Taquine, Alberto C.: Esophageal Pulse under Normal and Abnormal Conditions. Am. Heart J. *20:* 129, 1940.

3. Buckstein, J.: The Digestive Tract in Roentgenology. Philadelphia, J. B. Lippincott, 1948.

4. Templeton, Frederic, E.: X-ray Examination of the Stomach. Chicago, University of Chicago Press, 1944.

4a. Barclay, A. E.: The Digestive Tract. Cambridge, Cambridge University Press, 1936.

5. Zenker, F. A., and Von Ziemsen, H.: Krankheiten des Oesophagus. In: Handbuch der speziellen Pathologie und Therapie (Ziemsen) Vol. 7, p. 1 (Anhang). Leipzig, F. C. W. Vogel, 1877.

6. Keith, Sir A.: A Demonstration of Diverticula of the Alimentary Tract of Congenital or of Obscure Origin. Brit. M. J. *1:* 376, 1910.

7. Udaondo, B. C., Resano, H., and D'Alotto, V.: Plummer-Vinson Syndrome. Prensa Med. Argent. *36:* 257–261, 1949.

8. Plass, E. D.: Congenital Atresia of the Esophagus with Tracheo-esophageal Fistula: Associated with Fused Kidney. Bull. Johns Hopkins Hosp. *18:* 259, 1919.

9. Ysander, Fredrik: Zur Frage der Genese der Oesophagus-atresien. Upsala Lakareforenings. Forhandlinger, N. Y. Feljd *30:* 195, 1924–1925.

10. Gruenwald, Peter: A Case of Atresia of the Esophagus Combined with Tracheo-esophageal Fistula in a 9 mm. Human Embryo and its Embryological Explanation. Anat. Rec. *78:* 193, 1940.

11. Rokitansky, C.: Handbuch der pathologischen Anatomie, Vol. 3. Vienna, Braumueller u. Seidel, 1842–46, p. 160.

12. Farrel, J. T., Jr.: Roentgenology of the Gastro-intestinal Tract. Springfield, Ill. Charles C Thomas, 1946.

12a. Neuhauser, E. B. D., and Berenberg, W.: Cardioesophageal Relaxation as a Cause of Vomiting in Infants. Radiology *48:* 480, 1947.

13. Aurelius, J. R.: Peptic Ulcer of the Esophagus. Am. J. Roentgenol. *26:* 696, 1931.

14. Chacul, H., and Adam, A.: Die Schleimhaut des Verdauungskanals im Röntgenbild; eine

normale und pathologische Röntgenanatomie der Innenwand des Verdauungskanals. Berlin and Vienna, Urban & Schwartzenberg, 1931.

15. DVORAK, H. J.: Sarcoma of the Esophagus. Arch. Surg. *22:* 794, 1931.

16. KRIEGLSTEIN, FR.: Ein gestielter, polyposer Tumor des Oesophagus. Ztschr. f. Pathol. *50:* 1, 1936.

17. HAENISCH, F.: Beitrag zur Röntgendiagnostik des Oesophagus—benigner Oesophagus-tumor. Fortsch. a. d. Geb. d. Rontgenstrahlen *32:* 432, 1924.

18. SCOTT, W. G., AND S. MOORE: A Method of Roentgen Diagnosis of Non Opaque Foreign Bodies in the Esophagus. J.A.M.A. *106:* 906, 1936.

19. GOLDEN, R.: Diagnostic Roentgenology, Vol. 1. New York, T. Nelson & Sons, 1948, p. 340T.

20. FITZGIBBON, J. H.: Diagnosis of Lesions near the Cardia. J.A.M.A. *142:* 453–458, 1950.

21. DREYFUS, J. R., AND WILLCOS, R. G.: The

22. TERRACOL, J., AND SWEET, R. H.: Diseases of the Esophagus. Philadelphia, W. B. Saunders Co., 1958, pp. 173–198.

23. MACHELLA, T. E.: Functional Disturbances of the Gastrointestinal Tract. Radiology *73:* 379–397, 1959.

24. RITVO, M., AND MCDONALD, E. J.: The Value of Nitrites in Cardiospasm. (Achalasia of the Esophagus): Preliminary Report. Am. J. Roentgenol. *43:* 500–508, 1940.

25. KRAMER, P., AND INGELFINGER, F. J.: Esophageal Sensitivity to Mecholyl in Cardiospasm. Gastroenterology *19:* 242–253, 1951.

26. GAY, B. B.: A Roentgenologic Method for Evaluation of the Larynx and Pharynx. Am. J. Roentgenol. *79:* 301–305, 1958.

27. Personal Communication, Dr. Sol M. Unger, Chief Radiologist, Veterans Administration Hospital, Kingsbridge Road, New York City.

Elevator Esophagus. Radiology *75:* 914–918, 1960.

Chapter V—Examination of the Stomach

1. AKERLUND, A.: Der "Spiralblendenkompressor," Spezialapparat für Detailbilder bei Kontrastuntersuchungen. Acta Radiol. *10:* 421–426, 1929.

2. FORSSELL, G.: Studies of the Mechanism of Movement of the Mucous Membrane of the Digestive Tract. Am. J. Roentgenol. *10:* 87, 1923.

3. BARCLAY, A. E.: The Digestive Tract. Cambridge, Cambridge University Press, 1936.

4. TEMPLETON, FREDERIC E.: X-Ray Examination of the Stomach. Chicago, University of Chicago Press, 1944.

4a. GOLDEN, ROSS: J.A.M.A. *109:* 1497–1500, 1937.

5. SHANKS, S. C., KERLEY, P., AND TWINING, E. W.: A Textbook of X-ray Diagnosis, Vol. 2. London, H. K. Lewis & Co., 1938–1939.

5a. RUSSELL, WALTER A., WEINTRAUB, SIDNEY, AND TEMPLE, HAROLD A.: An Analysis of X-Ray Findings in 405 Cases of Benign Gastric and Pyloric Ulcer. Radiology *51:* 790–797, 1948.

6. HARRIS, M.: Place of Fluoroscopy in Diagnosis of Peptic Ulcer. Radiology *52:* 781–785, 1949.

7. KIRLKIN, B. R.: A Technique for Roentgenoscopic Examination of the Stomach and Duodenum. Radiology *26:* 521–530, 1936.

8. BOLTON, C., AND SALMOND, R. W. A.: Lancet *1:* 1230, 1927.

9. COLE, L. G.: Diagnosis of Post Pyloric (Duodenal) Ulcer by Means of Serial Radiography. Lancet *1:* 1239–1244, 1914.

10. LEWALD, L. T.: Am. J. Roentgenol. *4:* 76, 1917.

11. CARMAN, R. D.: Roentgen Diagnosis of Diseases of the Alimentary Canal, ed. 2. Philadelphia, W. B. Saunders, 1920.

12. FELDMAN, M.: Clinical Roentgenology of the Digestive Tract, ed. 3. Baltimore, Williams and Wilkins, 1948.

13. KONJETZNY, G. E.: Zur Pathologie und chirurgischen Behandlung des Ulcus duodeni. Deutsche Ztschr. f. Chir. *184:* 85, 1924. Entzundliche Genese des Magen-Duodenalgeschwürs. Arch. f. Verdauungskr. *36:* 189, 1926.

14. BOCKUS, H. L.: Arteriomesenteric Occlusion of the Duodenum with Dilatation and Stasis. Pennsylvania M. J. *32:* 618, 1929.

15. WIDMANN, B. P.: The Roentgen-Ray Diagnosis of Chronic Duodenal Stasis. Pennsylvania M. J. *32:* 631–635, 1929.

16. RENDICH, R. A.: The Roentgenographic Study of the Mucosa in Normal and Pathologic States. Am. J. Roentgenol. *10:* 526–537, 1923.

17. HAMPTON, A. O.: A Safe Method for Roentgen Demonstration of Bleeding Duodenal Ulcers. Am. J. Roentgenol. *38:* 565–570, 1937.

18. MEYER, RALPH R.: Air Contrast Studies of the Duodenal Bulb. Radiology *58:* 393–400, 1952.

19. SHERMAN, ROBERT S.: Roentgen Diagnosis of the Cardiac Region of the Stomach. In: PACK, GEORGE T.: Cancer of the Oesophagus and Cardia. St. Louis, C. V. Mosby, 1949.

20. ZDANSKY, E.: Antiperistalsis of the Stomach in Extragastric Non-stenosing Lesions. Schweiz. med. Wchnschr. *87:* 1423, 1957.

21. SCHATZKI, R., AND GARY, J. E.: Face-on Demonstration of Ulcers in the Upper Stomach in a Dependent Position. Am. J. Roentgenol. *79:* 772–780, 1958.

22. BITNER, W. P.: Arteriomesenteric Occlusion of the Duodenum. Am. J. Roentgenol. *79:* 807–814, 1958.

23. WILHELM, G., AND SCHARF, G.: Radiology Clinics *28:* 160–174, 1959.

24. WOHL, G. T., AND SHORE, L.: Lesions of the Cardiac End of the Stomach Simulating Carcinoma. Am. J. Roentgenol. *82:* 1048–1057, 1959.

Chapter VI—Examination of the Small Bowel

1. BARCLAY, A. E.: The Digestive Tract. Cambridge, Cambridge University Press, 1936.

2. ALVAREZ, W.: Nervousness, Indigestion and Pain. New York, Harper, 1954.

3. McLAREN, J. W., ARDRAN, G. M., AND SUTCLIFFE, J.: Radiographic Studies of the Duodenum and Jejunum in Man. J. Fac. Radiol. *2:* 148: 1951.

4. GOLDEN, R.: Radiologic Examination of the Small Bowel. Philadelphia, Lippincott, 1945; J. A. M. A. *120:* 903–908, 1942.

5. PUESTOW, C. B.: Intestinal Motility and Postoperative Distention. Experimental and Clinical Studies. J. A. M. A. *120:* 903–908, 1942.

6. HENDERSON, S. G.: The Gastro-Intestinal Tract in the Healthy Newborn Infant. Radiology *39:* 253, 1942.

7. SCAMMON, R. E.: A Summary of the Anatomy of the Infant and Child. Abt's Pediatrics *1:* 309, 1923.

8. BOUSLOG, J.: The Normal Stomach and Small Intestine in the Infant. Radiology *39:* 253, 1942.

9. SUSSMAN, M. L., AND WACHTEL, E.: Factors Concerned in the Abnormal Distribution of Barium in the Small Bowel. Radiology *40:* 128–138, 1943.

10. ASTLEY, R., AND FRENCH, J. M.: The Small Intestine Pattern In Normal Children and in Coeliac Disease. Brit. J. Radiol. *24:* 221–238, 1951.

11. FRAZER, A. C., FRENCH, J. M., AND THOMPSON, N. D.: Radiographic Studies Showing Induction of Segmented Pattern in Small Intestine in Normal Human Subjects. Brit. J. Radiol. *22:* 123–126, 1949.

12. BERRIDGE, F. R.: The Small Intestine in Undernutrition. Brit. J. Radiol. *24:* 251, 1951.

13. PENDERGRASS, E. P., RAVDIN, T. S., JOHNSTON, C. G., AND HODGES, P. Z.: Studies of the Small Intestine. Radiology *26:* 651, 1936.

14. BERRIDGE, F. R.: Small Intestine in Undernutrition. Symposium, 6th International Congress of Radiology in London; 251–256, 1950.

15. MARSHAK, R. H., WOLF, B. S., AND ADLERSBERG, D.: Roentgen Studies of the Small Intestine in Sprue. Am. J. Roentgenol. *72:* 382–400, 1954.

16. FRIEDMAN, J.: Effects on the Small Intestine from Emotional Disturbances. Am. J. Roentgenol. *72:* 367–379, 1954.

17. PENDERGRASS, E. P., AND CHAMBERLIN, G. W.: Roentgen Diagnosis of Lesions Involving the Ileum, Cecum, and Proximal Ascending Colon. Am. J. Roentgenol. *48:* 16–26, 1942.

18. GOLDEN, R.: Amyloidosis of the Small Intestine. Am. J. Roentgenol. *72:* 401–408, 1954.

19. ABBOTT, W. D., AND PENDERGRASS, E. P.: Intubation Studies of the Human Small Intestine. V. The Motor Effects of Single Clinical Doses of Morphine Sulphate in Normal Subjects. Am. J. Roentgenol. *35:* 289–299, 1936.

20. BÜLBRING, EDITH, AND BURN, J. H.: The Interrelation of Prostigmine, Adrenaline and Ephedrine in Skeletal Muscle. J. Physiol. *101:* 224–245, 1942.

21. ADLERSBERG, D., AND SOBOTKA, H.: Influence of Lecithin Feeding on Fat and Vitamin A Absorption in Man. J. Nutrition *25:* 255–263, 1943.

22. ARAE, K.: Experimentelle Untersuchungen uber die Magen-Darmbewegungen bei akuter Peritonitis. Arch. f. exper. Path. u. Pharmakol. *94:* 149–189, 1922.

23. PANSDORF, H.: Die Fractionurte Ihre klinische Bedeutung. Fortschr, a.d. Geb. d. Roentgen. *56:* 627–634, 1937.

24. WEBER, H. M., AND KIRKLIN, B. R.: Roentgenologic Investigation of the Small Bowel. M. Clin. North America *22:* 1059, 1938.

25. WEINTRAUB, S., AND WILLIAMS, R. G.: A Rapid Method of Roentgenologic Study of the Small Intestine. Am. J. Roentgenol. *61:* 45, 1949.

26. MARTIN, J. F., AND FRIEDELL, H.: Partial Obstruction of the Small Intestine. Radiology *55:* 49–62, 1952.

27. SWENSON, P. C., AND HIBBARD, J. S.: Roentgenographic Manifestations of Intestinal Obstruction. Arch. Surg. *25:* 20, 1933.

28. SHANKS, S. C., AND KERLEY, P.: A Textbook of

X-ray Diagnosis, Vol. 3. Philadelphia, W. B. Saunders, 1950, pp. 301–302.

29. Pendergrass, E. P., Ravdin, I. S., Joynstone, C. G., and Hodes, P. F.: Studies of the Small Intestine; Effects of Foods on Various Pathological States in Gastric Emptying of the Small Intestinal Pattern. Radiology 26: 651–652, 1936.

30. Ardran, G. M., French, J. M., and McLaren, J. W.: Movements of the Jejunum. J. Fac. Radiol. 5: 267–275, 1954.

31. Goin, L. S.: Some Obscure Factors in the Production of Unusual Small Bowel Patterns. Radiology 53: 177–184, 1952.

32. Astley, R., and Gerrard, J. W.: The X-Ray Diagnosis of Celiac Disease. Brit. J. Radiol. 27: 484–490, 1954.

33. Nathan, M. H.: Clinical and Roentgenologic Correlation of Physiology of the Colon. Am. J. Roentgenol. 81: 650–660, 1959.

34. Golden, R.: Technical Factors in Radiologic Examination of the Small Intestine. Ann. de Radiol. 4: 559–569, 1961.

35. Morton, J. L.: Notes on a Small Bowel Examination. Am. J. Roentgenol. 86: 76–85, 1961.

36. Grayson, C. E.: Enlargement of the Ileocecal Valve. Am. J. Roentgenol. 79: 823–836, 1958.

37. Fleischner, F. G., and Bernstein, C.: Roentgen Anatomical Studies of the Normal Ileocecal Valve. Radiology 54: 43–58, 1950.

Chapter VII—Examination of the Colon

1. Feldman, Maurice: Clinical Roentgenology of the Digestive Tract, ed. 3. Baltimore, Williams and Wilkins, 1948.

2. Buckstein, J.: Digestive Tract in Roentgenology. Philadelphia, J. B. Lippincott, 1948.

2a. Ehrenpreis, T.: Megacolon in the Newborn. Acta Chir. Scandinav., Suppl. 112, 1946.

3. Uspensky, A.: Die pathogenetische Bedeutung des Symptomkomplexes der interpositic Colonis. Fortschr. a.d. Geb. d. Röntgenstrahlen 37: 540, 1928.

4. Jordan, A. C.: The Congenital Undescended Cæcum. Brit. J. Radiol. 10: 743, 1937.

5. Kantor, J. L.: A Clinical Study of Some Common Anatomical Abnormalities of the Colon: II. The Low Cecum. Am. J. Roentgenol. 14: 207, 1925.

6. Sabotta, Johannes: Atlas of Human Anatomy, Edited from the 7th German Edition by James Playfair McMurrich, 3 Vol. New York, G. E. Stechert Co., 1930. (Vol. 2, p. 51.)

7. Holzknecht, G.: Die normale Peristaltik des Kolon. München Med. Wchnschr. 56: 2401, 1909.

8. Stierlin, E.: Der Einfluss der Sennainfusionauf die Verdauungshemmungen beim Menschen. München Med. Wchnschr. 57: 1434, 1910.

9. Case, J. T.: X-ray Observation on Colonic Peristalsis and Antiperistalsis with Special Reference to the Function of the Ileocolic Valve. M. Rec. 85: 415, 1914.

10. Jacobj, C.: Pharmakalogische Untersuchungen über das Colchicumgift. Arch. f. exper. Path. u. Pharmakol. 27: 119, 1890.

11. Rieder, H.: Radiologische Untersuchungen des Magens und Darmes beim lebenden Menschen. München med. Wchnschr. 51: 119, 1890.

12. Schule, A.: Über die Sondierung und Radiographie des Dickdarms. Arch. f. Verdauungskr. 10: 111, 1904.

13. Stevenson, C. A., Moreton, R. D., and Seedorf, E. E.: Conduct of the Roentgenologic Examination of the Colon. Pamphlet, Scott White Clinic, Temple, Texas.

14. Gage, H. C.: A Case of Sarcoma of the Stomach. Brit. J. Radiol. 5: 718–719, 1932.

15. Stevenson, C. A., Moreton, R. D., and Cooper, E. M.: The Nature of Fictitious Polyps in the Colon. Am. J. Roentgenol. 43: 89–94, 1950.

15a. Pendergrass, Robert C.: Extrinsic Deformities of the Colon. Radiology 51: 320–325, 1948.

16. Hirschsprung, H.: Stuhltragheit Neugeborner in Folge von Dilatation und Hypertrophie des Colons. Jahrb. f. Kinderh. 27: 1, 1888.

17. Jackson, W. R.: Diverticulitis of the cecum. New York State J. Med. 106: 638, 1917.

18. Cooke, A. G.: When Appendicitis is not Appendicitis—A Case of Diverticulitis of the Cecum. J.A.M.A. 78: 579, 1922.

19. Pereira, H.: Diverticulitis of the cecum. Brit. M. J. 1: 279, 1927.

20. Jonas, A.: Solitary Cecal Diverticulitis. J.A.M.A. 115: 194, 1940.

21. Bergen, J. A., and Weber, H. M.: Clinical and Roentgenological Aspects of Chronic Ulcerative Colitis. Radiology 17: 1153, 1931.

22. Golden, R.: Diagnostic Roentgenology, Vol. 1. New York, T. Nelson & Sons, 1948.

23. Vallarino, J. J.: Preliminary Report on the Value of the Roentgen Ray in Estimating the Extent of Amebic Infection of the Large Intestine. International Conference of Health Problems in Tropical America, Boston, United Fruit Co., 1924.

24. Vallarino, J. J.: Report of Further Observations on the Value of Roentgen Rays in Estimating the Extent of Amebic Infection of the Large Intestine. Tr. Roy. Soc. Trop. Med. & Hyg. 22: 209, 1928.

25. HENDERSON, W. F.: Amebiasis of the Colon: Its Radiologic Aspects. Texas State J. Med. *27:* 363, 1931.

26. BELL, J. C.: The Roentgen Ray Examination of the Colon in the Study of Amebiasis. South. M. J. *29:* 462, 1936.

27. JONES, L. L.: The Roentgenologic Aspect of Colitis. Texas State J. Med. *14:* 244, 1918.

28. CRANE, A. W.: A Roentgenologic Sign of Mucous Colitis. Am. J. Roentgenol. *17:* 416, 1927.

29. BARGEN, J. A.: Conditions Commonly Called Colitis. Am. J. Roentgenol. *25:* 308, 1931.

30. ROKITANSKY, C.: A Manual of Pathological Anatomy, Vol. 2. Philadelphia, Blanchard & Lea, 1855.

31. STIERLIN, E.: Die radiographische Diagnostik der ileocecaltuberculose und anderer ulcerativer und indurirender Dickdarmprozesse. Verhandl. d. deutsch, Gesellsch. f. Chir. *40:* 170, 1911.

32. BROWN, L., AND H. L. SAMPSON: Intestinal Tuberculosis: Its Importance, Diagnosis and Treatment. Philadelphia, Lea & Febiger, 1926.

33. MELENEY, H. E.: Discussion of the paper by Bell (reference 26).

34. GUNN, H., AND HOWARD, N. J.: Amebic Granulomas of the Large Bowel, Their Clinical Resemblance to Carcinoma. J.A.M.A. *97:* 166, 1931.

35. PATTON, C. L., AND R. J. PATTON: Endometriosis of Sigmoid as a Cause of Acute Intestinal Obstruction. Am. J. Surg. *53:* 265, 1941.

36. JENKINSON, E. L., AND BROWN, W. H.: Endometriosis, Study of 117 Cases with Special Reference to Constricting Lesions of the Rectum and Sigmoid Colon. J.A.M.A. *122:* 349, 1943.

37. SHANKS, S. C., KERLEY, P., AND TWINING, E. W.: A Text Book of X-ray Diagnosis, Vol. 2. London, H. K. Lewis & Co., 1938–1939.

37a. STORCH, C. B., REDNER, B., AND TURIN, R.: Small Bowel Obstruction in Infancy and Childhood. J. Pediat. *35:* 366, 1949.

38. McLAREN, J. W.: Modern Trends in Diagnostic Radiology. London, Butterworth & Co., 1948.

39. HELLMER, HANS: The Roentgenologic Diagnosis and Treatment of Intussusception in Children. Acta Radiol. *24:* 235–258, 1943.

40. NORDENTOFT, JENS M.: The Value of the Barium Enema in the Diagnosis and Treatment of Intussusception in Children. Acta Radiol., Suppl. 51, 1943.

41. HELLMER, HANS: Intussusception in Children: Diagnosis and Therapy with Barium Enema. Acta Radiol., Suppl. 65, 1948, p. 120.

42. WILLIAMS, E. R.: Intussusception—A Radiological Study. Brit. J. Radiol. n.s. *13:* 51, 1940.

43. STEINBACH, H. L., AND BURHENNE, H. J.: Performing the Barium Enema: Equipment, Preparation, and Contrast Medium. Am. J. Roentgenol. *87:* 644–654, 1962.

44. RITAN, J. L.: Preparation of the Colon for Barium Enema Examination. Am. J. Roentgenol. *87:* 690–692, 1962.

45. STATMAN, A. J.: Effectiveness of X-Prep as as Bowel Evacuant Prior to Roentgenography of Gastro-Intestinal Tract. Am. J. Gastroenterol. *33:* 740–742, 1960.

46. NATHAN, M. H.: Clinical and Roentgenologic Correlation of Physiology of the Colon. Am. J. Roentgenol. *81:* 650–660, 1959.

47. BRAU, B. D.: The Value of Multiple Barium Enema Studies. Am. J. Roentgenol. *81:* 661–674, 1959.

48. LEVENE, G.: Rates of Venous Absorption of Carbon Dioxide and Air Used in Double-Contrast Examination of the Colon. Radiology *69:* 571–575, 1957.

49. LEVENE, G.: Low Temperature Barium-Water Suspensions for Roentgenologic Examination of the Colon. Radiology *77:* 117–118, 1961.

50. PRATT, J. H., AND JACKMAN, R. J.: Perforations of Rectal Wall by Enema Tips. Proc. Staff Meet., Mayo Clin, *20:* 277–283, 1945.

51. WALKING, A.: Rupture of Sigmoid by Hydrostatic Pressure. Ann. Surg. *102:* 471–472, 1935.

52. BURT, C. A. V.: Pneumatic Rupture of Intestinal Canal with Experimental Data Showing Mechanism of Perforation and Pressure Required. Arch. Surg. *22:* 875–902, 1931.

53. NATHAN, M. H., AND KOHEN, R.: The Bardex Tube in Performing Barium Enemas. Am. J. Roentgenol. *84:* 1121–1124, 1960.

54. NATHAN, M. H., AND NEWMAN, A.: A New Method of Air Contrast Examination of the Colon for Routine Application. Am. J. Roentgenol. *81:* 675–677, 1959.

55. PETERSON, C. A., AND CAYLER, G. G.: Water Intoxication. Am. J. Roentgenol. *77:* 69–70, 1957.

56. HILL, L. F.: Enema Can Be Fatal. Pediatrics *12:* 253–257, 1953.

57. MACHELLA, T. E.: Functional Disturbances of the Gastrointestinal Tract. Radiology *73:* 379–397, 1959.

58. NORDENTOFT, J. M.: Current Status of the Treatment of Intussusception: Use of the Roentgen Method in Reducing Intussusception in Children by Means of Hydrostatic Pressure. Fortschr. a. d. Geb. d. Rontgenstrahlen *94:* 181–198, 1961.

59. TEMPLETON, A. W.: Colon Sphincters Simulating Organic Disease. Radiology *75:* 237–241, 1960.

60. ARENDT, J.: The Significance of Cannon's Point in the Normal and Abnormal Functions of the Colon. Am. J. Roentgenol. *54:* 149–155, 1945.

61. BALL, R.: The Sphincter of the Colon. Radiology *33:* 372–376, 1939.

62. DeLORIMER, A. A., MOEHRING, H. G., AND HANNAN, J. R.: Clinical Roentgenology, Vol. IV. Springfield, Ill., Charles C Thomas, 1956, p. 261.

63. MEYERS, P. H.: Contamination of Barium Enema Apparatus during Its Use. J.A.M.A. *173:* 1589–1590, 1960.

64. STEINBACH, H. L., ROUSSEAU, R., McCORMACK, K. R., AND JAWETZ, E.: Transmission of Enteric Pathogens by Barium Enemas. J.A.M.A. *174:* 1207–1208, 1960.

65. ATKINSON, A. J., ADLER, H. F., AND IVY, A. C.: Motility of Human Colon; Normal Pattern, Dyskinesia and Effect of Drugs. J.A.M.A. *121:* 646–652, 1943.

66. BARCLAY, A. E.: Direct X-ray Cinematography with Preliminary Note on Nature of Nonpropulsive Movements of Large Intestine. Brit. J. Radiol. *8:* 652–658, 1935.

67. BEST, C. H., AND TAYLOR, N. B.: The Physiological Basis of Medical Practice: A Text in Applied Physiology, ed. 5. Baltimore, Williams and Wilkins Co., 1950, pp. 230–252; also pp. 496–501.

68. KERN, F. JR., ALMY, T. P., ABBOTT, F. K., AND BOGDONOFF, M. D.: Motility of Distal Colon in Non-Specific Ulcerative Colitis. Gastroenterology *19:* 492–503. 1951.

Chapter VIII—Intestinal Obstruction

1. LEVITAN, J.: Scout Film of the Abdomen. Radiology *47:* 10–29, 1946.

2. KLOIBER, H.: Roentgenographic Examination in Ileus. Münch. Med. Wchnschr. *63:* 1181, 1921.

3. STORCH, C., REDNER, B., AND TURIN, R.: Small Bowel Obstruction in Infancy and Childhood. J. Pediat. *37:* 380–386, 1950.

4. DENNIS, C.: Current Procedures in Management of Obstruction of Small Intestine. J.A.M.A. *154:* 463–468, 1954.

5. GOLDEN,, R.: Some Problems in Abnormal Intestinal Physiology Associated with Peritoneal Adhesions and Ileus. Am. J. Roentgenol. *56:* 555–568, 1946.

6. WANGENSTEIN, O. H.: Therapeutic Problems in Bowel Obstruction. Springfield, Charles C Thomas, 1937.

7. FRIMANN-DAHL: Roentgen Examination in Acute Abdominal Diseases. Springfield, Charles C Thomas, 1951.

8. SHANKS, S. C., AND KERLEY, P.: A Textbook of X-ray Diagnosis, Vol. III. Philadelphia, W. B. Saunders, 1950.

9. SAMUEL, E.: Radiology of Vascular Abdominal Catastrophes. J. Fac. Radiol. *6:* 27–37, 1954.

10. RENDICH AND HARRINGTON, L. A.: Roentgenologic Observations in Mesenteric Thrombosis. Am. J. Roentgenol. *52:* 317, 1944.

11. RABIN, C.: Personal communication.

12. FRIMANN-DAHL, J.: The Administration of Barium Orally in Acute Obstruction. Acta Radiol. *42:* 285–295, 1954.

13. ABBOTT, W. O., AND MILLER, T. G.: Intubation Studies of the Human Small Intestine. III. Technic for Collection of Pure Intestinal Secretion and for the Study of Intestinal Absorption. J.A.M.A. *106:* 16–18, 1936.

14. EINHORN, M.: An Intestinal Tube. New York State J. Med. **110:** 456–459, 1919.

15. SCHELTEMA, G.: Permeation in the Examination and Treatment of the Stomach and Intestines. Arch. Roentgen Ray *13:* 144–149, 1908–1909.

16. MILLER, T. G.: Intestinal Intubation, a Practical Technique. Am. J. M. Sc. *187:* 595–599, 1934.

17. WANGENSTEIN, O. H.: Intestinal Obstruction, ed. 3. Springfield, Charles C Thomas, 1955, pp. 745–769.

18. CANTOR, M. O.: Intestinal Intubation. Springfield, Charles C Thomas, 1949, pp. 147–159.

19. MacPHERSON, R. A.: J. Canad. A. Radiol. *3:* 54–56, 1952.

20. GOLDEN, R.: Radiologic Examination of the Small Intestine. Philadelphia, Lippincott, 1945.

21. GOLDEN, R., LEIGH, O., AND SWENSEN, P.: Roentgen Ray Examination with Miller-Abbott Tube. Radiology *35:* 521–533, 1940.

22. NOER, R. J., AND JOHNSTOWN, C. G.: Decompression of the Small Bowel in Intestinal Obstruction. Am. J. Dig. Dis. *6:* 46, 1939.

23. PENDERGRASS, E. P., AND CHAMBERLAIN, G. W.: Roentgen Diagnosis of Lesions Involving the Cecum, Ileum, and Proximal Ascending Colon. Am. J. Roentgenol. *48:* 16–26, 1942.

24. LEFSTROM, J. E., AND NOER, R. J.: The Use of Intestinal Intubation in the Localization of Lesions of the Gastro-Intestinal Tract. Am. J. Roentgenol. *42:* 321–331, 1939.

25. CANTOR, M. O.: Radiological Criteria for Re-

moval of Intestinal Decompression Tube. Radiology *54:* 535–540, 1950.

26. CANTOR, M. O.: Swallowed Intestinal Decompression Tube. Am. J. Dig. Dis. *18:* 250–254, 1951.

27. BERGER, L., AND ACHS, S.: Perforation of the Small Intestine by the Miller-Abbott Tube. Surgery *22:* 648–656, 1947.

28. HARRIS, F. I.: New Rapid Method of Intubation with Miller-Abbot Tube. J.A.M.A. *125:* 784–785, 1944.

29. MAYER, H., JR.: Passage of the Miller-Abbott Tube through Pylorus with the Aid of Electro Magnet. U. S. Naval Med. Bull. *43:* 463–466, 1944.

30. MESCHAN, I.: Roentgen Signs in Clinical Diagnosis. Philadelphia and London, W. B. Saunders Co., 1956.

31. FIGIEL, L. S., AND FIGIEL, S. J.: Coiling of the Long Tube in the Small Intestine. Am. J. Roentgenol. *87:* 721–723, 1962.

Chapter IX—The Gallbladder

1. GRAHAM, E. A., COLE, W. H., AND COPHER, G. H.: Visualization of the Gallbladder by the Sodium Salt of Tetrabromphenolphthalein. J.A.M.A. *82:* 613, 1924.

2. GRAHAM, E. A., COLE, W. H., AND COPHER, G. H.: Cholecystography: Development and Application. Am. J. Roentgenol. *14:* 487, 1925.

3. BUCKSTEIN, J.: Digestive Tract in Roentgenology. Philadelphia, Lippincott, 1953.

4. SANDSTROM, C.: Fraktionierte perorale. Cholecystographic. Acta Radiol. *12:* 9, 1931.

5. STEWART, W. H., AND ILLICK, H. E.: Advantages of Oral Cholecystography. Am. J. Roentgenol. *33:* 624, 1935.

6. KIRKLIN, B. R.: Cholecystography. Brit. J. Radiol. *18:* 170, 1945.

7. SCHINZ, H. R., BAENSCH, W. E., FRIEDL, E., AND UEHLINGER, E. (transl. by James T. Case): Roentgen-Diagnostics, Vol. IV. New York, Grune & Stratton, 1954.

8. IVY, A. C.: The Physiology of the Gall Bladder. Physiol. Rev. *14:* 1–102, 1934.

9. BREWER, A. A.: Physiological Stasis, a Cause of Cholecystographic Error. Am. J. Roentgenol. *53:* 106–111, 1947.

10. CURL, H.: High Fat Diet Preceding Cholecystography. Review of Literature and Experimental Studies on Filling a Normal Gallbladder. J.A.M.A. *119:* 607–610, 1942.

11. SHAPIRO, R.: Cholecystography. A Critical Review. Radiology *62:* 245–247, 1954.

12. HINES, L. E.: Cholecystography in the Presence of Achylia Gastrica. J.A.M.A. *90:* 2099–2100, 1928.

13. IVY, A. C., AND OLDBERG, E.: A Hormone Mechanism for Gallbladder Contraction and Evacuation. Am. J. Physiol. *86:* 613, 1928.

14. OLSSON, O.: Das Stillen—Eine Fehlerquelle bei der Cholecystographie. Acta Radiol. *24:* 289–494, 1943.

15. COLLETT, H. S., TIRMAN, W. S., AND CAYLOR, H. D.: Roentgen Demonstration of Common Duct Entering Duodenal Diverticulum. Radiology *55:* 72, 1950.

16. ELSEY, E. C., AND JACOBS, D. L.: Floating Gallbladder Stones. Am. J. Roentgenol. *65:* 73–76, 1951.

17. ETTER, LEWIS E.: Left-sided Gallbladder. Am. J. Roentgenol. *70:* 987–990, 1953.

18. DRECHSEL, J.: Anomalie des Recessus umbilicalis mit Linkslage der Gallenblase. Ztschr. f. d. ges. Anat. (Abt. 1). *91:* 638–643, 1930.

19. J.A.M.A. June 2, 1962.

20. LANG, J. J.: Nonoperative Biliary Tract Roentgenography. G. P. *21:* 86–98, 1960.

20a. PALMER, J. J.: Gastroenterology, 2nd Edition. New York, Hoeber, 1957.

21. RILEY, J. R.: Cholecystography and Cholangiography Today. Texas State J. Med. *50:* 108–111, 1960.

22. McCONNELL, F.: Malignant Neoplasm of the Gallbladder: Roentgenological Diagnosis. Radiology *69:* 720–725, 1957.

23. FELDMAN, M.: Clinical Roentgenology of the Digestive Tract, ed. 2. Baltimore, Williams and Wilkins Co., 1945, p. 619.

24. SCHINZ, H. R. ET AL.: Roentgen-Diagnostics. First American edition (based on 5th German edition), edited by J. T. Case. New York, Grune & Stratton, 1954, Vol. IV, pp. 3714–3715.

25. TWIGG, H. C., AND ZELNA, A.: Stratification in Intravenous Cholangiography. Radiology *80:* 774–775, 1963.

26. McLAREN, J. W.: Modern Trends in Diagnostic Radiology, 3rd Series. New York, Hoeber, 1960, p. 60–65.

Index